THE TOXICITY OF ANTICANCER DRUGS

THE TOXICITY OF ANTICANCER DRUGS

Edited by
Garth Powis, D. Phil.
Department of Pharmacology
Mayo Clinic
Rochester, Minnesota

Miles P. Hacker, Ph.D.
Department of Pharmacology
University of Vermont
Burlington, Vermont

PERGAMON PRESS
Member of Maxwell Macmillan Pergamon Publishing Corporation
New York • Oxford • Beijing • Frankfurt
São Paulo • Sydney • Tokyo • Toronto

Pergamon Press Offices:

U.S.A.	Pergamon Press, Inc., Maxwell House, Fairview Park, Elmsford, New York 10523, U.S.A.
U.K.	Pergamon Press plc, Headington Hill Hall, Oxford OX3 0BW, England
PEOPLE'S REPUBLIC	Pergamon Press, Xizhimenwai Dajie, Beijing Exhibition Centre, Beijing 100044, People's Republic of China
FEDERAL REPUBLIC OF GERMANY	Pergamon Press GmbH, Hammerweg 6, D-6242 Kronberg, Federal Republic of Germany
BRAZIL	Pergamon Editora Ltda, Rua Eça de Queiros, 346, CEP 04011, Paraiso, São Paulo, Brazil
AUSTRALIA	Pergamon Press Australia Pty Ltd., P.O. Box 544, Potts Point, NSW 2011, Australia
JAPAN	Pergamon Press, 8th Floor, Matsuoka Central Building, 1-7-1 Nishishinjuku, Shinjuku-ku, Tokyo 160, Japan
CANADA	Pergamon Press Canada Ltd., Suite No. 271, 253 College Street, Toronto, Ontario, Canada M5T

Library of Congress Cataloging in Publication Data

The toxicity of anticancer drugs / edited by Garth Powis and Miles P. Hacker.
p. cm.
Includes index.
ISBN 0-08-040302-6 (hardcover)
1. Antineoplastic agents--Toxicology. I. Powis, Garth. II. Hacker, Miles P.
[DNLM: 1. Antineoplastic Agents--toxicity. QV 269 T755]
RC271.C5T67 1990
616.99'4061--dc20
DNLM/DLC
for Library of Congress 90-7260
CIP
Rev.

Printing: 1 2 3 4 5 6 7 8 9 Year: 1 2 3 4 5 6 7 8 9 0

Printed in the United States of America

™ The paper used in this publication meets the minimum requirements of American National Standard for Information Sciences -- Permanence of Paper for Printed Library Materials, ANSI Z39.48-1984

Contents

List of Contributors

Robert B. Diasio
The University of Alabama at Birmingham
Division of Clinical Pharmacology
Birmingham, Alabama

William B. Ershler
Department of Medicine and Human Oncology
University of Wisconsin Center for Health Sciences
Madison, Wisconsin

Martin E. Gore
Division of Oncology
Cancer Research Unit
University of Newcastle Upon Tyne
Newcastle, England

Charles K. Grieshaber
Division of Clinical Pharmacology
Office of Research Resources
U.S. Department of Health and Human Services
Rockville, Maryland

Larry D. Grant
Department of Medicine and Human Oncology
University of Wisconsin Center for Health Sciences
Madison, Wisconsin

Miles P. Hacker
Department of Pharmacology
University of Vermont
Burlington, Vermont

Paul R. Kaesberg
Department of Medicine and Human Oncology
University of Wisconsin Center for Health Sciences
Madison, Wisconsin

David R. Newell
Division of Oncology
Cancer Research Unit
University of Newcastle Upon Tyne
Newcastle, England

Garth Powis
Department of Pharmacology
Mayo Clinic and Foundation
Rochester, Minnesota

Charles B. Pratt
St. Jude Children's Research Hospital
Memphis, Tennessee

Ching-Hon Pui
St. Jude Children's Research Hospital
Memphis, Tennessee

David J. Sweeny
The University of Alabama at Birmingham
Division of Clinical Pharmacology
Birmingham, Alabama

CHAPTER 1

Toxicity of Anticancer Drugs to Humans: A Unique Opportunity to Study Human Toxicology

Garth Powis, D. Phil.

CANCER, A WORLDWIDE PROBLEM

Cancer is a global problem and not one, as is sometimes thought, limited to the industrial nations. There are an estimated 5.9 million new cases of cancer worldwide a year. However, there is great variation in the patterns of cancer occurrence in different regions of the world (Table 1-1). As the age structure of the population in developing countries changes as a result of a reduction in infectious disease mortality, and as these nations adopt a more "Western" life-style so the risk of cancer increases. The positive impact of chemotherapy on survival of cancer patients can be seen from the survival rates for cancer patients which in the United States (U.S.A.) today is approaching 50%, compared to 40% in the early 1960s before the widespread use of chemotherapy (DeVita, 1989). Chemotherapy can be curative in about 12% of human cancers including choriocarcinoma, acute lymphocytic leukemia, Wilm's tumor, Hodgkin's disease, and testicular cancer; most human cancers remain resistant to chemotherapy. Because increasing numbers of people will receive chemotherapy for the

Table 1-1. Estimate of the Worldwide Frequency of Major Cancers*

	NEW CASES PER YEAR (in thousands)†					
	MOUTH/ PHARYNX	OESOPHAGUS	STOMACH	COLON/ RECTUM	LIVER	BRONCHUS/ LUNG
Africa	21.3	8.0	14.4	11.9	33.4	7.6
North America	26.3	8.2	22.3	110.9	5.3	103.6
China	58.3	168.0	205.5	76.6	110.2	74.9
Japan	2.9	5.9	75.1	18.2	11.3	18.3
Europe	42.9	22.8	147.6	166.9	24.2	204.0
U.S.S.R.	20.7	16.9	104.5	33.4	15.8	64.3
Total	339.5	296.3	682.4	506.9	259.2	591.0

	BREAST/ CERVIX	PROSTATE/ BLADDER	LYMPHATIC TISSUE	LEUKEMIA	ALL SITES
Africa	50.7	24.8	31.4	8.8	331.7
North America	121.0	97.7	35.9	22.4	752.7
China	185.9	21.7	25.5	37.2	1211.3
Japan	21.2	6.0	5.3	4.7	207.0
Europe	209.0	129.4	51.2	37.5	1402.9
U.S.S.R.	62.6	23.0	8.8	12.6	435.0
Total	1000.6	367.8	220.9	175.7	5870.3

*Adapted from Parkin et al. (1984).
†Based on cases in 1975.

treatment of their cancer, thus, more people will experience the toxic effects of these drugs.

DRUGS USED TO TREAT CANCER

There has been a steady growth in the number of available anticancer drugs since they were first introduced into clinical use over 40 years ago. There are currently 42 clinically approved anticancer drugs in the U.S.A., excluding hormonal agents (Fig. 1-1). Other countries have similar lists of approved anticancer drugs, with a greater or lesser number of agents. There are also many anticancer drugs in different stages of preclinical and clinical development and the list of available drugs will continue to grow. Not all anticancer drugs are widely used and some have specialized uses for only a few types of cancer. For example, the main use of procarbazine is in the treatment of Hodgkin's disease (a type of lymphoma), L-asparaginase is indicated only in the induction of treatment of acute lymphocytic leukemia and busulfan is used almost exclusively to treat chronic myelogenous leukemia.

ORIGINS OF MODERN CANCER CHEMOTHERAPY

It was through toxic effects that the early anticancer drugs were discovered and the modern era of chemotherapy started. Toxicity has continued to have a major influence on the way anticancer drugs are used. The first anticancer agent introduced into clinical trial was nitrogen mustard (methyl-bis[chloroethyl]amine hydrochloride) (Einhorn, 1985). Sulfur mustard was originally synthesized in 1854 and was used in World War I as an offensive weapon when it was found that very low concentrations could effectively incapacitate unprotected combat

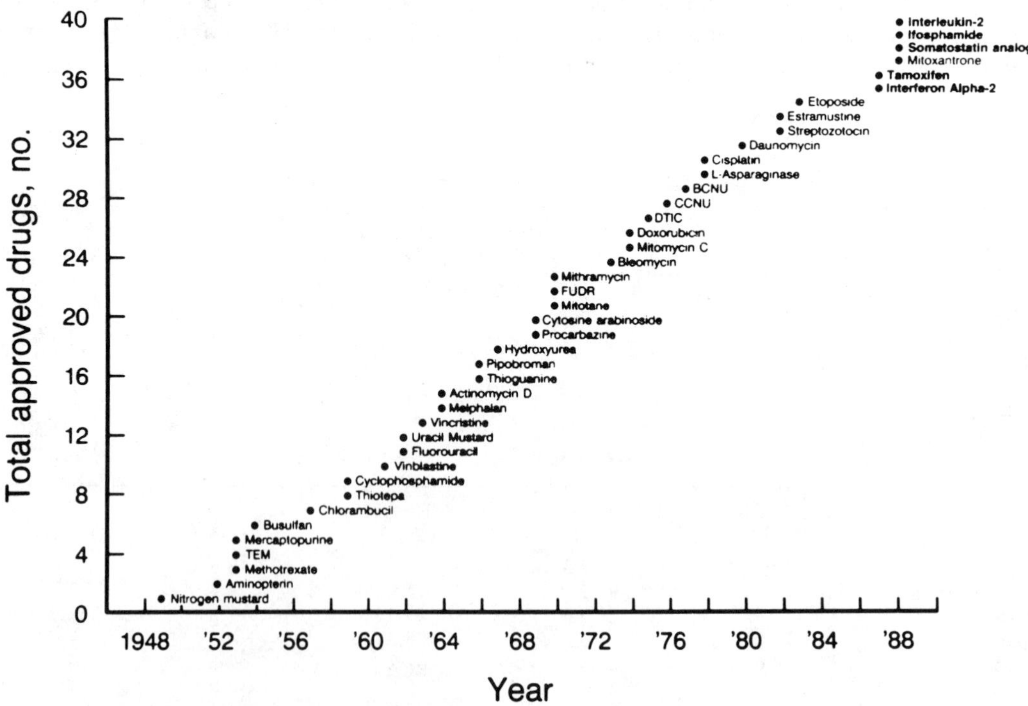

FIGURE 1-1. Anticancer drugs approved for use in the U.S.A. This list does not include hormonal agents such as adrenal cortical steriods (cortisone and prednisone), androgens (testosterone), estrogens (diethylstilbestrol), progesterone, and adrenocorticotropic hormone (ACTH) that are used to treat some hormonally dependent tumors.

troops by causing severe irritation of the respiratory tract and eye. It was soon recognized that sulfur mustard also had effects on the rapidly dividing cells of the gastrointestinal tract and blood forming organs. As early as 1935 Berenblum had recorded that mustard gas could impede the development of chemically induced tumors in animals. However, the question of whether the mustard agents might be used to destroy a tumor before it destroyed the host was first formulated by two young pharmacologists at Yale University, Alfred Gilman and Louis S. Goodman. They conducted animal studies of the toxicity and pharmacokinetics of intravenous (IV) nitrogen mustard and showed that it could produce remission of murine lymphoma. The first clinical trial of nitrogen mustard was by Gustav Lindskog at Yale in 1942 on a patient with rapidly progressive malignant lymphoma who achieved a complete although transient remission. Several clinical trials soon confirmed the effectiveness of nitrogen mustard in the treatment of malignant lymphoma as well as some epithelial tumors and the era of modern cancer chemotherapy was born.

TOXICITY AND CANCER CHEMOTHERAPY

Significant patient toxicity continues to be closely associated with the use of all the effective anticancer drugs. The major potentially lifethreatening organ toxicities of anticancer drugs (and their frequencies) are gastrointestinal (92%), bone marrow (88%), hepatic (52%), renal (40%), cardiovascular (40%), neuromuscular (28%), and respiratory (20%) (Rozencweig et al., 1981). Other toxicities, although nonlifethreatening, can seriously affect the quality of the life of the patient. The most common nonlifethreatening toxicities are nausea and vomiting, and alopecia which in some degree affect nearly all patients receiving chemotherapy. Another side effect of the way anticancer drugs are usually given, by the IV route, is that they can accidentally extravasate and produce localized and sometimes severe necrosis in up to 6% of patients (Svingen et al., 1981).

Anticancer drugs are one of the few classes of therapeutic agents that are routinely given to patients at doses producing moderate to severe toxicity. When drugs are given to patients at a fixed dose close to the toxic dose individual variability inevitably ensures that some patients experience little toxicity whereas other patients become severely intoxicated. Clinicians are well used to titrating the dose of anticancer drugs because of individual variation in toxicity, but deaths still occur. This unfortunate side effect and hazard of anticancer drug therapy is tolerated because of the belief that the higher the dose of anticancer drugs given, the more likelihood there is of a favorable therapeutic response. Only recently with the introduction of immunomodulatory agents, the so-called biological response modifiers (BRMs), has the universality of this concept been challenged (Herberman, 1987). It is evident from work with the interferons that the dose of BRM having the optimal immunomodulatory effect may be considerably lower than the maximum tolerated dose. Thus, large toxic doses of BRMs may not be necessary for effective therapy. However, for conventional anticancer drugs there is good evidence that higher doses offer a greater likelihood of a therapeutic response. The therapeutic effect of anticancer drugs against sensitive tumors, such as leukemias, the lymphomas, testicular cancer, and small cell lung cancer, shows a clear dose dependency (DeVita, 1989; Frei and Canellos, 1980; Gehan, 1984). When very high doses of anticancer drugs are used, such as in patients undergoing bone marrow transplantation, or high local concentrations given by isolation perfusion or regional infusion, there is a substantial increase in tumor response rates. The clinical evidence indicates that the dose–response relationship for antitumor activity is steep. Unfortunately, so is the dose–response relationship for toxicity and significant patient morbidity is almost invariably associated with attempts at curative therapy. It should not be forgotten in the discussion of anticancer drug toxicity that patients with benign disorders may receive anticancer drugs, for example, patients with collagen-vascular diseases, transplant patients, and individuals on immunosuppressive chemotherapy.

COMBINATIONS OF ANTICANCER DRUGS

It is common clinical practice, to limit the lethal toxicity of anticancer drugs while maintaining the highest therapeutic effect, to give the drugs in combination so that toxic effects are spread among different organs. This approach, known as subadditive host toxicity, leads to a wider range of side effects and greater discomfort to a patient but minimizes the risk of lethal effect of the drugs. Drugs that lack bone marrow toxicity, such as bleomycin (a lung toxic drug), prednisone (that causes osteoporosis), vincristine (causing peripheral neurotoxicity), and L-asparaginase (causing liver toxicity), are particularly useful for combining with myelosuppressive anticancer drugs. Factors often considered desirable in developing a new drug combination in this manner are: (a) each drug should be active when used alone against the tumor in question, (b) the drugs should have different mechanisms of antitumor action (as far as is known), (c) the toxic effects of the drugs should not overlap so that each drug can be given at, or near its maximum tolerated dose. An example of this approach is the MOPP regimen (Mechlorethamine/Oncovin/Procarbazine/Prednisone) used to treat Hodgkin's disease as shown in Table 1-2. In the era of single agent chemotherapy responses to Hodgkin's disease were usually of short duration (2 to 6 months) and the disease was incurable. Today the MOPP regimen produces complete remission in 81% of patients and in approximately one-half of all cases remissions persistent for up to 10 years and these patients can be considered cured (DeVita et al., 1978).

There are other rationales that are sometimes used for combining anticancer drugs (Mihich and Grindey, 1977). The cytokinetic rationale relies on the fact that some anticancer drugs are more active against cells in one phase of the cell cycle than another, the so-called cell cycle phase-specific drugs, whereas other anticancer drugs are cell-cycle nonspecific. Most combinations of chemotherapeutic agents used clinically involve cell-cycle phase specific drugs, for example, vincristine, methotrexate or cytosine arabinoside, combined with drugs that are cell-cycle phase nonspecific, for example, 5-fluorouracil, alkylating agents, and anticancer antibiotics. The MOPP regimen contains both cell-cycle phase specific and nonspecific drugs. The biochemical rationale for combining drugs attempts to make use of known biochemical mechanisms as the basis for giving drugs in combination, for example, methotrexate preceding or given together with 5-fluorouracil, both of which inhibit thymidilate synthesis; 5-fluorouracil by the binding of its nucleotide 5-FdUMP to thymidilate synthetase and methotrexate by depleting the intracellular reduced folate pool. With such drug combination subadditive host toxicity is usually a secondary consideration.

Table 1-2. Toxicities of Drugs Used in the Treatment of Hodgkin's Disease

DRUG	MECHANISM	ACTIVITY % COMPLETE RESPONSE	MAJOR TOXICITY
nitrogen mustard (Mechlorethamine)	Alkylating agent	20	Marrow toxicity, nausea, vomiting
vincristine (Oncovin)	Mitotic inhibitor	< 10	Neuropathy, alopecia, constipation
procarbazine	Alkylating agent	< 10	Marrow toxicity, nausea, vomiting
prednisone	Unknown	< 5	Osteoporosis, hypertension, diabetes, peptic ulcer
MOPP regimen (mechlorethamine, oncovin, procarbazine, prednisone)		> 80	All of the above

TOXICITIES OF ANTICANCER DRUGS

The toxicities found to occur with anticancer drugs have been reported to affect almost every organ system and tissue (Table 1-3). The most commonly affected organs and tissues are those with rapidly dividing cells, particularly the bone marrow, gastrointestinal tract, germinal epithelium, lymphoid tissue, and hair follicles. This occurs because most currently used anticancer drugs were initially selected for their ability to kill rapidly dividing cells. The most widely used animal models for detecting antitumor activity, until recently, were the mouse leukemias P-388 and L1210 which are rapidly growing tumors. Many other toxic effects of anticancer drugs are seen, but unlike toxicities affecting rapidly dividing cells these are often delayed and cumulative dose-dependent. Furthermore, unlike toxicity to rapidly dividing cells where there is a capacity for stem cell renewal the toxicities to other organs tend to be irreversible, or only partially reversible after drug treatment is stopped. It then becomes a matter of clinical judgement as to how much drug toxicity a patient can tolerate before their well-being and life quality are irreparably degraded, weighed against the possibility of therapeutic benefit to their disease. As we become adept at handling the reversible toxicities of anticancer drugs and higher doses of drugs are given, it is perhaps inevitable that new and potentially more serious irreversible toxicities will be increasingly evident. Myelosuppression is less of a problem than it once was due to effective clinical management through antibiotic therapy, thrombocyte replacement, and autologous bone marrow transplantation. However, without this barrier to the use of higher drug doses other, often irreversible toxicities have become apparent for many anticancer drugs.

FACTORS AFFECTING CANCER DRUG TOXICITY

Schedule Dependence

There are important principals to be learned from the clinical toxicities of anticancer drugs. First, the way in which anticancer drugs are given can greatly affect the toxicity seen. For a number of anticancer drugs toxicity is related to the integral of the serum or blood drug concentration (C) $\times$ time (t) measured from time zero to infinity (Powis, 1987). $C \times t$ is the same as the area under the plasma, serum, or blood drug concentration time curve from time zero to infinity (area under the curve, AUC) and is inversely related to total body drug clearance (Cl) by the relationship

$$C \times t = \text{Dose}/\text{Cl}$$

A similar relationship appears to hold between species. For a number of anticancer drugs a general correlation has been found between the AUC at the maximum tolerated human therapeutic dose and the AUC at the dose causing death of 10% of mice (Collins et al., 1986). However, there are a number of exceptions to this relationship (EORTC PAM Group, 1987).

Intermittent bolus administration of doxorubicin every three weeks was originally adopted, in part, because of the long biologic half-life of doxorubicin (Benjamin et al., 1973). Evidence then accumulated that weekly administration of doxorubicin produced less cardiotoxicity, although the incidence of other toxicities was unchanged and therapeutic efficacy was maintained (Chlebowski et al., 1980; Weiss et al., 1976). More recently it has been reported that giving doxorubicin every three weeks, by 48 hr or 96 hr continuous infusion produces less cardiotoxicity and less nausea and vomiting than bolus administration, whereas mucositis and myelosuppression are unchanged (Legha et al., 1982). Because of decreased cardiotoxicity, larger total doses of doxorubicin could be given by infusion than by bolus which may be responsible for an apparent small increase in therapeutic activity of the infusion schedule of doxorubicin administration. Pharmacokinetic studies showed similar plasma $C \times t$ values for bolus administration of doxorubicin and infusion schedules, but

Table 1-3. Organ or Tissue Directed Toxicities of Commonly Used Anticancer Drugs

ORGAN	DRUG
Heart	doxorubicin, daunomycin
Kidney	cisplatin, methotrexate, nitrosourea (delayed)
Peripheral nervous system	vincristine, cisplatin
Central nervous system	procarbazine, L-asparaginase, 5-fluorouracil, mitomycin C, methotrexate (given intrathecally)
Ototoxicity	cisplatin
Gastrointestinal	
Nausea and vomiting	most agents, but especially cisplatin, DTIC, nitrogen mustard, mitomycin C, nitrosoureas
Mucositis	methotrexate, 5-fluorouracil, vinca alkaloids
Diarrhea	vincristine, 5-fluorouracil
Liver	methotrexate, 6-mercaptopurine, cytosine arabinoside, nitrosoureas, L-asparaginase
Bladder	cyclophosphamide
Lung	bleomycin, busulfan, carmustine, methotrexate
Testes	alkylating agents
Ovary	busulfan, chlorambucil, cyclophosphamide, vinblastine
Fetus (Teratogenesis)	methotrexate, 6–mercaptopurine
Bone	methotrexate, corticosteriods
Bone marrow	most agents *except* vincristine, bleomycin, cisplatin, and L-asparaginase
Skin and Blood Vessels	
Alopecia	doxorubicin, cyclophosphamide, nitrosoureas, 5-fluorouracil
Phlebitis	nitrogen mustard, anthracyclines, actinomycin D, vinblastine, mitomycin C, DTIC
Hypersensitivity	L-asparaginase, cisplatin, procarbazine
Hyperpigmentation/ Photosensitization	busulfan, anthracyclines, actinomycin D, 5-fluorouracil, methotrexate

with peak plasma concentrations of doxorubicin up to 13-fold higher following bolus administration. These findings suggest that high peak plasma concentrations of doxorubicin are a contributory factor in increased cardiotoxicity associated with bolus administration.

Another example of schedule-dependent anticancer drug toxicity is found with the administration of 5-fluorouracil by schedules which avoid high plasma drug concentrations to reduce the incidence of myelosuppression. Moertel et al. (1969) compared the effect of the same dose of 5-fluorouracil administered over several days by IV bolus injection and by slow IV infusion and found the incidence of leukopenia to be decreased from 83% to 6% with slow infusion, although there was no difference in the objective response rate. Interestingly, other studies have reported an increase in response rate for 5-fluorouracil administered by infusion (Seifert et al., 1975).

The acute toxicity of anticancer drugs may be determined by the extent to which a drug time threshold rather than a concentration threshold is exceeded. Goldie et al. (1972) found that methotrexate infusions giving peak plasma concentrations of 5×10^{-4} M resulted in significant myelosuppression only when leucovorin rescue, which reverses the effects of methotrexate, was delayed more than 36 hr after the start of methotrexate infusion. Bleyer (1978) has estimated the toxicity concentration and time thresholds of methotrexate for bone marrow and gastrointestinal epithelium to be 2×10^{-8} M and 42 hr, respectively.

Individual Variability in Toxicity

A frequent clinical finding is one of great variability in the toxic response to anticancer drugs between patients. Factors which might cause differences in toxic responses are the age of the patient, the severity of the disease, concomitant renal or hepatic dysfunction, and previous chemotherapy. An example of how age can affect toxicity occurs with methotrexate which is eliminated primarily by the kidneys. The clearance of methotrexate is decreased in elderly subjects over 70 years of age because of decreased renal function in this age group (Kristensen, 1975). This results in higher plasma concentrations of methotrexate in the elderly with an increased potential for toxicity.

As a major factor causing individual variability we are just now beginning to appreciate the importance of genetics to toxic responses to anticancer drugs. A good example is the demonstration that inherited deficiencies in the levels of thiopurine methyltransferase lead to increased toxicity of thiopurine drugs (Weinshilboum, 1988). Thiopurine methyltransferase catalyzes the *S*-methylation of aromatic and heterocyclic sulfhydryl compounds, including 6-mercaptopurine, azathioprine (a prodrug form of 6-mercaptopurine), and 6-thioguanine, using *S*-adenosyl-L-methionine as a methyl donor. The toxicity of thiopurines is caused by conversion to 6-thioguanine nucleotides and incorporation into DNA, and methylation of thiopurines decreases their cytotoxicity. The red blood cells contain thiopurine methyltransferase that reflects the levels of the enzyme in kidney and liver, the major sites of thiopurine metabolism in the body. The use of red blood cells allows large scale population studies to be conducted relatively easily. Thiopurine methyltransferase levels show a trimodal frequency distribution with 88.6% of the population having high thiopurine methyltransferase activity, 11.1% having intermediate activity, and 0.3% having no detectable enzyme activity (Weinshilboum and Sladek, 1980). Family inheritance studies have shown that a single genetic locus with two alleles, one for low and one for high enzyme activity, is responsible for the trimodal frequency distribution. It was suspected that differences in the levels of thiopurine methyltransferase activity might be responsible for differences in the toxic responses to thiopurines. This was demonstrated in a retrospective study of acute azathioprine-induced bone marrow suppression where five patients who developed severe myelosuppression while taking azathioprine were found to have extremely low red blood cell thiopurine methyltransferase activities (Lennard et al., 1989). Furthermore, red blood cell concentrations of 6-thioguanine nucleotide in children with acute lymphoblastic leukemia receiving 6-mercaptopurine chemotherapy were shown to be inversely correlated with the neutrophil count and to the level of red blood cell thiopurine methyltransferase activity (Lennard et al., 1987). Based on these observations screening for individuals with genetically low or absent thiopurine methyltransferase activity before commencing thiopurine therapy is recommended so that they may be given much lower doses of thiopurine drug, or changed to alternate modes of therapy (Lennard et al., 1989).

THE FUTURE

We should not forget that toxicity is not an inevitable consequence of cancer treatment. We do not want to be in the state of 18th century physicians, many of whom denied there was such a thing as mercury poisoning in patients taking mercury for syphilis (Mathias, 1816). Mercury was so widely used for treating syphilis for over 400 years (although it was eventually proven to be ineffective) that physicians rarely saw a patient who had not knowingly or unknowingly, through a quack or secret remedy, taken mercury (Goldwater, 1972). Consequently, physicians were unable to distinguish the effects of the disease from the treatment. To the public today there is a tendency to associate with cancer the disease, wasting, hair loss, infection, and bleeding that is, in fact, caused by the drugs used to treat the disease. This need not be the case and great advances have been made in limiting and controlling the toxicities of anticancer drugs. A good example is the toxicity of cisplatin (see Chapter 6). The major dose-limiting toxicities of cisplatin when it was first introduced were severe nausea and vomiting, and nephrotoxicity. The use of antiemetics, hydration, diuresis, and prolonged infusions to avoid high concentrations of the drug in plasma have greatly reduced the severity of these toxicities. Unfortunately, bone marrow suppression and neurotoxicity have become major complications of high dose cisplatin therapy (Lokich, 1980).

Studies in animals can provide much useful information on the toxicity of anticancer drugs although it is clear that some toxicities in humans are not well predicted by animal models (see Chapter 2). Most of our information on the toxicities of less toxic classes of drugs and chemicals to which we are exposed in our food, in the work place or home, or in the environment comes from studies of animals. Just how useful this information is in extrapolating the risk of toxicity to humans is very difficult to judge. There are not usually large numbers of exposed individuals and even so, the dose and time of their exposure to the agents is usually not known.

Anticancer drugs are one of the few classes of truly toxic compounds administered to relatively large numbers of humans under controlled conditions where the dose, drug concentration in the body, and toxic response can be correlated. We can learn much of mechanisms of toxicity in humans by the study of anticancer drug toxicity that may be applicable to other toxic agents. In a few years, it is hoped, we will have more effective and less toxic ways of treating cancer and the drugs currently in use will not be used, or at least their toxicities will be modified so as not to be a problem. We may then look back on this period as the dark ages of cancer treatment, when our ignorance of the basic causes of cancer and the biology of the cancer cell led us to use toxic mixtures of randomly selected chemicals, more in the hope than in the expectation of a cure for the disease. This may be an overly pessimistic interpretation of the present state of cancer treatment and there are several bright spots and some cancers that we can now cure. However, it remains a fact that for most common cancers there is no effective treatment. Perhaps, in looking back from future years some of the most useful information to have been derived from the present phase of cancer chemotherapy will be a knowledge of human toxic responses. We are presented with a unique window in time in which to study these toxic responses to anticancer drugs and while it is the fervent hope of us all that more effective cancer treatments will soon become available, we should not neglect the useful knowledge of toxicity that is currently being gained from these drugs. There have been some excellent recent reviews on organ directed toxicities of anticancer drugs (Hacker et al., 1987; Perry, 1982; Perry and Yarbro, 1984) but there is no work that covers the basic mechanisms of toxicity of anticancer drugs in humans. It is to fill this gap that the following chapters have been written to provide information on the basic mechanisms of some of the major toxicities of anticancer drugs in human subjects.

REFERENCES

Benjamin RS, Riggs CE, and Bachur NR Pharmacokinetics and metabolism of adriamycin. Clin Pharmacol Ther 1973 14:592–600.

Berenblum I Experimental inhibition of tumour induction by mustard gas and other compounds. J Path Bact 1935 40:549–558.

Bleyer WA The clinical pharmacology of methotrexate. Cancer 1978 41:36–51.

Chlebowski RT, Paroly WS, Pugh RP, Hueser J, Jacobs EM, Pajak TF, and Bateman R Adriamycin given as a weekly schedule without a loading course: Clinical effective with reduced incidence of cardiotoxicity. Cancer Treat Rep 1980 64:47–51.

Collins JM, Zaharko DS, Dedrick RL, and Chabner BA Potential roles for preclinical pharmacology in Phase I clinical trials. Cancer Treat Rep 1986 76:73–80.

DeVita VT Principles of chemotherapy. In: Cancer Principles and Practice of Oncology DeVita VT, Hellman S, and Rosenberg SA Eds 3rd ed., Lippincott, Philadelphia 1989 pp. 276–300.

DeVita VT, Lewis BJ, Rozencweig M, and Muggia FM The chemotherapy of Hodgkin's disease. Past experience and future directions. Cancer 1978 42:979–990.

Einhorn J Nitrogen mustard: The origin of chemotherapy for cancer. Int J Radiat Oncol Biol Phys 1985 11:1375–1378.

EORTC Pharmacokinetics and Metabolism Group Commentary and proposed guidelines on "Pharmacokinetically-Guided Dose Escalation in Phase I Clinical Trials". Eur J Cancer Clin Oncol 1987 23:1083–1087.

Frei E and Canellas GP Dose: A critical factor in cancer chemotherapy. Am J Med 1980 69:585–594.

Gehan EA Dose response relationship in clinical oncology. Cancer 1984 54:1204–1207.

Goldie JH, Price LA, and Harrap KR Methotrexate toxicity: Correlation with duration of administration plasma levels dose and excretion pattern. Eur J Cancer 1972 8:409–414.

Goldwater LJ Mercury. A History of Quicksilver. York Press, Baltimore, MD 1972.

Hacker MP, Lazo JS, and Tritton TR Organ Directed Toxicities of Anticancer Drugs, Martinus Nijhoff Publishing, Boston, MA 1987.

Herberman RB Cancer therapy by biological response modifiers. Arzn Forsch 1987 37:246–250.

Kristensen LO, Weismann K, and Hutters L Renal function and rate of disappearance of methotrexate from serum. Eur J Clin Pharmacol 1975 8:439–444.

Legha SS, Benjamin RS, MacKay B, Ewer M, Wallace S, Valdivieso M, Rasmussen SL, Blumenschein GR, and Freireich EJ Reduction of doxorubicin cardiotoxicity by prolonged continuous intravenous infusion. Ann Intern Med 1982 96:133–139.

Lennard L, Van Loon JA, Lilleyman JS, and Weinshilboum RM Thiopurine pharmacogenetics in leukemia: Correlation of erythrocyte thiopurine methyltransferase activities and 6-thioguanine nucleotide concentrations. Clin Pharmacol Ther 1987 41:18–25.

Lennard L, Van Loon JA, and Weinshilboum RM Pharmacogenetics of acute azathioprine toxicity: Relationship to thiopurine methyltransferase genetic polymorphism. Clin Pharmacol Ther 1989 46:149–154.

Lokich JJ Phase I study of cis-diamminedichloroplatinum (II) administered as a constant 5 day infusion. Cancer Treat Rep 1980 64:905–908.

Mathias A The Mercurial Disease: An inquiry into the history and nature of the disease produced in the human condition by the use of mercury 3rd ed., J Callow, London 1816.

Mihich E and Grindey GB Multiple basis of combination chemotherapy. Cancer 1977 40:534–543.

Moertel CG, Reitemeir RJ, and Hahn RG Considerations regarding optimal method of administration of fluorinated pyrimidines. In: Advanced Gastrointestinal Cancer/Clinical Management and Chemotherapy Moertel CG and Reitemeir RJ Eds Chapter 14, Harper and Row, New York 1969 pp. 108–118.

Parkin DM, Stjernsward J, and Muir CS Estimates of the worldwide frequency of twelve major cancers. Bull WHO 1984 62:163–182.

Perry MC Toxicity of chemotherapy. Semin Oncol 1982 9:1–154.

Perry MC and Yarbro JW Toxicity of Chemotherapy, Grune and Stratton, Orlando, FL 1984.

Powis G Metabolism of anthracyclines. In: Metabolism and Action of Anti-Cancer Drugs Powis G Ed Taylor and Francis, London 1987 pp. 211–260.

Rozencweig M, Von Hoff DD, Staquet MJ, Schein PS, Penta JS, Goldin A, Muggia FM, Freireich EJ, and DeVita VT Animal toxicology for early clinical trials with anticancer agents. Cancer Clin Trials 1981 4:21–28.

Seifert P, Baker LH, Reed M, and Vaitkevicius VK Comparison of continuously infused 5-fluorouracil with bolus injection in treatment of patient with colorectal adenocarcinoma. Cancer 1975 36:123–128.

Svingen BA, Powis G, Appel PL, and Scott M Protection against adriamycin-induced skin necrosis in the rat by dimethyl sulfoxide and α-tocopherol. Cancer Res 1981 41:3395–3399.

Weinshilboum RM Pharmacogenetics of methylation: Relationship to drug metabolism. Clin Biochem 1988 21:201–210.

Weinshilboum RM and Sladek SL Mercaptopurine pharmacogenetics: Monogenic inheritance of erythrocyte thiopurine methyltransferase activity. Am J Human Genet 1980 32:651–662.

Weiss AJ, Metter GE, Fletcher WS, Wilson WL, Grage TB, and Ramirez G Studies on adriamycin using a weekly regimen demonstrating its clinical effectiveness and lack of cardiac toxicity. Cancer Treat Rep 1976 60:813–822.

CHAPTER 2

Prediction of Human Toxicity of New Antineoplastic Drugs from Studies in Animals

Charles K. Grieshaber, Ph.D.

The vast majority of the important chemotherapeutic drugs used today to treat neoplastic diseases display one common phenomenon, toxicity, regardless of their mechanism of anticancer action. This undesirable, yet to date unavoidable, phenomenon is so critically important that dosages at which these drugs are administered to patients are defined not by their antitumor potential, the intended pharmacologic effect, but by their potential to induce toxicity. In early experimental treatment of neoplastic disease with investigational drugs, toxic events are the absolute rule rather than the exception. Thus, to place investigational new drugs into clinical trials, dose levels posing only minimal threats to a patient's well-being must be initially established. To date, there is no known universal dose level for all investigational anticancer agents at which toxicity will not be produced, that can serve as a moral or ethical starting dose for clinical trials. Therefore, an estimated safe starting dose for human trials must be ascertained in carefully designed and controlled preclinical toxicology studies in experimental animals. This alternative depends, of course, upon the generally accepted assumption that there is a high degree of correlation between effects in animals and humans.

The importance of toxicity in clinical use of anticancer chemotherapeutic agents and the requirement for establishing safe initial human doses highlights the benefit, to the clinician and the patient, of knowing the toxic potential of each chemotherapeutic agent, be it clinically available or a newly discovered investigational drug. This chapter will focus in general terms on the clinical toxicity prediction of investigational agents from studies performed in experimental species. Full and complete details illustrating the species differences in toxicity of the clinically available anticancer agents will not be individually documented here but are included in the chapters dedicated to individual drugs or drug classes and their specific toxicities. Species differences in toxicity will be noted in this chapter for some experimental drugs, to show how notice of interspecies variations in sensitivity contributes to these agents.

Toxicology is the scientific study of poisons, their biological effects, and the means of treating these effects. As one of the specific disciplines in preclinical studies for anticancer drug development, toxicology is more specifically defined as the detection of, and the description of, adverse effects associated with treating a mammalian organism with a potential new antineoplastic chemotherapeutic drug. For the most part, anticancer chemotherapeutic drugs are chemical toxins, usually of synthetic or natural origin. To more fully appreciate the role of preclinical animal toxicology studies in the development of a new anticancer agent, the reader should be familiar with the overall preclinical drug development process through which investigational anticancer chemotherapeutic agents proceed. The drug development scheme depicted in Fig. 2-1 highlights two major components of the preclinical portion of drug development, discovery of a potentially pharmacologically active agent, and its development into a drug for safe and effective investigational human use. The discovery component

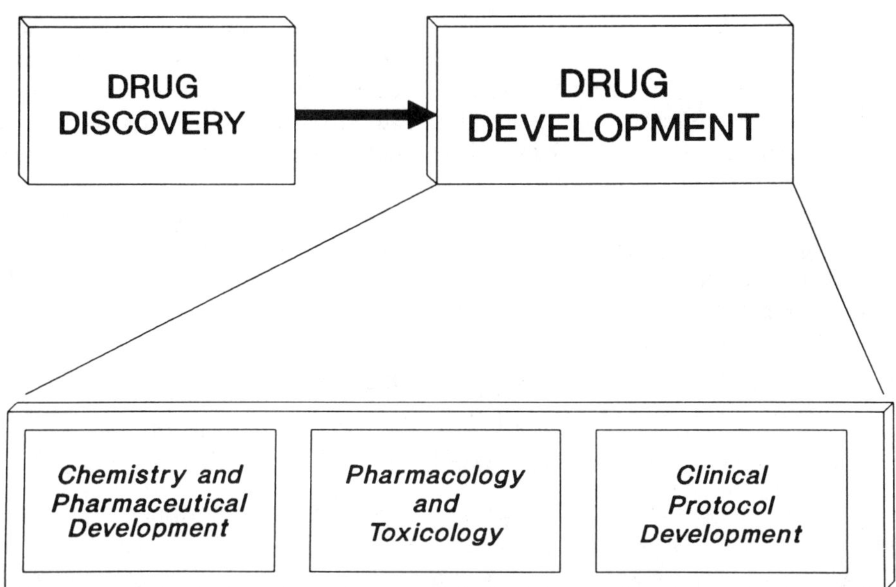

FIGURE 2-1. Components of the Preclinical Drug Development Process. The two major components of the preclinical drug development system are illustrated as major blocks. The preclinical drug discovery component is comprised of the screens and tumor systems for which potential new agents are identified. The preclinical drug development component consists of three interrelated units to provide a finished clinical product. The pharmaceutical chemistry portion whose task centers on the production of bulk drug and formulation research; the pharmacology and toxicology portion whose tasks center on efficacy and toxicity studies; and clinical product development portion whose tasks involve production of the clinical dosage form for final toxicology studies and Phase I clinical trials comprise the three major elements of the preclinical development component.

of the process represents the detection of agents with defined pharmacologic potential for cytotoxicity to, or cytostasis of, cancer cells through investigations in murine tumors (Goldin and Venditti, 1980; Venditti, 1981; Venditti, 1983; Driscoll, 1984; Zubrod, 1984) or human xenografts in vivo (Bogden et al., 1979), or clonogenic (Hamberger and Salmon, 1977; Shoemaker et al., 1985) and growth inhibitory studies in vitro (Alley et al., 1988; Scudiero et al., 1988; Shoemaker et al., 1988). Preclinical drug development, on the other hand, is the process wherein a clinical pharmaceutical product, safe for human use, is produced from the pharmacologically active agents with recognized antitumor activity. These products are usually made for intravenous (IV) administration for the first human studies.

The critical elements of the preclinical drug development process are often subdivided into pharmaceutical and pharmacological disciplines. In the first steps the newly discovered agent is synthesized or isolated from its source in sufficient quantity for formulation into a clinically functional product. The product, in either experimental or final form, must then be evaluated for toxicity prior to human use by a more or less rigidly defined series of studies in experimental animals. The latter represent the toxicity studies central to this chapter. Note that anticancer efficacy is not the central issue in these preclinical studies, safety of the clinical trial starting dose and description of potential organ toxicity are the key points. Both critical elements of the preclinical development process are governed, in the United States, by the Food and Drug Administration (FDA) through the Current Good Manufacturing Practice Regulations for drug manufacture (Federal Reg., 1978) and Good Laboratory Practice Regulations for conduct of the toxicology studies (Federal Reg., 1978; 1987). Compliance with these regulations, in large part, assures that bulk drug production, clinical product manufacture and toxicity studies are carried out using quality procedures with unparalleled integrity.

To critically examine the ability of toxicology tests carried out in animals to predict for toxic effects in a clinical situation, the so-called clinical toxicity correlations, the purpose of preclinical toxicity testing on these agents and the role these specialized studies play in the overall scheme of preclinical drug development must be fully appreciated. The role is best defined in terms of the main objectives of preclinical toxicology studies for new anticancer agents. Table 2-1 highlights, in rather simplistic terms, the three basic goals of preclinical toxicology studies for antineoplastic drugs: to establish a safe dose at which to initiate clinical trials, to predict the toxic reactions likely to be encountered in these human trials, and to determine the reversibility of induced adverse affects. The procedures and protocols used to accomplish these goals follow.

EVOLUTION OF PROCEDURES FOR PRELIMINARY TOXICOLOGIC EVALUATION OF EXPERIMENTAL CANCER CHEMOTHERAPEUTIC AGENTS IN ANIMALS

Studies in animals on the toxicity of new drugs for treatment of any human disease indication are intended to forecast untoward effects of the new agent at dose levels scheduled for human use thereby minimizing patient risk. As previously highlighted, preclinical toxicology studies have the same purpose and objectives whether performed for regulatory requirements or to facilitate an initial clinical trial. Over the past two to three decades a number of preclinical procedures or protocols have been employed using animal species to determine the potential risk involved in treating patients with new antineoplastic chemotherapeutic agents. The evolution of preclinical toxicity studies for new antineoplastic agents is suitably studied by examination of the protocols developed under the auspices of the National Cancer Institute (NCI). It was recognized 30 years ago, as it is generally acknowledged today, that the application of findings in experimental animals to clinical use depends on the probable correlation between the response of laboratory animals and humans to the effects of the agents tested. The Cancer Chemotherapy National Service Center (CCNSC) of the NCI outlined protocols for the preclinical toxicologic characterization of candidate anticancer compounds in the 1950s and early 1960s (CCNSC, 1959; CCNSC, 1961; CCNSC, 1964). These first toxicology protocols consisted of three basic toxicity studies which included the appropriate gross and microscopic pathology evaluations. The first, a single-dose toxicity study in which the LD_{50} (dose producing lethality in 50% of treated animals) was approximated in mice and rats, was followed by a lethality study in dogs. Second, the local irritant action and corrosive properties of each agent were determined in rabbits and guinea pigs. Last, repeated dose toxicity studies were carried out in rats, dogs, and monkeys by treating the animals with the test compound daily for four consecutive weeks. The route of administration was predicated on the proposed route for clinical trials. Body weights and full-scale pathology examinations served as the basis for toxicologic characterizations.

The protocol for candidate anticancer chemotherapeutic agents was refined by the Drug Research and Development Program of the NCI in 1973 (Prieur et al., 1973). This revised comprehensive protocol is presented in Table 2-2. The objective of these toxicology studies was the same as for all previous and future studies, to establish a safe clinical starting dose

Table 2-1. Traditional Goals for Preclinical Toxicology Studies on New Antineoplastic Agents

Establish a safe clinical trial entry dose—quantative phase
Determine the acute hazard of the entry level dose
Determine potential end-organ toxicity—qualitative phase
Establish both acute and delayed effects
Determine reversibility of acute end-organ injury

Table 2-2. Toxicology Protocol Studies Designed in 1973*

- Single dose – dogs
- Five consecutive daily treatments – dogs
- Five consecutive daily treatments – monkeys
- Five consecutive daily treatments, nine days rest, repeated for three treatment periods – dogs
- Schedule dependency studies – dogs
  (using at least one of the following)
  – 48 hr IV infusion once per week for six weeks
  – Treatment every six hr for 42 hrs once per week for six weeks
  – Single dose once per week for six weeks
  – Ten consecutive daily treatments

*Adapted from Prieur et al., 1973.

and to predict, in mammalian species closely related to man, the primary organ systems at risk of toxicity. To these ends, an LD was established in dogs and monkeys from which nonlethal, progressively less toxic doses were derived. Doubling the highest dose at which toxicity did not occur (HNTD) yielded a dose that produced minimal hematologic, chemical, or pathologic lesions, designated the lowest toxic dose (TDL). Doubling the TDL produced a dose level at which the toxic manifestations were much more severe, the toxic dose high (TDH). Finally, doubling the TDH produced a lethal dose, the LD. These studies established the acute toxic effects of new agents in multiple biologic systems. Longer term effects and effects of repeated administration were assessed solely in dogs. Animals were sacrificed for full-scale pathologic evaluation at variously scheduled times following completion of the drug administration schedule. Hematology and clinical chemistry parameters were measured along with cage side observations to complement the pathology findings in a complete and detailed description of the adverse effects of the experimental drugs. Safe starting doses for clinical trials were estimated by calculating one-third the TDL for the most sensitive species, either monkeys or dogs, if the long-term and schedule-dependency studies predicted no serious toxicity at these dose levels.

The NCI protocols served as the industry standard for toxicology studies carried out prior to the filing of an Investigational New Drug Application with the FDA, and initiation of the first human trials. In 1980, preclinical toxicology protocols were produced by the Division of Cancer Treatment of the NCI incorporating recommendations of the FDA Oncologic Drugs Advisory Committee made one year earlier. The 1979 recommendations were based on the finding that one-tenth the LD_{10} in mice expressed on a square meter body surface basis ($MELD_{10}$) and computed from statistically reliable studies would serve well as the starting dose for clinical trials for new anticancer agents based on a retrospective study of toxicology data and clinical results with several drugs (Rozencweig et al., 1981). The Advisory Committee also proposed dogs, not monkeys, as the species to test the safety of the one-tenth $MELD_{10}$ prior to clinical trial. Monkeys were excluded as a result of reviews of older data, in combination with an update of the report by Schein et al. (1970), wherein similar toxicities were seen in beagle dogs and monkeys leading to the conclusion that there was not significant justification for inclusion of subhuman primates in routine protocol toxicity studies. The high cost of monkeys relative to dogs also contributed greatly to the decision. In sum, the 1980 protocol for toxicology called for acute lethality studies in mice to estimate the clinical starting dose and acute toxicity studies in dogs and mice to assess the qualitative toxicities of the new agents (Lowe and Davis, 1987; Lowe, 1987). Each drug was to be administered on a single dose and five consecutive day regimen with sacrifices in the acute toxicity studies at various time points shortly after dosing was completed and at one to two months post dosing. Complete pathology, hematology, and clinical chemistry evaluations were made on each animal on study (Grieshaber and Marsoni, 1986; Lowe and Davis, 1987; Lowe, 1987). In 1983 rats replaced mice for the acute toxicity studies in rodents to provide a larger animal for blood collection in clinical laboratory studies (Grieshaber and Marsoni, 1986). The current standardized protocols in use since the early 1980s for preclinical toxicology studies on new antineoplastic agents are presented in Table 2-3. In addition to serving the drug development effort at the NCI, these protocols also served the anticancer drug development community as the standard studies to be performed on each new agent taken to Phase I clinical trial, at the time they were established and continue to be used presently. In fact, properly conducted and analyzed studies will satisfy the requirements promulgated jointly by the FDA and the NCI in 1979 (Lowe and Davis, 1987).

ANIMAL TOXICOLOGY IN THE PREDICTION OF ANTINEOPLASTIC DRUG TOXICITY IN HUMANS

The attention paid to the preclinical toxicology protocols over the years by scientists and clinicians involved in experimental cancer chemotherapy clearly acknowledges the importance these protocols play in the overall preclinical drug development process for antineoplastic agents. The alterations and modifications made to the NCI initiated protocols over the past 25 to 30 years of their evolutionary course is a reflection of that attention as well as an educated concern for the toxic potential of these agents.

There long has been the implication that preclinical drug safety and toxicity studies based on sound scientific principles carried out in experimental animals have predictive value for findings in man. In truth, this is the sole legitimately ethical and moral reason for performing such studies. This hypothesis has generally been accepted, with constraints, and has been critically evaluated and proven over the years for anticancer chemotherapeutic agents. Almost all scientists and clinicians agree that extrapolating toxicity findings from animals to humans makes some sense, but almost all disagree on precisely how much sense it makes.

From the clinical perspective, the priority toxicology studies are those which provide quantitative data on interspecies dose relationships. The Phase I clinician is mainly, and to a point exclusively, interested in knowing a starting dose for human trial which is relatively safe along with an estimate of the maximally tolerated dose (MTD) regardless of the actual dose-limiting toxicity (DLT). The effectiveness of preclinical toxicology studies in predicting risk to humans is reviewed here with exclusive emphasis on studies in which the NCI participated as the major or exclusive sponsor. Numerous retrospective reviews of these clinical correlations have appeared over the past two to three decades dealing with either quantitative or qualitative toxicity. Some have already been cited in the preceding section (Prieur et al., 1973; Rozencweig et al., 1981; Grieshaber and Marsoni, 1986).

Quantitative Correlations

Comparative quantitative correlations between experimental animal species and humans have been made for three decades in a noble attempt to precisely estimate a dose at which a Phase I clinical trial for an antineoplastic drug can safely be initiated yet be sufficiently near

Table 2-3. The Current NCI Preclinical Toxicology Protocols

Single-dose lethality study in mice
Five daily-dose lethality study in mice
Single-dose toxicity study in dogs
Five daily-dose toxicity study in dogs
Single-dose toxicity study in rodents*
Five daily-dose toxicity study in rodents*

*Optional studies for filing an INDA.

the MTD in humans so not to require a large number of dose escalations to attain a representative dose for Phase II trials. As stated previously, the prime objective of preclinical, animal toxicology studies with anticancer drugs is to identify the elusive entry level dose for human trials. A brief review of the information acquired over the years indicates clearly that data from animals, on individual drugs, can and does accurately predict the potential MTD in humans and therefore, a safe dose for initiation of studies in humans.

Freireich et al. (1966) published their classic retrospective work in which quantitative toxicity data from mice, rats, hamsters, dogs, monkeys, and humans were compiled for 18 selected antineoplastic drugs. Relationships were established among and between the various species, including humans, wherein dose levels based on body surface area provided a more direct interspecies correlation regarding toxicity than dose levels based on body mass. To standardize the analysis, all data were converted to a uniform schedule of once daily for five days. Regression analysis after logarithmic transformation of the data demonstrated a linear relationship between the MTD in humans, the LD_{10} in rodents and the highest nonlethal dose (defined as the MTD) in dogs or monkeys. Their data established for the first time that the MTD for antineoplastics in humans is about the same as that in each experimental species. From these data the conclusion was drawn that each of the experimental test species used to evaluate the toxicity of anticancer agents can provide information relating to potential dose levels in the clinical setting. This analysis provided the rationale for using a specific fraction of the MTD in the most sensitive specie as the clinical trial entry level dose. In fact, the authors suggested that clinical trials could be safely initiated at doses equivalent to one-third the MTD in animals.

Homan (1972) confirmed and extended these comparative quantitative observations from dogs, monkeys, and humans based on results with 37 antitumor drugs. By applying regression analyses to the data of Freireich et al. (1966) and reviewing and reanalyzing the drugs covered by Schein et al. (1970) Homan determined the distributions of toxic doses in dogs and monkeys in relation to clinical MTDs. The MTD in animals was defined as the dose producing only minimal, reversible toxicity, an assumption which likely would underpredict the MTD in humans in the clinical setting. Homan concluded that there was a 6% probability of exceeding the human MTD if clinical trials were initiated at one-third the MTD for the more sensitive large animal species. Using only data from dogs or monkeys, but not both, the risk increased to 10%. Homan concluded that the risk from the more sensitive animal model was approximately 10-fold that of using one-tenth the MTD in mg/m^2.

To illustrate the contemporary significance of these classic attempts to equate doses between species, the data retrospectively analyzed by Freireich et al. (1966) was recently reexamined by Mordenti (1986). In her reevaluation, a power function $Y = aW^b$ was used to describe the relationship of body weight to equivalent dose, dosing schedule, and toxic dose. Her findings illustrate the adequacy of such a functional expression for describing the relationship between toxic dose and animal body weight indicating that accurate scaling for pharmacokinetic parameters by power functions should play an important role in the assessment of dosing regimens for interspecies toxicity comparisons. Travis and White (1988), recently, reanalyzed the data on 14 drugs from the Freireich et al. (1966) study and 13 additional drugs from the early study by Schein et al. (1970) to similarly ascertain whether a more accurate body weight scaling factor could be determined. Note that Freireich et al. (1966) used a power function to extrapolate doses between species wherein body weight was raised to the two-thirds power. They then based their comparative analysis on body surface area because this parameter is proportional to body weight to the two-thirds power. In their simple and elegant reanalysis, Travis and White (1988) determined that body weight to the three-fourths power may be the most appropriate interspecific scaling factor to use in risk assessment of direct-acting compounds. The utility and biological meaning of these reanalyses are unclear, however, in light of the fact that today we can count upon species specific toxicity and pharmacokinetic data to more meticulously define the interspecies relationships between dose and adverse drug effects. The critical importance of these reiterative studies resides in their power function descriptions which can easily be translated into pharmacokinetics and the concepts of pharmacokinetic equivalency.

In 1973, toxicology protocols were introduced wherein large animals were used to estimate a safe starting dose for clinical trials with new antitumor drugs (Prieur et al., 1973). By the mid to late 1970s the Prieur protocol for toxicology studies had been tested in the development of sufficient numbers of new drugs leading to two analytical reports on the clinical correlations of toxicity (Goldsmith et al., 1975 and Penta et al., 1979). In the former study, dose schedules used in animals were converted to the human schedules and comparisons made. If starting doses for Phase I clinical trials had been selected by calculating one-third TDL (see Prieur et al., 1973) in the most sensitive large animal species, five of 30 drugs would have produced significant toxicity in the first patient treated. The latter study retrospectively analyzed data on 12 agents of diverse origin. One-third the TDL in the more sensitive large animal species expressed in mg/m^2 served as a tolerable starting dose in humans under all administration schedules used. The number of dose escalation steps needed to reach the human MTD using a modified Fibonacci dose escalation scheme varied from two to 12. One-third the LD_{10} in mice, also expressed in mg/m^2, would have estimated a safe starting dose requiring fewer dose escalation steps to reach the human MTD.

Guarino et al. (1979) added to these retrospective surveys in an effort to assess both the advantages and problems associated with using toxicological data from mice in dose prediction in humans. These authors limited their analyses to 58 cytotoxic agents for which clinical data was available following IV administration on a single dose schedule, a weekly schedule or daily administration for five to seven days. The results stimulated caution in using murine lethality data without reviewing the strain of mouse used, the route and schedule of administration and the drug vehicle. Each variable contributes to the variation in results among and between species. The importance of this review lies in its assessment of the variables to consider in examining correlations between animal and human quantitative toxicity. Firm conclusions regarding the 58 reviewed drugs were precluded, according to the authors, because of the wide range of experimental variables. Nevertheless, adding this review to the preceding data analysis of Goldsmith et al. (1975) permits the conclusion that there are no overwhelming quantitative differences between large animal and rodent data which estimate safe clinical trial dose levels.

Rozencweig et al. (1981) investigated whether quantitative data from mice could be used to estimate the starting doses in Phase I clinical trials. Essentially, the MTD in humans for 21 anticancer agents was compared to the LD_{10} in mice and the TDL and TDH in dogs. As noted earlier in this chapter, this study of the comparative data obtained on preclinical and clinical MTDs convinced the anticancer drug development community that the streamlined approach to preclinical toxicity tests promulgated in 1979 would provide safe clinical starting doses and be easily completed in a relatively short time frame. In their analysis, Rozencweig and colleagues determined that one-sixth the murine LD_{10} or one-third the TDL found in dog studies would have yielded an acceptable starting dose for the 21 drugs considered. Importantly, the selection of the clinical dose by either method would have required no difference in the number of escalations in the Phase I trial. The authors further suggested that the selection of one-tenth the murine LD_{10} for clinical trial provided this dose proves tolerable to dogs. This alternative had the advantage of not requiring the determination of dose levels specifically toxic to dogs. Therein resided the efficiency of scale and the time advantage seized by the 1979 NCI preclinical toxicology protocols.

In 1986, Grieshaber and Marsoni (1986) evaluated the data from the first seven anticancer drugs for which preclinical toxicity studies were conducted according to the new protocol. One-tenth the murine LD_{10} established a safe human starting dose. Six of the seven drugs could have started at that level with no adverse effects. Because of moderate toxicity in beagle dogs at the estimated clinical starting dose, the actual entry dose was reduced to levels equivalent to one-thirtieth the $MELD_{10}$. Therefore, it was concluded that studies in beagle dogs did not effectively predict whether the one-tenth $MELD_{10}$ dose represented a risk to humans by overpredicting doses at which toxicity would occur. Interestingly, toxicity data in dogs seriously underpredicted the dose at which one drug, the purine nucleoside analog fludarabine (Fludara), would safely start clinical trial. In this case, no myelosuppressive effect was noted in beagle dogs at 20 times the projected starting dose. Unfortunately, severe myelosuppression occurred in patients at the entry dose, however, the outcome was more fortunate in that no patients were fatally compromised. The eventual human MTD turned out to be the originally estimated entry dose. Today, however, unlike at the time of clinical trial initiation, we are aware of the biochemical circumstances which led to this particular episode of species differential toxicity. Essentially, the purine nucleoside analog is phosphorylated to the triphosphate species more efficiently in human bone marrow cells than in dog or murine bone marrow cells. This, in effect, made the same dose yielding similar intracellular drug concentrations, more toxic to humans than lower animals since more "active" species would be formed in human cells. Fortunately no major human complications resulted from initiating the clinical trial at too high a dose. It should be emphasized that standard protocol toxicology studies are not designed to determine the pharmacologic basis for this interspecies discrepancy.

The sum and substance of these appraisals of data collected over two decades can be simply stated: The clinical starting dose for antineoplastic agents can be determined from animal studies wherein the route of administration and dosing schedule are the same as that projected for the clinical trial. Over time, these quantitative projections of drug tolerance and toxicity have provided a more or less acceptable prediction of a well-tolerated dose in humans. The most appropriate entry dose remains one-tenth the MTD in mice regardless of which power function one uses to describe interspecies scaling. There are, however, problems and uncertainties associated with using murine lethality data to estimate human clinical starting doses. The precision, or lack thereof, with which the study was carried out, the strain of mice used, the route of drug administration, and the schedule of administration all impact on the accuracy, precision and reliability of the data for clinical predictions (Guarino, 1979; Van Putten, 1983). Furthermore, the LD_{10} is a derived data point from lethality studies with a wide distribution range for the 95% confidence limits at this lower end of the dose–response curve.

More importantly, however, major uncertainties occur because of the designed end point of the lethality study itself. The measured end point is obviously death of a large number of animals, but the critical parameter to the toxicologist and clinician should be the cause of death. Essentially, immediate lethality, in minutes to a few hours, following drug administration is due most probably to very high peak plasma levels of the drug or vehicle leading to catastrophic neurologic or cardiovascular compromise and not to toxicity imparted by the cytotoxic pharmacologic effect of the agent which is a frequent source of toxicity in humans, especially to the gastrointestinal mucosa and bone marrow. In such cases, the LD_{50} or any LD derived therefrom will be essentially meaningless as an estimate of the MTD in human clinical trials. This is so since the traditional mathematical calculation of the human starting dose is based on body surface area which is proportional to the clearance of the drug rather than to peak drug concentration leading to substantial underprediction of the human MTD. This shortcoming in dose estimation is repeatedly observed in those Phase I clinical trials in which 10 to 20 dose escalations were required to reach the clinical MTD. In all likelihood, the $MELD_{10}$ was calculated from a study in which the mice died within a short time after drug administration. A more advantageous method of predicting the human MTD is to establish clearly the MTD and understand the DLT in experimental animals short of inducing lethality while investigating various administration schedules. It is instructional to note that certain pharmacokinetic relationships such as total body drug clearance are also important to species differences in toxicity. These critical parameters will be addressed later in this chapter.

Qualitative Correlations

Qualitative prediction for organ toxicity produced by anticancer agents in man represents the second major objective of animal toxicology studies. Qualitative toxicology data on new agents have traditionally been accepted as secondary information as they attempt to predict for the specific organ system(s) affected as the DLT. It has been claimed that animal toxicology studies should be performed to alert the Phase I clinician to potential human hazards of anticancer agents (Schein, 1977). Nevertheless there has been, and remains today, a perception that prediction of human DLTs from studies in experimental animals is fraught with uncertainty. There have been fewer reviews of the qualitative historical data than for quantitative comparisons.

The predictive value of qualitative findings has been assessed in three major retrospective studies. In the first and most thorough study, Schein et al. (1970) evaluated the usefulness of dogs and monkeys as the experimental species for predicting qualitative drug toxicity in man. They retrospectively concluded that a large animal toxicity screen involving the determination of acute lethality in dogs and subacute, repeated dose toxicity in dogs and monkeys detected a large portion of the total spectrum of toxic effects encountered in the clinical use of new anticancer drugs. A large series of individual toxicologic parameters (approximately 170) induced by 25 anticancer drugs were evaluated and determinations made regarding whether or not a particular parameter was observed in each specie. All serious organ system toxicities were well predicted. Qualitatively, dogs and monkeys predicted bone marrow depression, gastrointestinal disturbances, and hepatotoxicity for each drug producing these toxic effects clinically. For example, studies in dogs predicted correctly 80% of the time that a particular agent would cause significant human hematologic toxicity. The predictability was 83% for the same toxicity using monkeys. In overall usefulness, the preclinical toxicity studies predicted for 100% of hematologic toxicity, gastrointestinal toxicity, and hepatotoxicity, and 90% of the nephrotoxicity. As a shortcoming, the screen failed to quantify cardiovascular and neuromuscular toxicities. Moreover, the correct correlations were found at the expense of a high percentage of false positives resulting from the severely toxic doses required in animals to produce all observable toxic effects.

In their invaluable reanalysis of the 25 agents reviewed by Schein et al. (1970), Rozencweig et al. (1981) assessed the qualitative findings in preclinical models using a Baysian approach. The predictive value of qualitative testing was high for the common toxic effects produced by cytotoxic antineoplastic agents in man. In fact, the positive predictive value was actually greater than 85% for gastrointestinal toxicity and myelosuppression. The predictive value for unusually rare adverse affects was dramatically lower, ranging from five to 50%. The authors concluded that there was no clear superiority of findings in animals over the clinical experience with the prevalence of these findings in humans since myelosuppression, stomatitis, and mucositis are generally to be expected and usually observed.

In a more recent review, Grieshaber and Marsoni (1986) examined human DLTs with respect to qualitative predictions from animals for seven drugs on two administration schedules, a single dose and five consecutive daily doses. Maximally tolerated doses producing human DLTs are compared in Table 2-4 to doses evoking a corresponding toxic effect in beagle dogs. There is satisfactory correlation between the human MTD and the lowest dose in dogs at which similar toxicity was noted for three of five drugs (carboplatin, homoharringtonine, and triciribine) on a single dose schedule and for four of seven drugs (N-methylformamide, carboplatin, teroxirone, and homoharringtonine) on the five consecutive daily dose schedule. On the single dose schedule, the dose of teroxirone producing myelosuppression and phlebitis was sixfold lower than that in humans, a substantial underprediction of the MTD. Nevertheless, a margin of safety accompanies such an underprediction. Conversely, the dose of fludarabine producing myelosuppression in dogs was 20 to 50 times greater than

Table 2-4. Toxicity at Human Maximally Tolerated Dose Compared to Dose at Which Similar Toxicity Was Detected in Dogs*

ANTINEOPLASTIC AGENT	HUMAN DOSE LIMITING TOXICITY	HUMAN MTD ($mg/m^2/d$)		DOG DOSE ($mg/m^2/d$)	
		× 1	× 5	× 1	× 5
Carboplatin	Myelosuppression	400–500	99	312	60
Teroxirone	Myelosuppression	2250	400	360	160
	Phlebitis	2250	400	360	320
Homoharringtonine	Myelosuppression	9	5	6.4	2.9
	Hypotension	9	5	NA†	NA
Fludarabine	Myelosuppression	260	40	5200	2200
Triciribine	Hepatotoxicity	250	55	338	154
	Hyperglycemia	250	–	676	–
N-Methylformamide	Hepatotoxicity	–	1170	–	1324
Dihydroazacytidine	Myelosuppression	–	2500	–	223
	Chest pain	–	2500	–	NA
	Nausea and vomiting	–	2500	–	223

*Data from Grieshaber and Marsoni (1986).
†NA = not assessed in dogs.

the human MTD depending upon the schedule of administration. This discrepancy and its basis has been discussed in the section on quantitative correlations.

Dose level comparability in producing similar end-organ toxicity was reanalyzed by calculating ratios of the human MTD and the lowest dose at which comparable toxic effects occurred in dogs or mice. Table 2-5 illustrates these ratios and the passable success of qualitative prediction from dogs. The ideal MTD/LTD ratio is 1.0 indicating that studies in animals predict absolutely for drug dose and toxicity in humans. This is obviously not always the case, however, ratios between 1.0 and 3.0 can be acceptable. As noted with fludarabine and triciribine, ratios lower than 1.0 pose some degree of clinical risk. Predictably, the most frequently encountered DLT in humans in this study was myelosuppression with hepatotoxicity as limiting with two drugs. In summary then, this recent review illustrates that qualitative toxicology studies in dogs on seven new antitumor drugs predicted the human DLT 100% of

Table 2-5. Comparison of MTD in Man to Doses in Dogs and Mice at Which Corresponding Human Dose Limiting Toxicity Was Observed*

DRUG	DOSE-LIMITING TOXICITY	SCHEDULE	MTD MAN/LTD ANIMAL*	
			MAN/DOG	MAN/MICE
Triciribine	Hepatotoxicity	× 1	0.7	Not predicted
		× 5	0.4	Not predicted
N-Methylformamide	Hepatotoxicity	× 5	0.9	0.9
Fludaribine	Myelosuppression	× 1	0.05	0.11
		× 5	0.02	0.03
Carboplatin	Myelosuppression	× 1	1.4	Not predicted
		× 5	1.6	0.8
Homoharringtonine	Myelosuppression	× 1	1.4	0.7
		× 5	1.7	0.9
Dihydroazacytidine	Myelosuppression	× 5	2.3	2.2
Teroxirone	Myelosuppression	× 1	6.2	12.5
		× 5	2.5	5.0

*Data from Grieshaber and Marsoni (1986).
†Ratio calculated from doses at which clinical observation (man and animal) and histopathological findings (dog, mouse) showed consistent toxic effects. < 1.0 = toxicity occurred in humans at lower dose than in experimental animals; > 1.0 = toxicity occurred in experimental animals at lower doses than in humans.

the time whereas murine studies foretold the DLT 75% of the time. The major deficiencies noted are the lack of perfect correlation between human and animal doses at which these DLTs occur and the appearance of other, confounding toxicities in dogs at the dose levels judged to produce the toxicity similar to the human MTD. The authors, nevertheless, concluded that appropriately interpreted toxicity data from studies with beagle dogs can be a valuable asset in predicting the potential end-organ risk to humans even though the safety of the clinical entry level doses is occasionally underpredicted. As newer, more disease selective drugs are discovered to treat many malignancies, different, unexpected, and unpredictable toxicities are likely to be produced. A reevaluation and readjustment of our toxicology schemes are, therefore, essential.

GUIDELINES FOR PRECLINICAL ANIMAL PHARMACOLOGY AND TOXICOLOGY STUDIES FOR NEW DRUGS DESIGNED TO TREAT HUMAN DISEASES OF FATAL OUTCOME

The universal problem of correlating animal toxicology and pharmacology data to humans, in practical terms, has been exhaustively discussed in the literature and needs no detailed reiteration here. One prominent theme, however, consistently recurs: the importance of understanding species differences in the mechanisms which underlie pharmacokinetic and pharmacodynamic behavior of drugs. This theme may be more specifically restructured in terms of our present subject by noting that one of the primary reasons, if not the major reason, for the comparative toxicology problem with antineoplastic drugs resides in the universe of pharmacodynamics and pharmacokinetics.

Typically, little, if any, information is available on the pharmacodynamic, pharmacokinetic, or toxicologic properties of a newly discovered cytotoxic or cytostatic anticancer drug in either animals or man. Essentially, one initiates preclinical drug development (see Fig. 2-1) at ground zero knowing nothing factual about the toxicity of a specific agent, other than the general assumption that all cytotoxic drugs, regardless of mechanism of action, will be toxic to organs with dividing cell types such as hair follicles, the gastrointestinal tract, the bone marrow, and the lymphoid organs. Consequently, there has been a deeply seated obsession in both the drug development and regulatory communities to standardize preclinical toxicology and safety methodologies for all new anticancer drugs within inviolate protocols. The flaw in this strategy is historically obvious in the correlative deficiencies noted in the preceding section. Preclinical toxicology studies performed with little consideration of pharmacokinetics and pharmacodynamics cannot be expected to consistently correlate well with clinical findings for all drugs. Consequently, there are bound to be acute toxicities observed in humans which will not be observed in animals and vice versa due to species differences in pharmacologic handling of the individual drugs. Individualized, agent-directed preclinical pharmacology and toxicology studies can be designed and followed based on known biological and biochemical properties of each new drug, thereby preempting in large part the critical traps encountered in the past.

A number of the new antitumor agents developed recently by the NCI demonstrate species differences in toxicity due to pharmacokinetic or pharmacodynamic properties. Flavone acetic acid (NSC-347512), developed due to exciting preclinical activity versus colon cancer (Corbett et al., 1986; Plowman et al., 1986; O'Dwyer et al., 1987), serves as one example of a drug where marked species differences were observed in the doses at which toxicity was seen due primarily to interspecies pharmacokinetic differences. The single dose $MELD_{10}$ in mice, 1029 mg/m^2 (343 mg/kg), is strikingly similar to the MTD in rats (1032 mg/m^2; 172 mg/kg) based on body surface area, yet beagle dogs easily tolerated 4000 mg/m^2 (200 mg/kg) with no major sign of toxicity. These comparative toxicity differences are easily reconcilable when the interspecies pharmacokinetic differences are considered. Flavone acetic acid is cleared from plasma in a dose-dependent fashion in all species studied. It is noteworthy that the plasma clearance in dogs is at least two-fold greater at all doses tested (Zaharko et al., 1986), a fact that goes a long way toward explaining how dogs tolerate substantially greater drug doses than rodents. It is worthy of further note that the MTD in humans is 10 to 15 gm/m^2 depending on the schedule of administration and that serious, nonlethal toxicity (lethargy, hyperthermia, and gastrointestinal distress) was observed in dogs at 7 to 12 mg/m^2 after a single drug dose. The total body clearance in humans is similar to that in dogs at respective doses which most likely accounts for the similarities in the dosage level at which serious toxicity occurs in these two species.

A second new drug, 4-ipomeanol (NSC-349438), a naturally occurring furan selectively toxic to clara cells in the lung (Boyd, 1977; Falzon et al., 1986), is being developed as a potential agent to treat lung cancer (Christian et al., 1989). The single dose LD_{10} in mice is 23 mg/kg (69 mg/m^2), whereas the MTD in both dogs and rats is 12 mg/kg. Calculation of these latter dose levels on a body surface basis reveals an equality of the MTD in rats and mice, but the MTD in dogs is substantially greater at 240 mg/m^2. In each of the three experimental species studied in INDA-directed (investigational new drug application) toxicology tests (Smith et al., 1987), the DLT was similar, pulmonary fibrosis leading to respiratory distress followed by death if the dose was too high. One plausible explanation for the differential dose (mg/m^2) to toxicity response of ipomeanol lies in the pharmacodynamic relationship between drug uptake, P450 metabolism to a highly reactive intermediate and macromolecular binding, the cellular event producing necrosis, and subsequent toxicity. Several years ago Boyd and Burka (1978) demonstrated a dose-response relationship for binding of the reactive intermediate and toxicity, which indicates that the kinetics of the pharmacodynamic effect (drug metabolism and in situ macromolecular binding) is different among species at similar drug exposures producing an apparent dose-toxic response inconsistency.

A scheme for universal preclinical pharmacology and toxicology studies with new antineoplastic agents can be described in which the pharmacokinetic similarities or differences between species are established. Reasonably straightforward and efficient preclinical toxicity studies include measuring these parameters which are, or will be meaningful in the design and guidance of the human clinical trial. The design, then, of preclinical toxicology studies centers on how the drug will be used clinically, including route and schedule of administration, and what is reasonable and convenient to examine in animals. Rare or unusual toxic effects which will undoubtedly occur in man, such as cardiotoxicity with doxorubicin (Adriamycin), pulmonary toxicity with bleomycin (Blenoxane), or ototoxicity with cisplatin (Platinol) are not likely to be detected by generalized acute toxicity screening tests in animals. In fact, it is more than likely impossible to devise prospective tests in animals for undefined, rare toxic events in humans and furthermore, it is not practical to prospectively look for the unusual toxicity. Fortunately, these kinds of toxicities are, today, an infrequent cause of withdrawal of an anticancer drug from therapeutic usage.

As the standard for collecting more meaningful and clinically applicable data on the toxicity of potential antineoplastic agents, preclinical studies other than those based solely on doses producing lethality in mice are essential. Murine lethality studies collect only minimal information (i.e., mortality) with no definable toxicity. True toxicological information defining the limitations of dosing, therefore defining the MTD instead of the LD_{10}, would distinguish between acute peak plasma drug effects and actual organ-directed toxicity. Coupled with other data, most notably pharmacokinetics and schedule dependence of toxicity, information of this nature permits prediction of interspecies toxicity variations somewhat more precisely. Agent directed studies which can constitute a sound preclinical toxicology/pharmacology program for new anticancer drugs are presented in Table 2-6.

Methodologically, the first toxicology studies might be performed using the intravenous route in a few rodents wherein the MTD is approximated in terms of administration schedule and dose intensity (a measure of plasma concentration over time). This information is followed by, and coupled with, similar measures of kinetics and toxicity of the agent in dogs.

Table 2-6. Toxicology Studies Coupled with Pharmacology for Preclinical Appraisal of New Antineoplastic Agents

STAGE A – PRELIMINARY EXPERIMENTS

- Rodents:
  Estimate the maximally tolerated dose (MTD) and dose limiting toxicity (DLT).
  Determine pharmacokinetics on two administration schedules – single bolus and continuous infusion.
- Dogs:
  Determine pharmacokinetics on single administration.
  Assess preliminary toxicity of equivalent rodent MTD.

STAGE B – INDA-DIRECTED EXPERIMENTS

Fully define the toxicity profile in rodents and dogs at the respective MTD and the proposed clinical trial entry dose using the appropriate schedule of administration.
Characterize the pharmacokinetic profile in rodents and dogs relating toxicity to dose and plasma concentration intensity using the appropriate schedule of administration.

Note that such studies can be accomplished using very few rodents and two to four dogs. Neither study would use lethality as its end-point but place the main emphases on clinical observations, clinical chemistry, hematology, and histopathology as toxicity determinants. Data from these two studies characterize not only the MTD and DLT in rodents and dogs but also the foremost procedures for approaching the full-scale preclinical toxicology studies and the initial Phase I clinical trials. As a matter of record, these types of studies extend, to early preclinical drug development, those previously proposed (Bradner et al., 1980; Bradner and Schurig, 1981; Schurig et al., 1986; Schurig and Bradner, 1987) wherein simple, straightforward toxicology studies in mice were described as an aid to drug discovery. These authors advocated determination of the relative myelosuppressive effects (a typically encountered DLT) of newly discovered anticancer drugs and analogs to enable one, coupled with antitumor efficacy studies, to choose the most active, least toxic member of the analog series. The Stage B, INDA-directed preclinical toxicity/safety studies are then carried out using the most appropriate administration schedule in the most appropriate species wherein the toxicity to each organ system is defined in terms of pharmacokinetic parameters in addition to the dose levels administered. These studies are more detailed extensions of those performed in the preliminary stage. The conclusion of these two stages provides data on the schedule dependency of agent toxicity in two species and the relationship between toxic effects and plasma drug levels or areas under the concentration versus time curves; thereby indicating scheduling modifications through which the potential human toxicity of particular agents can be reduced or ameliorated without ablating the antitumor effect. A forerunner to this strategy was used in the preclinical studies with hexamethylene bisacetamide (HMBA), deoxyspergualin, merbarone, and flavone acetic acid (Table 2-7). The approach taken with these agents added pharmacokinetic studies in mice (Collins et al., 1986) or rats and dogs along with schedule

Table 2-7. Agent Directed Toxicity Studies—Design and Rationale

DRUG	NSC NO.	AGENT DIRECTED TOXICOLOGY DESIGN	RATIONALE
Hexamethylene bisacetamide	095589	Continuous infusion	Schedule dependent differentiating agent
Deoxyspergualin	356894	Continuous infusion	Schedule dependency of efficacy
Merbarone	336628	Continuous infusion	Schedule dependency of efficacy
Flavone acetic acid	347512	Daily continuous infusions × 3	Efficacy enhanced, toxicity reduced

dependency toxicity experiments (Collins et al., 1987) to the standardized protocols of the NCI. A brief review of each agent listed will demonstrate the rationale of study design as well as the value of the information provided for the preclinical-clinical interface. A description of the toxicology/pharmacology studies carried out with flavone acetic acid was discussed earlier in this section.

Hexamethylene bisacetamide is a polar-planar compound capable of inducing terminal differentiation in murine erythroleukemia cells (Fibach et al., 1977) and human promyelocytic leukemia cells (Collins et al., 1980) in vitro at concentrations of 2 to 5 mmol/L for three to five days. Preclinical toxicology studies on HMBA were performed using repeated intraperitoneal injections, every four hours for 12 injections, in rats and continuous infusions of 120 hr in dogs (Chun et al., 1986) to ascertain whether concentrations similar to those required in culture could be produced in vivo for the in vitro demonstrated period of time. Clinical signs of central nervous system (CNS) toxicity were judged to limit dosing in both species with dogs exhibiting convulsive activity at plasma steady state concentrations of 1 to 2 mM HMBA over 120 hr. These data convinced us that HMBA could be administered to humans in a manner producing plasma drug levels having the potential to induce the desired biological effect. Pharmacokinetic studies conducted in conjunction with Phase I trials demonstrated that plasma steady state HMBA concentrations were dose dependent and that 1 to 2 mM could be achieved with acceptable, dose-limiting CNS toxicity consisting of agitation, confusion, and occasional hallucinations. The MTD was reached in three dose escalations using plasma steady state drug levels as the guide. Interestingly, administration of sodium bicarbonate to overcome metabolic acidosis ameliorated CNS toxicity and led to plasma concentrations of 2 mM with thrombocytopenia as dose limiting.

Deoxyspergualin is the synthetic 15-deoxy analog of the antibiotic spergualin. Schedule dependency of maximal antitumor activity toward L1210 leukemia cells was observed in studies wherein the agent was administered by constant infusion for three days (Plowman et al., 1987). In standard toxicity studies, the major adverse effects in rats and dogs were neurologic in origin consisting of subconvulsive jerking, ataxia and bradypnea, and moderate myelosuppression. Continuous IV infusions over 120 hr in dogs altered the toxicity pattern whereby hemorrhagic cystitis and anemia as its sequelae became dose limiting with doses producing drug plasma levels greater than 7 to 10 μg/mL. Nevertheless, over 144 mg/kg/day (2.9 gm/m^2/d) could be administered producing a steady state blood level of approximately 22 μg/mL, well above the concentration expected for antitumor activity (7 μg/mL), yet below that propagating unacceptable toxicity. Clinical pharmacology studies were performed during the subsequent Phase I study with the 120 hr continuous infusion schedule as the only clinical regimen tested. At doses greater than 2000 mg/m^2/d, hypotension is dose limiting, however, plasma drug levels range at an acceptable 6 to 8 μg/mL (12–15 μM). Other toxicities noted include mild myelosuppression and mild diarrhea. No sign of toxic cystitis was observed in humans.

The antineoplastic agent, merbarone, a conjugate of thiobarbituric acid and aniline joined in amide linkage demonstrated a broad activity spectrum in several murine tumor models (Brewer et al., 1985). Evidence that antitumor activity was schedule dependent emerged from more detailed studies prompting a rethinking of the toxicology protocols (Glover et al., 1987). Treatment of rodents and dogs with merbarone under the standard toxicology protocol produced neurotoxicity as the limiting effect on both schedules with evidence for peak plasma effects since there was little evidence of cumulative toxicity. In studies with dogs using the continuous infusion schedule, hematologic and gastrointestinal toxicities were found directly related to the rate of drug infusion, and consequently to the steady state plasma level achieved. At plasma drug levels above 10 to 15 μg/mL clearance became concentration-dependent indicating saturation of elimination pathways. Clinically, the DLTs with a five day continuous infusion schedule of merbarone were myelosuppression and nephrotoxicity at doses greater than 1000 mg/m^2/d. The steady state plasma levels of merbarone were linearly correlated with dose and reached slightly over 40 μg/mL in one patient treated with the highest dose. Local phlebitis was seen in all patients receiving greater than 200 mg/m^2/d and was overcome by the use of a central venous line.

The overall utility of such preclinical toxicology and pharmacology studies wherein adverse effects were related to pharmacokinetics and schedule dependence of toxicity followed by pharmacologically based clinical dose escalations resides in a more enlightened design of human trials and a reduction in the numbers of patients required. Equally important, fewer patients were treated with these experimental drugs at potentially ineffective dose levels. These expanded preclinical studies in conjunction with the elegant clinical pharmacologic studies carried out on HMBA (Egorin et al., 1987a; 1987b), carboplatin (Egorin et al., 1984; 1985), and Menogaril (Egorin et al., 1986) will serve as the foundation for future preclinical and Phase I clinical studies. In these clinical trials, the plasma levels of each agent were correlated to an effect in patients, either an alteration in a physiologic function or a true toxic effect, thereby providing data on which prospective clinical judgments regarding dose levels for subsequent patients were made.

The advent of in vitro methods for drug screening currently under validation at the NCI (Alley et al., 1988; Scudiero et al., 1988; Shoemaker et al., 1988) will presumably select for new agents specific for particular disease types. As a result, preclinical pharmacology/toxicology studies can be designed to target specific efficacious drug exposure intensities (a plasma concentration for a specific duration) in different animal species based on the pharmacodynamically active in vitro exposure intensities and secondly, identifying drug exposure intensities which produce DLTs. The goal is to not only identify toxic effects but also to establish a preclinical therapeutic index thereby proving potentially helpful in designing the early clinical trials and determining appropriate dose escalation intervals. This novel drug discovery/preclinical development concept, coupled with the use of plasma drug AUC (area under the concentration times time curve) to guide dose escalations in Phase I trials (Collins et al., 1986) provide further stimuli for the redesign of preclinical pharmacokinetically based toxicology studies for experimental antineoplastic agents.

REFERENCES

Alley MC, Scudiero DA, Monks A, Hursey ML, Czerwinski MJ, Fine DL, Abbott BA, Mayo JG, Shoemaker RH, and Boyd MR Feasibility of drug screening with panels of human tumor cell lines using a microculture tetrazolium assay. Cancer Res 1988 48:589–601.

Bogden AE, Haskell PM, LePage DJ, Kelton DE, Cobb WR, and Esber HJ Growth of human tumor xenografts implanted under the renal capsule of normal immunocompetent mice. Exptl Cell Biol 1979 47:281–293.

Boyd MR Evidence for the Clara cell as a site of cytochrome P450-dependent mixed-function oxidase activity in lung. Nature (Lond.) 1977 269:713–715.

Boyd MR and Burka LT In vivo studies on the relationship between target organ alkylation and the pulmonary toxicity of a chemically reactive metabolite of 4-ipomeanol. J Pharmacol Exptl Ther 1978 207:687–697.

Bradner WT, Schurig JE, Huftalen JB, and Doyle GJ Evaluation of antitumor drug side effects in small animals. Cancer Chemother Pharmacol 1980 4:95–101.

Bradner WT and Schurig JE Toxicology screening in small animals. Cancer Treat Rev 1981 8:93–102.

Brewer AD, Minatelli JA, Plowman J, Paull KD, and Narayanan VL 5-(N-phenyl-carboxamido)-2-thiobarbituric acid (NSC 336628), a novel potential antitumor agent. Biochem Pharmacol 1985 34: 2047–2050.

Cancer Chemotherapy National Service Center (CCNSC) Specifications for preliminary toxicological evaluation of experimental cancer chemotherapeutic agents. Cancer Chemother Rep 1959 1:89–98.

Cancer Chemotherapy National Service Center (CCNSC) An outline of procedures for preliminary toxicologic and pharmacologic evaluation of experimental cancer chemotherapeutic agents. Cancer Chemother Rep 1960 9:120–139.

Cancer Chemotherapy National Service Center (CCNSC) An outline of procedures for preliminary toxicologic and pharmacologic evaluation of experimental cancer chemotherapeutic agents. Cancer Chemother Rep 1964 37:3–17.

Christian MC, Wittes RE, Leyland-Jones B, McLemore TE, Smith AC, Grieshaber CK, Chabner BA, and Boyd MR 4-Ipomeanol: A novel investigational new drug for lung cancer. J Nat Cancer Inst 1989 81:1133–1143.

Chun HG, Leyland-Jones B, Hoth D, Shoemaker DD, Wolpert-DeFilippes M, Grieshaber CK, Cradock J, Davignon JP, Moon R, Rifkind R, and Wittes R Hexamethylene Bisacetamide: A polar-planar compound entering clinical trials as a differentiating agent. Cancer Treat Rep 1986 70:991–996.

Corbett TH, Bissery M-T, Wozniak A, Plowman J, Polin L, Tapazoglou E, Dieckman J, and Valeriote F Activity of Flavone acetic acid (NSC 347512) against solid tumors of mice. Invest New Drugs 1986 4: 207–220.

Collins JM, Zaharko DS, Dedrick RL, and Chabner BA Potential roles for preclinical pharmacology in phase I clinical trials. Cancer Treat Rep 1986 70:73–80.

Collins JM, Leyland-Jones B, and Grieshaber CK Role of preclinical pharmacology in phase I clinical trials: Considerations of schedule-dependence. In: Concepts, Clinical Developments, and Therapeutic Advances in Cancer Chemotherapy Muggia FM Ed Martinus Nijhoff Publishers, Boston 1987 pp. 129–140.

Collins SJ, Bodner A, Ting R, and Gallo RC Induction of morphological and functional differentiation on human promyelocytic leukemia cells (HL-60) by compounds which induce differentiation of murine leukemia cells. Int J Cancer 1980 25:213–218.

Current Good Manufacturing Practice for Finished Pharmaceuticals (21 CFR Part 211). Fed Reg 1978 43:45077–45089.

Driscoll JS The preclinical new drug research program of the National Cancer Institute. Cancer Treat Rep 1984 68:63–76.

Egorin MJ, Van Echo DA, Tipping SJ, Olman EA, Whitacre MY, Thompson BW, and Aisner J Pharmacokinetics and dosage reduction of cis-diammine (1,1-cyclobutanedicarboxylato) platinum in patients with impaired renal function. Cancer Res 1984 44:5432–5438.

Egorin MJ, Van Echo DA, Olman EA, Whitacre MY, Forrest A, and Aisner J Prospective validation of a pharmacologically based dosing scheme for the cis-diamminedichloroplatinum (II) analogue diamminecyclobutanedicarboxylatoplatinum. Cancer Res 1985 45:6502–6506.

Egorin MJ, Van Echo DA, Whitacre MY, Forrest A, Sigman LM, Engisch KL, and Aisner J Human pharmacokinetics, excretion, and metabolism of the anthracycline antibiotic menogaril (7-OMEN, NSC 269148) and their correlation with clinical toxicities. Cancer Res 1986 46:1513–1520.

Egorin MJ, Sigman LM, Van Echo DA, Forrest A, Whitacre MY, and Aisner J Phase I clinical and pharmacokinetic study of hexamethylene bisacetamide (NSC-95880) administered as a five-day continuous infusion. Cancer Res 1987a 47:617–623.

Egorin MJ, Zuhowski EG, Cohen AS, Geelhaar LA, Callery PS, and Van Echo DA Plasma pharmacokinetics and urinary excretion of hexamethylene bisacetamide metabolites. Cancer Res 1987b 47: 6142–6146.

Falzon M, McMahon JB, Schuller HM, and Boyd MR Metabolic activation and cytotoxicity of 4-ipomeanol in human non-small cell lung cancer lines. Cancer Res 1986 46:3484–3489.

Fibach E, Reuben RC, Rifkind RA, and Marks PA Effect of hexamethylene bisacetamide on the commitment to differentiation of murine erythroleukemia cells. Cancer Res 1977 37:440–444.

Freireich EJ, Gehan EA, Rall DP, Schmidt LH, and Skipper HE Quantitative comparison of toxicity of anticancer agents in mouse, rat, hamster, dog, monkey, and man. Cancer Chemother Rep 1966 50: 219–244.

Glover A, Chun HG, Kleinman LG, Cooney DL, Plowman J, Grieshaber CK, Malspeis L, and Leyland-Jones B Merbarone: An antitumor agent entering clinical trials. Invest New Drugs 1987 5:137–143.

Goldin A and Venditti JM The new NCI screen and its implications for clinical evaluation. In: Recent Results in Cancer Research Vol 70 Carter SK and Sakurai Y Eds Springer-Verlag, New York 1980 pp. 5–20.

Goldsmith MA, Slavik M, and Carter SK Quantitative prediction of drug toxicity in humans from toxicology in small and large animals. Cancer Res 1975 35:1354–1364.

Good Laboratory Practice Regulations for Nonclinical Laboratory Studies (21 CFR Part 58). Fed Reg 1978 43:59986–59998.

Good Laboratory Practice Regulations for Nonclinical Laboratory Studies (21 CFR Part 58). Fed Reg 1987 52:33779–33782.

Grieshaber CK and Marsoni S Relation of preclinical toxicology to findings in early clinical trials. Cancer Treat Rep 1986 70:65–72.

Guarino AM Pharmacologic and toxicologic studies of anticancer drugs: Of sharks, mice, and men. In: Methods in Cancer Research, Vol 15 DeVita VT Jr and Busch H Eds Academic Press, Inc., New York 1979 pp. 91–174.

Guarino AM, Rozencweig M, Kline I, Penta JS, Venditti JM, Lloyd HH, Holzworth DA, and Muggia FM Adequacies and inadequacies in assessing murine toxicity data with antineoplastic agents. Cancer Res 1979 39:2204–2210.

Hamberger AW and Salmon SE Primary bioassay of human tumor stem cells. Science 1977 197:461–463.

Homan ER Quantitative relationships between toxic doses of antitumor chemotherapeutic agents in animals and man. Cancer Chemother Rep 1972 3:13–19.

Lowe MC Large animal toxicological studies of anticancer drugs. In: Fundamentals of Cancer Chemotherapy Hellmann K and Carter SK Eds McGraw-Hill, New York 1987 pp. 236–247.

Lowe MC and Davis RD The current toxicology protocol of the National Cancer Institute. In: Fundamentals of Cancer Chemotherapy Hillmann K and Carter SK Eds McGraw-Hill, New York 1987 pp. 228–235.

Mordenti J Dosage regimen design for pharmaceutical studies conducted in animals. J Pharm Sci 1986 75:852–857.

O'Dwyer PJ, Shoemaker DD, Zaharko DS, Grieshaber CK, Plowman J, Corbett T, Valeriote F, Cradock J, Hoth DF, and Leyland-Jones B Flavone acetic acid (LM-975, NSC-347512): A novel antitumor agent. Cancer Chemother Pharmacol 1987 19:670–678.

Penta JS, Rozencweig M, Guarino AM, and Muggia FM Mouse and large-animal toxicology studies of twelve antitumor agents: Relevance to starting dose for phase I clinical trials. Cancer Chemother Pharmacol 1979 3:97–101.

Plowman J, Narayanan VL, Dykes D, Szarvasi E, Briet P, Yoder OC, and Paull KD Flavone acetic acid: A novel agent with preclinical antitumor activity against the colon adenocarcinoma 38 in mice. Cancer Treat Rep 1986 70:631–635.

Plowman J, Harrison SD, Trader MW, Griswold DP, Chadwick M, McComish MF, Silveira DM, and Zaharko D Preclinical antitumor activity and pharmacologic properties of deoxyspergualin. Cancer Res 1987 47:685–689.

Prieur DJ, Young DM, Davis RD, Cooney DA, Homan ER, Dixon RL, and Guarino AM Procedures for the preclinical toxicologic evaluation of cancer chemotherapeutic agents: Protocols of the laboratory of toxicology. Cancer Chemother Rep 1973 4:1–30.

Rozencweig M, Von Hoff DD, Staquet MJ, Schein PS, Penta JS, Goldin A, Muggia FM, Freireich EJ, DeVita VT Jr Animal toxicology for early clinical trials with anticancer agents. Cancer Clin Trials 1981 4:21–28.

Schein PS Preclinical toxicology of anticancer agents. Cancer Res 1977 6:1934–1937.

Schein PS, Davis RD, Carter S, Newman J, Schein DR, and Rall DP The evaluation of anticancer drugs in dogs and monkeys for the prediction of qualitative toxicities in man. Clin Pharmacol Ther 1970 11:3–40.

Schurig JE, Florczyk AP, and Bradner WT The mouse as a model for predicting the myelosuppressive effects of anticancer drugs. Cancer Chemother Pharmacol 1986 16:243–246.

Schurig JE and Bradner WT Small animal toxicology of cancer drugs. In: Fundamentals of Cancer Chemotherapy Hellmann K and Carter SK Eds McGraw-Hill, New York 1987 pp. 248–261.

Scudiero DA, Shoemaker RH, Paull KD, Monks A, Tierney S, Nofziger TH, Currens MJ, Seniff D, and Boyd MR Evaluation of a soluble tetrazolium/formazan assay for cell growth and drug sensitivity in culture using human and other tumor cell lines. Cancer Res 1988 48:4827–4833.

Shoemaker RH, Wolpert-DeFillippes M, Kern D, Lieber M, Makuch R, Miller S, Salmon S, Venditti J, and Von Hoff D Application of a human tumor colony-forming assay to new drug screening. Cancer Res 1985 45:2145–2153.

Shoemaker RH, Monks A, Alley MC, Scudiero DA, Fine DL, McLemore TL, Abbott BJ, Paull KD, Mayo JG, and Boyd MR Development of human tumor cell line panels for use in disease-oriented drug screening. In: Prediction of Response to Cancer Chemotherapy T. Hall Ed Alan R. Liss Inc., New York 1988 pp. 265–286.

Smith AC, Barrett D, Stedham MA, El-hawari M, Kastello MD, Grieshaber CK, and Boyd MR Preclinical toxicology studies of 4-ipomeanol: A novel candidate for clinical evaluation in lung cancer. Cancer Treat Rep 1987 71:1157–1164.

Travis CC and White RK Interspecific scaling of toxicity data. Risk Analysis 1988 8:119–125.

Van Putten LM The preclinical evaluation of anticancer drug toxicity. In: Anticancer Drug Development Hilgard P and Hellmann K Eds J. R. Prous, Barcelona 1983 pp. 61–65.

Venditti JM Pre-clinical drug evaluation: Rationale and methods. Semin Oncol 1981 8:349–361.

Venditti JM The National Cancer Institute antitumor drug discovery program, current and future perspectives: A commentary. Cancer Treat Rep 1983 67:767–772.

Zaharko DS, Grieshaber CK, Plowman J, and Cradock JC Therapeutic and pharmacokinetic relationships of flavone acetic acid: An agent with activity against solid tumors. Cancer Treat Rep 1986 70: 1415–1421.

Zubrod CG Origins and development of chemotherapy research at the National Cancer Institute. Cancer Treat Rep 1984 68:9–20.

CHAPTER 3

Second Tumors After Treatment With Anticancer Drugs

Charles B. Pratt, M.D. and Ching-Hon Pui, M.D.

The objective of cancer treatment is cure. As chemotherapy has developed over the past 30 years, more complicated and aggressive schedules of agents have been used in combination, with or without radiation therapy, and survival has improved (Boice, 1988). Adjuvant chemotherapy has also increased the number of long-term survivors of the more common types of cancer in adults and children.

As the cure rates for primary cancers have improved with the use of intensive treatment, the number of therapy related second neoplasms has also increased. Reduction of the immediate, early, or late side effects of treatment should be considered in the context of patient comfort, quality of life, and the risk of serious complications, including treatment related second cancers.

ONCOGENIC POTENTIAL OF ANTICANCER AGENTS

The oncogenic potential of chemotherapeutic agents in humans was recognized when these agents were used for their immunosuppressive effects in organ transplant recipients (Casciato and Scott, 1979; Grunwald and Rosner, 1979; Harris, 1975, 1976; Hoover and Fraumeni, 1975; Kyle, 1982; Penn and Starzl, 1972; Reiche, 1984; Scheneck and Penn, 1971; Schmahl et al., 1982). First reports of the development of lymphomas in renal transplant recipients appeared in the 1970s (Penn and Starzl, 1972; Scheneck and Penn, 1971). There were reports of similar cancers in patients with collagen vascular diseases who received these agents for immunosuppression of the primary disease process. The oncogenic potential of anticancer agents was determined by their use in long-term studies involving laboratory animals.

The carcinogenic potential of anticancer agents has been difficult to assess for humans (Boice et al., 1988). Many patients died of their primary disease before the latency time for the second tumor was reached. Humans may be less sensitive to the oncogenic potential of these agents than animals, and second tumors caused by anticancer agents have not always been recognized or reported. The synergistic or additive effect of single agent chemotherapy and radiation therapy cannot be evaluated, because chemotherapeutic agents are generally used in combination, and the identification of a single carcinogenic agent is extremely difficult when a combination of agents is used (Schmahl et al., 1982).

Nonetheless, as the use of chemotherapy has become more extensive in recent years and has added to the success of treatments, long-term follow-up has permitted assessment of survivors for development of second malignant neoplasms.

The oncogenic potential of treatments is determined by comparing the incidence of new

Supported in part by Cancer Center Support (CORE) Grant CA-21765, Childhood Solid Tumor Program Project Grant CA-23099, and Childhood Leukemia Program Project Grant, CA-20180 from the National Cancer Institute and by the American Lebanese Syrian Associated Charities (ALSAC).

primary malignancies observed following treatment with the incidence in the general population. By comparing the rates derived from the total person–years of observation, adjusted for age, race, and sex with rates from the Surveillance Epidemiology and End Results (SEER) registry, the risk of second cancers can be calculated for each type of treatment delivered (Young et al., 1981). Ultimately, risk of each treatment modality will be assessed by the types of second malignancy produced (Lavey and Prosnitz, 1987).

Development of second malignant neoplasms has also been recognized to be commonly associated with certain types of primary cancers, such as Hodgkin's disease (Aisenberg, 1983; Arseneau et al., 1972; Baccarani et al., 1980; Bartolucci et al., 1983; Blayney et al., 1987; Boivin and O'Brien, 1988; Boivin and Hutchison, 1981; Cadman et al., 1977; Coleman, 1987; Coleman et al., 1977, 1987; Coltman and Dixon, 1982; Dorreen et al., 1986; Glicksman et al., 1982; Greene and Wilson, 1985; Hawkins et al., 1987; Henry-Amar, 1983; Kingston et al., 1987; Koletsky et al., 1986; Kushner et al., 1988; Meadows et al., 1977, 1985; Pedersen-Bjergaard et al., 1982, 1985, 1987; Schmahl et al., 1982; Selby and Horwich, 1980; Takaue et al., 1986; Terracini et al., 1987; Tester et al., 1984; Tucker et al., 1985, 1988; Valagussa et al., 1982, 1986, 1987; van der Velden et al., 1988), bowel cancer (Boice et al., 1980, 1983; Hyman et al., 1963), and retinoblastoma (Abramson et al., 1984; Hawkins et al., 1987; White et al., 1985), with and without prior treatment with anticancer agents or radiation therapy (Greene, 1984; Lavey and Prosnitz, 1987; Tucker et al., 1987).

DRUG INDUCED SECONDARY CANCERS

Although offering successful treatment for patients with many types of primary cancer, specific anticancer agents have been associated with the development of second cancers, primarily leukemias and lymphomas, and less frequently with other second malignancies (Schmahl et al., 1982).

Boivin and O'Brien (1988) compared the relative risk of solid cancers in 6513 patients with Hodgkin's disease after radiotherapy or after chemotherapy. A 2.1–fold increase in the risk of solid cancers of all sites occurred after any treatment, with a relative risk of 2.2 after radiotherapy and a relative risk of 1.1 after chemotherapy alone.

By the early 1980s, the literature began to describe second cancers developing after single-agent or combination chemotherapy of primary malignant or non-malignant conditions treated with or without irradiation (Schmahl et al., 1982; Reimer, 1982; Zarrabi et al., 1983). In the late 1980s, reports on the carcinogenic effect of combinations of agents or modalities used to treat specific types of cancer were published (Bhambhani et al., 1987; Boivin and O'Brien, 1988; Coleman, 1987; Davis et al., 1987; Geller et al., 1988; Heyn et al., 1986; Ingram et al., 1987; Lishner et al., 1987; Ochs and Mulhern, 1988; Osterlind et al., 1985; Pedersen-Bjergaard et al., 1985; Pratt et al., 1988; Ratain et al., 1987). Yet it may be too early to evaluate the risks associated with specific treatment, because the current methods of studying second neoplasms require large numbers of patients receiving similar treatments who are followed for long periods of time (Coleman, 1987; Curtis et al., 1989; Makuch and Simon, 1979). Although similar treatments are given, the cumulative dosage, dosage intensity, and schedule of delivery of a specific agent(s) should be considered (Greene et al., 1983).

ASSESSING THE RISK OF SECOND CANCERS

One of the more difficult problems associated with drug-induced carcinogenesis is assessing the contribution of each agent or combinations of agents in relation to genetic susceptibility (Abramson et al., 1984; Meadows et al., 1977, 1985; Wacholder and Boivin, 1987). Retinoblastoma furnishes the prototype of a cancer gene associated with both unilateral or bilateral involvement, unifocal or multifocal tumor, and sporadic or familial disease (Knudson, 1971). In 1971, Knudson reiterated the multiple-hit theory of carcinogenesis, which suggested that all retinoblastomas arise from at least two mutations. The second mutation always occurs after conception (postzygotically); the first mutation may be post-zygotic, as in sporadic cases, or prezygotic, as in hereditary cases. The association of retinoblastoma with secondary osteosarcoma has recently been explained by isolation of the human DNA segment with properties of the gene that suppresses retinoblastoma and osteosarcoma (Friend et al., 1986; Fung et al., 1987). Mutational inactivation of the tumor suppressing agent has been proposed as a crucial step in the development of these tumors. Indeed, the demonstration of suppression of the neoplastic phenotype by replacement of the gene in human cancer cells provided direct evidence for an essential role of the gene in tumorigenesis (Huang et al., 1988).

Some preexisting conditions, such as adenomatous polyps of the colon, may undergo malignant transformation. The associations between primary lymphoma and secondary colon carcinoma (Boice et al., 1980, 1983; Gastrointestinal Group Study, 1984) and between colon carcinoma and leukemia or lymphoma have long been recognized, but only recently have survivors of breast, ovarian, brain, and lung cancer been recognized to be at increased risk of developing secondary leukemias, usually associated with adjuvant chemotherapy (Coleman et al., 1987; Clark et al., 1984; Curtis et al., 1989; Fisher, et al., 1985; Greene et al., 1982; Haas et al., 1987; Herring et al., 1986; Horn and Thompson, 1988; Murohashi, 1985; Osterlind et al., 1985; Pedersen-Bjergaard et al., 1980; Reimer et al., 1977; Tucker et al., 1987; Valagussa et al., 1987).

Harris and Coleman (1989) have indicated that the statistics for relative risk are meaningful for epidemiologic purposes, but may overestimate the concern for an individual patient. The importance of any therapy induced second cancers underscores the need for well-designed and well-analyzed scientific research and for ways of rapidly translating new discoveries into practical applications.

Pedersen-Bjergaard and Philip (1989) recently have summarized the risk of treatment related acute nonlymphoblastic leukemia (ANLL) in cohorts of patients treated for ovarian, lung, breast, or gastrointestinal cancer. The cumulative risk for treatment related ANLL is 11.2 ± 2% by 10 years for patients treated with melphalan, and 5.4 ± 3.2% by 10 years for those treated with cyclophosphamide. For patients treated for lung cancer with busulfan, the risk is 5.8% by five years; with cyclophosphamide vincristine VP-16, the risk is 25 ± 13% by 3.1 years, and with semustine cyclophosphamide vincristine VP-16, the risk is 14 ± 6.9% by four years. For patients treated for breast cancer with melphalan, the risk is 1.7 ± 0.3% by 10 years, and for those treated for colorectal carcinoma with semustine/5-fluorouracil, the risk is 4 ± 2.2% by six years. These authors emphasize that the only positive associations of therapy related leukemia and tumors have been with alkylating agents.

CONTRIBUTIONS OF SPECIFIC AGENTS

Agents associated with later development of cancer include the radioisotopes, hormones, immunosuppressive and cytotoxic drugs, and miscellaneous agents such as arsenic and coal tar ointments known to be associated with the development of skin cancers (Fraumeni and Miller, 1972). The associations of phenytoin with lymphomas and chloramphenicol with aplastic anemia and leukemia and of polyvinyl chloride with liver tumors remain questionable, despite temporal exposure relationships.

Procarbazine has gained the reputation of being a potent carcinogenic chemotherapeutic agent; its contribution to the leukemias of patients with Hodgkin's disease remains questionable because those patients also received other alkylating agents (Table 3-1).

Dactinomycin is reputed to have protective abilities in preventing second malignancies in patients with Wilms' tumor (Breslow et al., 1988; D'Angio et al., 1976). The potential of

Table 3-1. Cancers After Single-Agent Chemotherapy

CLASS OF AGENT	TYPE OF SECOND CANCERS
Alkylating agents	
cyclophosphamide	Carcinoma of bladder, lymphoma, ANLL, squamous cell carcinoma of lung, skin, stomach, gallbladder, melanomas
melphalan	ANLL, melanoma, squamous cell carcinoma
thiotepa	ANLL
nitrogen mustard	ANLL
chlorambucil	ANLL
busulfan	ANLL, carcinoma of lung
carmustine, lomustine, semustine	ANLL
streptozotocin	? ANLL
procarbazine	ANLL
Antimetabolites	
5-fluorouracil	ANLL
6-mercaptopurine	?
azathioprine	Lymphoma, ANLL, carcinoma of tongue, lung, renal cell carcinoma
methotrexate	Head and neck, skin, liver, soft tissue sarcoma
Metal-containing compounds	
cisplatin	ANLL
carboplatin	?
bleomycin	?
Tubulin binders	
Vincristine	?
Vinblastine	?
VM-26	? ANLL
VP-16	? ANLL
Antibiotics	
dactinomycin	?
daunorubicin	?
doxorubicin	?
mitomycin	?
Enzyme inhibitors	
L-asparaginase	?

ANLL = acute nonlymphoblastic leukemia.

ifosfamide to cause bladder cancer may never be fully recognized because it is given with mesna, which protects the bladder mucosa, and prevents hemorrhagic cystitis.

Second cancers can occur after treatment with alkylating agents, antimetabolites, metal-containing anticancer agents, and tubulin-binding drugs (Table 3-1). Mechanisms of carcinogenesis of these cytotoxic agents, especially the alkylating agents, are described in subsequent chapters.

THERAPY RELATED SOLID TUMORS

Schmahl and associates (1982) compiled a list of 303 reported cases of second cancers in patients for whom the primary and secondary tumor type, the dosage of anticancer agent (or agents), and the latent period were known. Also included were patients who received immunosuppressive agents for treatment of their primary nonmalignant disease processes. Among the second diagnoses of these patients were 207 patients with leukemias, predominantly ANLL. The most frequent malignant solid tumors were bladder carcinomas ($n = 28$) and nonmelanoma skin cancers ($n = 13$). The median latent periods of second tumors after cytotoxic agents ranged from 44 to 62 months, in ascending order for nitrogen mustard, azathioprine, melphalan, thiotepa, cyclophosphamide, chlorambucil, and busulfan. For the 97 patients who received cyclophosphamide, the median total dose was 4.7 g. For patients who developed ANLL as a second cancer after cyclophosphamide, the median latent period was 49 months; for carcinoma of the urinary bladder, it was 81 months, and for squamous cell carcinoma of the skin, 18 months.

Patients who received long-term treatment with cyclophosphamide are at increased risk for both bladder cancer and leukemia (Pedersen-Bjergaard, et al., 1988). There is an increased frequency of solid tumors after treatment of hematopoietic malignancies (Krause et al., 1985; Tucker et al., 1985). Among 26 solid tumors in 2262 patients with primary neoplasms treated between 1970 and 1982, there were seven lung, six colon, four gastric, three bladder, three esophageal, two anorectal, and one pancreatic carcinoma, compared with one lung and one chronic lymphocytic leukemia among 3055 cases treated between 1957 and 1969.

Tucker and colleagues (1987, 1988) from the National Cancer Institute and Meadows and colleagues (1977, 1985) of the Late Effects Study Group delineated the risks of second cancers in children with various childhood tumors or leukemia (Abramson et al., 1984; Bhambhani et al., 1987; D'Angio et al., 1976; Gutjahr, 1985; Hawkins et al., 1987; Heyn et al., 1986; Ingram et al., 1987; Ironside, 1987; Kingston et al., 1987; Kushner et al., 1988; Li, 1977; McKenzie et al., 1988; Ochs and Mulhern, 1988; Olsen, 1986; Orazi et al., 1988; Spector et al., 1979; Strong et al., 1979, 1987; Weh et al., 1986; Zarrabi et al., 1983). The risk of secondary bone sarcomas, for example, increased if alkylating agents were delivered in conjunction with doses of radiation therapy exceeding 3000 cGy (Tucker et al., 1987). Tucker et al. (1985) have also described second cancers following melanoma, brain, thyroid and connective tissue, bone, and eye.

Among 1916 patients treated at St. Jude Children's Research Hospital for acute lymphoblastic leukemia (ALL), 13 developed radiation associated tumors, two developed chemotherapy associated bladder carcinomas, and 21 developed nonradiation associated solid tumors and ANLL (Pratt et al., 1988). Approximately 9% of children treated for ALL will develop a second malignancy within 15 years from the original diagnosis, a risk that approaches the risk of second tumors after Hodgkin's disease. The nonradiation associated solid tumors included ependymoma of the spinal cord, paraganglioma, melanoma, Hodgkin's disease, hepatocellular carcinoma, and carcinoma of the cervix.

Fourteen of the 45 second malignant neoplasms seen in more than 2800 patients with primary solid tumors at St. Jude Children's Research Hospital have not been associated with prior radiation therapy (Pratt, C. B., unpublished data, 1989). The primary tumors of these patients were Hodgkin's disease, osteosarcoma, adrenocortical carcinoma, rhabdomyosarcoma, non-Hodgkin's lymphoma, retinoblastoma, and neuroblastoma. Types of second cancers in these patients were non-Hodgkin's lymphoma, melanoma, malignant fibrous histiocytoma, medulloblastoma, osteosarcoma, Ewing's sarcoma, colon carcinoma, ALL, and ANLL.

For children and adults, survival after development of a second malignant neoplasm is related to the type and extent of the second tumor or leukemia and the available treatment options (Meadows et al., 1985; Pratt et al., 1988).

THERAPY RELATED LEUKEMIA

Therapy related leukemia is a clinicopathologically distinct late complication of chemotherapy or radiotherapy (Kantarjian and Keating, 1987; Levine and Bloomfield, 1986; Pedersen-Bjergaard et al., 1987). In almost every instance, therapy related leukemia is nonlymphoblastic. It is a pluripotent stem cell disease involving the myeloid, erythroid, and megakaryocytic series and it often is preceded by a preleukemic phase (myelodysplastic syndrome), characterized by pancytopenia, anisopoikilocytosis, large platelets with decreased granulation, hypogranular leukocytes with pseudo-Pelger-Huët nuclei, basophilia in the blood, and trilineage dysplasia in the bone marrow (Anderson et al., 1981; Cadman et al., 1977; Foucar et al., 1979). Although patients with the myelodysplastic syndrome will progress to acute leukemia within several months, many patients succumb to the infections or hemorrhagic complications of severe pancytopenia before developing acute leukemia (Michels et al., 1985). Because of the trilineage involvement, therapy related leukemia frequently presents problems in classification by French–American–British criteria. Among the cases that could be classified, most had M2 or M4 leukemia (Groupe Français de Cytogénétique Hématologique, 1984; Michels et al., 1985).

Epidemiology

Therapy related leukemia was first reported in patients with Hodgkin's disease (Arseneau et al., 1972). Because of intensive chemotherapy and prolonged survival of patients with cancers, an increased risk of therapy related leukemia has been found in patients with a wide spectrum of tumors. Although therapy related leukemia is relatively infrequent in children (Pui et al., 1990), it accounts for 10 to 15% of adults with ANLL (Murohashi, 1985). In adults, this complication has been reported in patients with malignant lymphomas (Aisenberg, 1983; Arseneau et al., 1972; Bartolucci et al., 1983; Blayney et al., 1987; Boivin and Hutchison, 1981; Greene et al., 1983; Henry-Amar, 1983; Koletsky et al., 1986; Pedersen-Bjergaard and Larsen, 1982; Pedersen-Bjergaard et al., 1987; van der Velden et al., 1988), multiple myelomas (Bersagel et al., 1979; Gonzales et al., 1977), breast cancer (Curtis et al., 1989; Fisher et al., 1988), ovarian cancer (Pedersen-Bjergaard et al., 1985; Reimer et al., 1977), germ cell tumor (Redman et al., 1984), lung cancer (Markman et al., 1982; Ratain et al., 1987), gastrointestinal cancer (Boice et al., 1983), polycythemia vera (Berk et al., 1981), other cancers (Groupe Français de Cytogénétique Hématologique, 1984; Le Beau et al., 1986; Michels et al., 1985; Tucker et al., 1985), and some benign diseases (Grunwald and Rosner, 1979).

In children, therapy related leukemia has been associated with the treatment of Hodgkin's disease (Kushner et al., 1988; Meadows et al., 1985; Tucker et al., 1987; Pui et al., 1990), non-Hodgkin's lymphoma (Ingram et al., 1987; Pui et al., 1990), brain tumor (Meadows et al., 1985; Pui et al., 1990), Wilms' tumor (Tucker et al., 1987; Meadows et al., 1985), soft tissue sarcoma (Meadows et al., 1985; Strong et al., 1987), neuroblastoma (Weh et al., 1986; Pui et al., 1990), osteogenic sarcoma (Meadows et al., 1985), Ewing's sarcoma (Meadows et al., 1985; Tucker et al., 1987) and retinoblastoma (Meadows et al., 1984).

The cumulative risk of therapy related leukemia varies substantially, depending on age at diagnosis, the type of primary malignancy and the intensity and duration of therapy used (Kantarjian and Keating, 1987; Pui et al., 1990). Children have a much lower risk of developing therapy related leukemia than adults. In our single institution study involving 3365 consecutive children and adolescents treated for malignant solid tumors, the estimated risk of this complication was 1.2% overall and 0.4% for patients remaining in complete remission (Pui et al., 1990). Patients who received salvage chemotherapy for relapse appeared to have an increased risk of therapy related leukemia (Pedersen-Bjergaard et al., 1985; Pui et al., 1990). Among various primary malignancies, Hodgkin's disease is most frequently associated with subsequent leukemia, accounting for approximately half of the reported cases (Kantarjian and Keating, 1987); the reason for this increased risk may be related to its associated immunosuppression and the frequent use of alkylating agents in relatively high cumulative doses (Pui et al., 1990).

Etiology

The challenge in identifying risk factors for second cancers lies in determining the relative pathogenetic contributions of the disease, the associated immune deficiency, underlying genetics, environmental factors, and intensive chemotherapy and radiotherapy.

The relationship between radiotherapy and development of therapy related leukemia is not well understood. The quality of radiation, total dose, fraction size, dose rate, treatment field, and other exposure variables can influence the risk of therapy related leukemia (Curtis et al., 1989; Greene et al., 1983; Le Beau et al., 1986; Meadows et al., 1985; Murohashi, 1985; Pedersen-Bjergaard, 1985; Tucker et al., 1987). It is beyond the scope of this review to address this controversial issue.

Because destruction of tumor cells by a chemotherapeutic agent follows first-order kinetics, the drug destroys slightly less than 100% of the susceptible cells. The leukemogenic effect of alkylating agents may affect the remaining cells. By cross-linking DNA during the resting phase, alkylating agents damage DNA, causing mutations resulting in a malignant clone (Saffhill et al., 1985). Immunosuppression from alkylating agents may also play a role in leukemogenesis (Kantarjian and Keating, 1987). An increased risk of the development of ANLL has been observed after treatment with most alkylating agents, including mechlorethamine (Pedersen-Bjergaard and Larsen, 1982), busulfan (Stott et al., 1977), chlorambucil (Berk et al., 1981), dihydroxybusulfan (Pedersen-Bjergaard et al., 1980), carmustine (Glicksman et al., 1982), lomustine (Aisenberg, 1983; Glicksman et al., 1982; Pedersen-Bjergaard et al., 1985), semustine (Boice et al., 1983), melphalan (Greene et al., 1986; Wahlin et al., 1982), and cyclophosphamide (Pedersen-Bjergaard et al., 1985; Schmahl et al., 1982). Among alkylating agents, nitrosoureas and procarbazine appear to have the highest leukemogenic potential (Kantarjian and Keating, 1987).

Therapy related leukemia has rarely been reported in patients receiving other chemotherapeutic agents with a direct action of DNA such as adriamycin and cisplatin (Pedersen-Bjergaard et al., 1985; Valagussa et al., 1982). Recently, epipodophyllotoxins have been suggested to be leukemogenic (Ratain et al., 1987; Pui et al., 1989b). Four of 119 patients with advanced nonsmall cell carcinoma of the lung developed ANLL 13 to 35 months after the start of treatment with etoposide and cisplatin combination chemotherapy (Ratain et al., 1987). These cases had clinical and cytogenetic features of ANLL de novo that were distinct from alkylating-agent induced ANLL. Similar leukemias have been reported in other patients with neuroblastoma, non-Hodgkin's lymphoma, or lung cancer after combination chemotherapy that included an epipodophyllotoxin (Ingram et al., 1987; Pedersen-Bjergaard et al., 1988; Weh et al., 1986). Epipodophyllotoxins cause DNA strand breaks by forming a ternary complex with topoisomerase II (Long et al., 1985; Ross et al., 1984). These agents may also cause DNA damage by dehydrogenase-induced free radical intermediates (Wozniak et al., 1984). Because of these properties and because the topoisomerase II inhibitors produce many sister chromatid exchanges and other chromosomal aberrations in vitro (DeMarini et al., 1987; Singh and Gupta, 1983), epipodophyllotoxins may prove to be another class of drugs with leukemogenic potential.

A dose–response relationship between the cumulative dose of alkylating agents and the risk of developing leukemia is well established (Aisenberg, 1983; Berk et al., 1981; Greene et al., 1982, 1983, 1986; Pedersen-Bjergaard et al., 1980, 1985, 1987; Tucker et al., 1987). The latency period before the development of therapy related leukemia was found to be inversely proportional to the intensity of treatment (Cadman et al., 1977). Similarly, a positive correlation between the dose intensity and the development of ANLL has been suggested in patients receiving etoposide for lung cancer (Ratain et al., 1987). In patients with Hodgkin's disease, the risk was shown to decrease gradually two to three years after cessation of chemotherapy and level out after seven to eight years (Pedersen-Bjergaard et al., 1987).

Several host factors have been associated with increased risk of therapy related leukemia. These include being in an older age group (de Vathaire et al., 1989; Pui et al., 1990), and having an advanced or relapsed malignancy (Aisenberg, 1983; Kantarjian and Keating, 1987; Pedersen-Bjergaard et al., 1987; Pui et al., 1990). Impaired immune status of the host probably contributes to the increased risk.

Cytogenetic Findings

Complete loss, or deletions in the long arm of chromosome 7 or 5 (-7/7q-, -5/5q-), is a relatively consistent chromosomal alteration in patients who developed ANLL after treatment with alkylating agents or radiotherapy (Table 3-2) (Fourth International Workshop on Chromosomes in Leukemia, 1984; Group Français de Cytogénéntique Hématologique, 1984; Kantarjian and Keating, 1987; Le Beau et al., 1986; Michels et al., 1985; Pedersen-Bjergaard et al., 1984; Rowley et al., 1981; Sandberg et al., 1982; Whang-Peng et al., 1988). Depending on the patient populations, treatment regimens, and the quality of the banded chromosome preparations, chromosome 7 and(or) 5 abnormalities were reported in 50% to 90% of the patients. Abnormalities of chromosomes 3, 5, and 17 also appear to be preferentially involved in these cases (Fourth International Workshop on Chromosomes in Leukemia, 1984; Pedersen-Bjergaard et al., 1984; Sandberg et al., 1982; Whang-Peng et al., 1988). Compared with cases of de novo ANLL, these chromosomal changes are significantly more frequent in therapy related leukemia. Although chromosome 5 or 7 abnormalities have been observed in de novo ANLL, these patients generally had a history of carcinogenic exposure (Mitelman et al., 1978).

The close correlation between loss of DNA material from the long arms of chromosomes 5 or 7 and therapy related ANLL suggests a possible explanation of the pathophysiologic process. Leukemogenesis may result from the loss of a tumor-suppressing gene localized in these sites or from the expression of a recessive mutant gene residing on the remaining homologous chromosome. Several presently known proto-oncogenes and growth regulatory genes have been mapped to these regions (Kantarjian and Keating, 1987; Le Beau et al., 1986).

Several cases of ANLL associated with treatment that included an epipodophyllotoxin were found to have t(9;11)(p21;q23) (Ingram et al., 1987; Pedersen-Bjergaard et al., 1988; Ratain et al., 1987; Weh et al., 1986), a specific translocation for myelomonoblastic or monoblastic leukemia. There also have been scattered reports of therapy related leukemia with specific "favorable" cytogenetic abnormalities, such as t(15;17), t(8;21), inv(16), and del(16)(q22) (Kantarjian and Keating, 1987). Interestingly, these specific chromosomal alterations generally associated with de novo ANLL were found frequently in children with therapy related leukemia (Pui et al., 1990).

Therapy for Secondary Leukemia

The treatment response of therapy related leukemia is usually poor. Even if complete remission is achieved, long-term disease-free survival is seldom maintained with the most aggressive chemotherapy (Duane et al., 1985; Larson et al., 1988; Preisler et al., 1983; Pui et al., 1990). Low-dose cytarabine or 13-cis-retinoic acid have been similarly unsuccessful (Cheson et al., 1986; Koeffler et al., 1988; Kantarjian and Keating, 1987). Recently, promising results have been achieved with bone marrow transplantation. Approximately 40% of these patients may enjoy long-term disease-free survival when treated with marrow ablative therapy followed by marrow transplantation (Geller et al., 1988; Guinan et al., 1989; O'Donnell et al., 1987).

SECONDARY LEUKEMIA IN ACUTE LEUKEMIA

Most investigators have emphasized the stability of leukemic clones in acute leukemia, reporting only minor variations in phenotypes in cases studied at diagnosis and relapse. With the use of intensified chemotherapy in recent clinical trials, coupled with improved detection of cell lineage-associated phenotypic markers, there has been an apparent increase in the num-

Table 3-2. Clinical and Cytogenetic Findings of Therapy-Related Leukemia

REFERENCES	NO. OF PATIENTS	TREATMENT			CHROMOSOMAL ABNORMALITIES		MEDIAN LATENCY PERIOD (MO.)	MEDIAN SURVIVAL (MO.)
		CT	RT	CT + RT	NUMERICAL	STRUCTURAL		
Whang-Peng et al., 1988	68	22	15	31	−7, −5, −8, −17	5q-,7q-, 3,9,22	48 (2–252)	5 (1–34)
LeBeau et al., 1986	63	21	11	31	−7, −5, −12, −16, −18	5q-,7q-, 1,4,12,14,18	56 (10–192)	7 (0–57+)
Michels et al., 1985	65	25	14	26	−7, −5	5q-,7q-	58 (11–912)	4 (1–38)
Kantarjian et al., 1986	112	37	26	49	−7, −5	5q-,7q-	71 (7–331)	7
4th IWS, 1984	56	17	15	24	−7, −5, −17	5q-,7q- 17,1	60 (12–204)	5
French, 1984	55	20	10	25	−7, −5, −17	5q-,7q-	72 (24–288)	3 (1–17)
Pedensen-Bjergaard et al., 1984	55	25	8	22	−7, −5	5q-,7q-, 3,17	48 (12–131)	7
Rowley et al., 1981	26	7	15	4	−7, −5	5q-	49 (21–100)	9 (3–23)
Sandberg et al., 1982	18	6	1	11	−7, −5	5q-,7q-, 3,17	78 (7–120)	3 (1–107)

CT = chemotherapy, RT = radiotherapy, 4th IWS = Fourth International Workshop on Chormosomes in Leukemia, French = Groupe Français de Cytogénétique Hématologique.

ber of cases with lineage shifts (i.e., lymphoid to myeloid or the reverse) (DeCuia et al., 1989; Emami et al., 1983; Hershfield et al., 1984; Marcus et al., 1985; Pui et al., 1986; Stass et al., 1984; van Lierde et al., 1989; Zarrabi et al., 1983). In most instances, cases converted from ALL to ANLL. The rare occurrence of a lineage shift from ANLL to ALL may be due to fewer long-term survivors at risk with ANLL.

In a recent study of 733 children receiving intensive chemotherapy for ALL, an estimated 5% of patients were predicted to develop ANLL (Pui et al., 1989). The median time from diagnosis of ALL to the development of ANLL was 3 years. A constellation of presenting features related to T-cell ALL was associated with the development of secondary ANLL, suggesting a biologic predisposition in patients with T-cell ALL (Pui et al., 1989b). According to univariate analysis, treatment with either an epipodophyllotoxin or irradiation was significantly related to the development of ANLL. In multivariate analysis, neither factor was independently related to the complication. However, the determination of the relative importance of these treatment components in the pathogenesis of secondary ANLL was confounded by the fact that all patients with T-cell leukemia received epipodophyllotoxin and radiation therapy. Sequential cytogenetic studies of these cases of secondary leukemia revealed several probable mechanisms of pathogenesis, including clonal evolution and clonal selection in some of the cases (Stass et al., 1984; Pui et al., 1986; Pui et al., 1989b). In most instances, the original karyotype was completely replaced at the time of appearance of ANLL, suggesting induction of a second, independent malignancy (Pui et al., 1989b). The apparently independent clonal nature of the myeloid leukemic cell populations seen at relapse should be confirmed by studies with X-chromosome inactivation markers in heterozygous female patients (Pui et al., 1989a).

In most cases of secondary ANLL, the chromosomal abnormalities involve the 11q23 region (Pui et al., 1989b), suggesting malignant transformation of a pluripotent stem cell (Pui et al., 1987). The relationship of the lineage conversion with the mixed-lineage expression in some leukemia (Pui et al., 1984) is uncertain, and because of the relatively few cases studied, it is also unclear if secondary leukemia in these cases is therapy related. However, progressive lineage conversion to ANLL has been reported in patients who received 2′-deoxycoformycin for relapsed ALL (Hershfield et al., 1984; Stass et al., 1984).

The clinical outcome of retreatment with chemotherapy in patients with secondary ANLL has been disappointing (Pui et al., 1989b). Alternative treatment with ablative chemotherapy followed by bone marrow transplantation should be tested in these patients.

THE FUTURE

Much of the success of treatment of adults and children with solid tumors and leukemias is due to combination chemotherapy which usually included alkylating agents. Chemotherapy has become more intensive as well as more effective during the past 30 years. Unless therapy can be safely decreased or highly selective in terms of agents used, which is not possible for most cancers and leukemias, more second neoplasms must be expected in the future as more patients become long-term survivors of their primary cancer. Separation of the causes of these second cancers—in relation to environmental factors, immunosuppression, genetic predisposition, viral infection, radiation exposure, and exposure to chemotherapy (single or combination of agents)—will only become more complicated.

REFERENCES

Abramson DH, Ellsworth RM, Kitchin FD, Tung G Second non-occular tumors in retinoblastoma survivors: Are they radiation induced? Opthalmology 1984 91:1351–1355.

Aisenberg AC Acute nonlymphocytic leukemia after treatment for Hodgkin's disease. Am J Med 1983 75:449–454.

Anderson R, Bagby G, Richert-Boe K, Magenis RE, and Koler RD Therapy-related preleukemic syndrome. Cancer 1981 47:1867–1871.

Arseneau JC, Sponzo RW, Levin DL, Schnipper LE, Bonner H, Young RC, Canellos GP, Johnson RE, and DeVita VT Nonlymphomatous malignant tumors complicating Hodgkin's disease: Possible associations with intensive therapy. N Engl J Med 1972 287:1119–1122.

Baccarani M, Bosi A, and Papa G Second malignancy in patients treated for Hodgkin's disease. Cancer 1980 46:1735–1740.

Bartolucci AA, Liu C, Durant JR, and Gams RA, for the Southeastern Cancer Study Group. Acute myelogenous leukemia as a second malignant neoplasm following successful treatment of advanced Hodgkin's disease. Cancer 1983 52:2209–2213.

Bergsagel DE, Baily AJ, Langley GR, MacDonald RN, White DF, and Miller AB The chemotherapy on plasma-cell myeloma and the incidence of acute leukemia. N Engl J Med 1979 301:743–748.

Berk PD, Goldberg J, and Silverstein M Increased incidence of acute leukemia in polycythemia vera associated with chlorambucil therapy. N Engl J Med 1981 304:441–447.

Bhambhani K, Bollinger R, and Ravindranath Y Late effects following successful treatment of childhood acute lymphoblastic leukemia (ALL). Proc Ann Meet Am Soc Clin Oncol 1987 6:A626.

Blayney DW, Longo DL, Young RC, Greene MH, Hubbard SM, Postal MG, Duffey PL, and DeVita VT Jr Decreasing risk of leukemia with prolonged follow-up after chemotherapy and radiotherapy for Hodgkin's disease. N Engl J Med 1987 316:710–714.

Boice JD Jr, Greene MH, Killen JY Jr, Ellenberg SS, Keehn RJ, McFadden E, Chen TT, and Fraumeni JF Jr Leukemia and preleukemia after adjuvant treatment of gastrointestinal cancer with semustine (methyl-CCNU). N Engl J Med 1983 309:1079–1084.

Boice JD Jr Carcinogenesis: A synopsis of human experience with external exposure in medicine. Health Phys (USA) 1988 55:621–630.

Boice JD, Greene MH, Keehn RJ, Higgins GA, and Fraumeni JF Late effects of low-dose adjuvant chemotherapy in colorectal cancer. J NCI 1980 64:501–511.

Boivan JF and Hutchison GB Leukemia and other cancers after radiotherapy and chemotherapy for Hodgkin's disease. JNCI 1981 67:751–760.

Boivin JF and O'Brien K Solid cancer risk after treatment of Hodgkin's disease. Cancer 1988 61:2541–2546.

Breslow NE, Norkool PA, Olshan A, Evans A, and D'Angio GJ Second malignant neoplasms in survivors of Wilms' tumor: A report from the National Wilms' Tumor Study. JNCI 1988 80:592–595.

Cadman E, Capizzi R, and Bertino J Acute nonlymphocytic leukemia. A delayed complication of Hodgkin's disease therapy. Analysis of 109 cases. Cancer 1977 40:1280–1296.

Casciato D and Scott JL Acute leukemia following prolonged cytotoxic agent therapy. Medicine 1979 58:32–37.

Cheson BD, Jasper DM, Simon R, and Friedman MA A critical appraisal of low-dose cytosine arabinoside in patients with acute non-lymphocytic leukemia and myelodysplastic syndromes. J Clin Oncol 1986 4:1857–1864.

Clark LY, Sikic BI, Tucker MA, Hans RC Jr, and Cox RS Increased incidence of acute nonlymphocytic leukemia following therapy in patients with small cell carcinoma of the lung. J Clin Oncol 1984 2: 385–390.

Coleman CN Secondary malignancies after treatment of Hodgkin's disease: An evolving picture. J Clin Oncol 1987 4:821–824.

Coleman CN, Williams CJ, Flint A, Glatstein EJ, Rosenberg SA, and Kaplan HS Hematologic neoplasia in patients treated for Hodgkin's disease. N Engl J Med 1977 297:1249–1252.

Coleman MP, Bell CMJ, and Fraser P Second primary malignancy after Hodgkin's disease, ovarian cancer and cancer of the testis: A population-based cohort study. Br J Cancer 1987 56:349–355.

Coltman CA and Dixon DO Second malignancies complication Hodgkin's disease: A Southwest Oncology Group 10-year follow-up. Cancer Treat Rep 1982 66:1023–1033.

Curtis RE, Boice JD Jr, Stovall M, Flannery JT, and Moloney WC Leukemia risk following radiotherapy for breast cancer. J Clin Oncol 1989 7:21–29.

D'Angio GJ, Meadows A, Mike V, Harris C, Evans A, Jaffe N, Newton W, Schweisguth O, Sutow W, and Morris Jones P Decreased risk of radiation-associated second malignant neoplasms in actinomycin D-treated patients. Cancer 1976 37:1177–1185.

Davis JW, Weiss NA, and Armstrong BK Second cancers in patients with chronic lymphocytic leukemia. JNCI 1987 78:91–94.

DeCuia, MR, Alimena G, Gastaldi R, Spiriti MAA, Giona F, Mancini M, and Mandelli F Acute myeloblastic leukemia with t(8;21) following Philadelphia positive acute lymphoblastic leukemia. Leukemia 1989 3:310–313.

DeMarini DM, Brock KH, Doerr CL, and Moore MM Mutagenicity and clastogenicity of teniposide (VM-26) in L5178Y/TK$^{+/-}$ −3.7.2C mouse lymphoma cells. Mutat Res 1987 187:141–149.

Dorreen MS, Gregory WM, Wrigley PFM, Stansfeld AG, and Lister TA Second primary malignant neoplasms in patients treated for Hodgkin's disease at St. Bartholomew's hospital. Hematol Oncol (UK) 1986 4:149–161.

Duane SF, Peterson BA, Bloomfield CD, Michels SD, and Hurd DD Response of therapy-associated acute nonlymphocytic leukemia to intensive induction chemotherapy. Med Pediatr Oncol 1985 13: 207–213.

Emami A, Kaplan J, Ravindranath Y, Lusher JM, and Inoue S Phenotypic change of acute monocytic leukemia to acute lymphoblastic leukemia on therapy. Am J Pediatr Hematol Oncol 1983 5:341–343.

Fisher B, Rockette H, Fisher ER, Wicherham L, Redmond C, and Brown A Leukemia in breast cancer patients following adjuvant chemotherapy or postoperative radiation: The NSABP experience. J Clin Oncol 1985 3:1640–1658.

Foucar K, McKenna R, Bloomfield C, Bowers TK, and Brunning RD Therapy related leukemia: A panmyelosis. Cancer 1979 43:1285–1296.

Fourth International Workshop on Chromosomes in Leukemia, 1982. Secondary leukemias associated with neoplasia: Treated and untreated. Cancer Genet Cytogenet 1984 11:319–321.

Fraumeni JF Jr and Miller RW Drug-induced cancer. JNCI 1972 48:1267–1270.

Friend SH, Bernards R, Rogelj S, Weinberg RA, Rapaport JM, Alberg DM, and Dryja TP A human DNA segment with properties of the gene that predisposes to retinoblastoma and osteosarcoma. Nature 1986 323:643–646.

Fung Y-KT, Murphree AL, T'Ang A, Qian J, Horrich SH, and Benedict WF Structural evidence for the authenticity of the human retinoblastoma gene. Science 1987 236:1657–1661.

Gastrointestinal Study Group. Adjuvant therapy of colon cancer—results of a prospectively randomized trial. N Engl J Med 1984 310:737–743.

Geller RB, Vogelsang GB, Wingard JR, Yeager AM, Burns WH, Santos GW, and Saral R Successful marrow transplantation for acute myelocytic leukemia following therapy for Hodgkin's disease. J Clin Oncol 1988 6:1558–1561.

Glicksman AS, Pajak TF, Gottlieb A, Nissen N, Stutzman L, and Cooper MR Second malignant neoplasms in patients successfully treated for Hodgkin's disease: A Cancer and Leukemia Group B study. Cancer Treat Rep 1982 66:1035–1044.

Gonzales, F, Trujillo J, and Alexanian R Acute leukemia in multiple myeloma. Ann Intern Med 1977 86: 440–443.

Greene MH Interaction between radiotherapy and chemotherapy in human leukemogenesis. In: Radiation Carcinogenesis: Epidemiology and Biological Significance. Boice JD Jr and Fraumeni JF Jr Eds Raven Press, New York 1984 pp. 199–210.

Greene MH, Boice JD, Greet BE, Blessing JA, and Dembo AJ Acute nonlymphocytic leukemia after therapy with alkylating agents for ovarian cancer: A study of five randomized clinical trials. N Engl J Med 1982 307:1416–1421.

Greene MH, Young RC, Merrill JM, and DeVita VT Evidence of a treatment dose-response in acute nonlymphocytic leukemia which occur after therapy of non-Hodgkin's lymphoma. Cancer Res 1983 43:1891–1898.

Greene MH and Wilson J Second cancer following lymphatic and hematopoietic cancers in Connecticut, 1935–82. NCI Monogr (USA) 1985 68:191–217.

Greene MH, Harris EL, Gershenson DM, Malakasian GD, Melton LJ III, Dembo AJ, Bennett JM, Moloney WC, and Boice JD Melphalan may be a more potent leukemogen than cyclophosphamide. Ann Intern Med 1986 105:360–367.

Groupe Français de Cytogénétique Hématologique. Chromosome analysis of 63 cases of secondary nonlymphoid blood disorders: A cooperative study. Cancer Genet Cytogenet 1984 12:95–104.

Grunwald H and Rosner F Acute leukemia and immunosuppressive drug use: A review of patients undergoing immunosuppressive therapy for non-neoplastic diseases. Arch Intern Med 1979 139: 461–466.

Guinan EC, Tarbell NJ, Tantravahi R, and Weinstein HJ Bone marrow transplantation for children with myelodysplastic syndromes. Blood 1989 73:619–622.

Gutjahr P Nonleukemic second malignancies following childhood acute lymphocytic leukemia: A report of 19 cases from the Federal Republic of Germany. Paediatr Acta 1985 40:449–459.

Haas JF, Kittelmann B, Mehnert WH, Staneczek W, Möhner M, Kaldor JM, and Day NE Risk of leukaemia in ovarian tumour and breast cancer patients following treatment by cyclophosphamide. Br J Cancer 1987 55:213–218.

Harris CC Immunosuppressive anticancer drugs in man, their oncogenic potential. Radiology 1975 114:163–166.

Harris CC The carcinogenicity of anticancer drugs: A hazard in man. Cancer 1976 37:1014–1023.

Harris JR and Coleman CN Estimating the risk of second primary tumors following cancer treatment. J Clin Oncol 1989 7:5–6.

Hawkins MM, Draper GJ, and Kingston JE Incidence of second primary tumours among childhood cancer survivors. Br J Cancer (UK) 1987 56:339–347.

Henry-Amar M Second cancers after radiotherapy and chemotherapy for early stages of Hodgkin's disease. JNCI 1983 71:911–916.

Herring MK, Buzdar AU, Smith TL, Hortobagyi GN, and Blumenschein GR Second neoplasms after adjuvant chemotherapy for operable breast cancer. Am J Clin Oncol 1986 9:269–275.

Herschfield MS, Kurtzberg J, Harden E, Moore JO, Whang-Peng J, and Haynes BF Conversion of a stem cell leukemia from a T-lymphoid to a myeloid phenotype induced by the adenosine deaminase inhibitor 2′-deoxycoformycin. Proc Natl Acad Sci 1984 81:253–257.

Heyn R, Newton WA, Ragab A, Tefft M, Mauer HM, and Beltangady M Second malignant neoplasms in patients treated on the Intergroup Rhabdomyosarcoma Study I-II (abstract). Proc Assoc Soc Clin Oncol 1986 5:215.

Hoover R and Fraumeni JF Drugs in clinical use which cause cancer. J Clin Pharmacol 1975 15:16–23.

Horn PL and Thompson WD Exposure to chemotherapeutic agents and the risk of a second breast cancer: Preliminary findings. Yale J Biol Med 1988 61:223–231.

Huang H-JS, Yee J-K, Shew J-Y, Chen, P-H, Bookstein R, Friedmann T, Lee EY-HP, and Lee W-H Suppression of the neoplastic phenotype by replacement of the RB gene in human cancer cells. Science 1988 242:1563–1566.

Hyman GA, Ultmann JE, and Slanetz CA Chronic lymphocytic leukemia or lymphoma and carcinoma of the colon. JAMA 1963 186:87–90.

Ingram L, Mott MG, Mann JR, Raafat F, Darbyshire PJ, and Morris-Jones PH Second malignancies in children treated for non-Hodgkin's lymphoma and T-cell leukaemia with UKCCSG regimens. Br J Cancer 1987 53:463–466.

Ironside JAD Second malignant neoplasms after childhood cancer: A report of three cases of osteogenic sarcoma. Clin Radiol (UK) 1987 38:195–199.

Kantarjian HM and Keating MJ Therapy-related leukemia and myelodysplastic syndrome. Semin Oncol 1987 14:435–443.

Kingston JE, Hawkins MM, Draper GJ, Marsden HB, and Kinnier Wilson LM Patterns of multiple primary tumours in patients treated for cancer during childhood. Br J Cancer 1987 56:331–338.

Koeffler HP, Heitjan D, Mertelsmann R, Kolitz JE, Schulman P, Itri L, Gunter P, and Besa E Randomized study of 13-cis-retinoic acid v placebo in the myelodysplastic disorders. Blood 1988 71: 703–708.

Koletsky AJ, Bertino JR, Farber LR, Prosnitz LR, Kapp DS, Fischer D, and Portlock CS Second neoplasms in patients with Hodgkin's disease following combined modality therapy—the Yale experience. J Clin Oncol 1986 4:311–317.

Knudson AG Jr Mutation and cancer: Statistical study of retinoblastoma. Proc Natl Acad Sci USA 1971 68:820–823.

Krause JR, Ayuyang HQ, and Ellis LD Secondary non-hematopoietic cancers arising following treatment of hematopoietic disorders. Cancer 1985 55:512–515.

Kushner BJ, Zauber A, and Tan CTC Second malignancies after childhood Hodgkin's disease. The Memorial Sloan-Kettering Cancer Center experience. Cancer 1988 62:1364–1370.

Kyle RA Second malignancies associated with chemotherapeutic agents. Semin Oncol 1982 9:131–142.

Larson RA, Wernli M, LeBeau MM, Daly KM, Pape LH, Rowley JD, and Vardiman JW Short remission durations in therapy-related leukemia despite cytogenetic complete responses to high-dose cytarabine. Blood 1988 72:1333–1339.

Lavey R and Prosnitz L Impact of the combined use of radiotherapy (RT) and chemotherapy (CT) on the risk for a second malignancy. Proc Ann Meet Am Soc Clin Oncol 1987 6:A760.

Le Beau MM, Albain KS, Larson RA, Vardiman JW, Davis EM, Blough RR, Golomb HM, and Rowley JD Clinical and cytogenetic correlations in 63 patients with therapy-related myelodysplastic syndromes and acute nonlymphocytic leukemia: Further evidence for characteristic abnormalities of chromosomes no. 5 and 7. J Clin Oncol 1986 4:325–345.

Levine EG and Bloomfield CD Secondary myelodysplastic syndromes and acute leukaemias. Clin Haematol 1986 15:1037–1080.

Li FP Second malignant tumors after cancer in childhood. Cancer 1977 40:1899–1902.

Lishner M, Prokocimer M, Ron E, and Shaklai M Primary malignant neoplasms associated with chronic lymphocytic leukaemia. Israel Postgrad Med J 1987 63:253–256.

Long BH, Musail ST, and Brattain MG Single- and double-strand DNA breakage and repair in human lung adenocarcinoma cells exposed to etoposide and teniposide. Cancer Res 1985 45:3106–3112.

Makuch R and Simon R Recommendations for the analysis of the effect of treatment on the development of second malignancies. Cancer 1979 44:250–253.

Marcus RE, Matutes E, Drysdale H, and Catovsky D Phenotypic conversion of TdT+ adult AML to CALLA+ ALL. Scand J Haematol 1985 35:343–347.

Markman M, Pavy M, and Abeloff M Acute leukemia following intensive therapy for small-cell carcinoma of the lung. Cancer 1982 50:672–675.

McKenzie SE, August CS, Bunin G, Evans A, and D'Angio G Benign and malignant tumors after bone marrow transplantation (BMT) in childhood. Proc Ann Meet Am Assoc Cancer Res 1988 29:A730.

Meadows AT, D'Angio GJ, Mike V, Banfi A, Harris C, Jenkin RDT, and Schwartz A Patterns of second malignant neoplasms in children. Cancer 1977 40:1903–1911.

Meadows AT, Baum E, Fossati-Bellani F, Green D, Jenkin RDT, Marsden B, Nesbit M, Newton W, Oberlin O, Sallan SG, Siegel S, Strong LC, and Voute PA Second malignant neoplasms in children: An update from the Late Effect Study Group. J Clin Oncol 1985 3:532–538.

Michels SD, McKenna RW, Arthur DC, and Brunning RD Therapy-related acute myeloid leukemia and myelodysplastic syndrome: A clinical and morphologic study of 65 cases. Blood 1985 65:1364–1372.

Mitelman F, Brandt L, and Nilsson P Relation among occupational exposure to potential mutagenic/carcinogenic agents, clinical findings and bone marrow chromosomes in acute nonlymphocytic leukemia. Blood 1978 52:1229–1237.

Murohashi I Leukemia in patients following radiotherapy for malignant neoplasms in the pelvic region. Leuk Res 1985 9:1201–1208.

O'Donnell MR, Nademanee AP, Synder DS, Schmidt GM, Parker PM, Bierman PJ, Fahey JL, Stein AS, Krance RA, Stock AD, Forman SJ, and Blume KG Bone marrow transplantation for myelodysplastic and myeloproliferative syndromes. J Clin Oncol 1987 5:1822–1826.

Ochs J and Mulhern RK Late effects of antileukemic treatment. Pediatr Clin N Am 1988 35:815–833.

Olsen JH Risk of second cancer after cancer in childhood. Cancer 1986 57:2250–2254.

Orazi A, Sozzi G, Delia D, Morandi F, Rottoli L, and Cattoretti G Acute monoblastic leukemia as a second malignancy following chemotherapy for osteogenic sarcoma: A case report. Pediatr Hematol Oncol 1988 5:39–46.

Osterlind A, Olsen JH, Lynge E, and Ewertz M Second cancer following cutaneous melanoma and cancers of the brain, thyroid, connective tissue, bone, and eye in Denmark, 1943–80. NCI Monogr (USA) 1985 68:361–388.

Pedersen-Bjergaard J, Nissen NI, Sørensen HM, Hou-Jensen K, Larsen MS, Ernst P, Ersbøll J, Knudtzon S, and Rose C Acute non-lymphocytic leukemia in patients with ovarian carcinoma following long-term treatment with Treosulfan (= dihydroxybusulfan). Cancer 1980 45:19–29.

Pedersen-Bjergaard J and Larsen SO Incidence of acute nonlymphocytic leukemia, preleukemia, and acute myeloproliferative syndrome up to 10 years after treatment of Hodgkin's disease. N Engl J Med 1982 307:965–971.

Pedersen-Bjergaard J, Philip P, Pedersen NT, Hou-Jensen K, Svejgaard A, Jensen G, and Nissen NI Acute nonlymphocytic leukemia, preleukemia, and acute myeloproliferative syndrome secondary to treatment of other malignant disease. II. Bone marrow cytology, cytogenetics, results of HLA typing, response to antileukemia chemotherapy and survival in a total series of 55 patients. Cancer 1984 54:452–462.

Pedersen-Bjergaard J, Ersbøll J, Sorensen HM, Keiding N, Larsen SO, Philip P, Larsen MS, Schultz H, and Nissen NI Risk of acute nonlymphocytic leukemia and preleukemia in patients treated with cyclophosphamide for non-Hodgkin's lymphomas: Comparison with results obtained in patients treated for Hodgkin's disease and ovarian carcinoma with other alkylating agents. Ann Intern Med 1985 103:192–200.

Pedersen-Bjergaard J, Rørth M, Avnstrøm S, Philip P, and Hou-Jensen K Acute nonlymphocytic leukemia following treatment of testicular cancer and gastric cancer with combination chemotherapy not including alkylating agents: Report of two cases. Am J Hematol 1985 18:425–429.

Pedersen-Bjergaard J, Specht L, Larsen SO, Ersbøll J, Struck J, Hansen MM, Hansen HH, and Nissen NI Risk of therapy-related leukaemia and preleukaemia after Hodgkin's disease: Relation to age, cumulative dose of alkylating agents, and time from chemotherapy. Lancet 1987 2:82–88.

Pedersen-Bjergaard J, Ersbøll J, Hansen VL, Sorensen BL, Christoffersen K, Hou-Jensen K, Nissen NI, Knudsen JB, and Hansen MM Carcinoma of the urinary bladder after treatment with cyclophosphamide for non-Hodgkin's lymphoma. N Engl J Med 1988 381:1028–1032.

Pedersen-Bjergaard J, Philip P, Ravn V, Hansen SW, and Nissen NI Therapy-related acute nonlymphocytic leukemia of FAB type M4 of M5 with early onset and t(9;11) (p21;q23) or a normal karyotype: A separate entity? J Clin Oncol 1988 6:395–397.

Pedersen-Bjergaard J and Philip P Therapy related malignancies: A review. Eur J Haematol 1989 42: 39–47.

Penn I and Starzl TE Malignant tumors arising de novo in immunosuppressed organ transplant recipients. Transplantation 1972 14:406–417.

Pratt CB, George SL, Hancock ML, Hustu HO, Kun LE, and Ochs J Second malignant neoplasms (SMNs) in survivors of childhood acute lymphocytic leukemia. Pediatr Res 1988 23:345a.

Preisler HD, Early AP, Razar A, Vlahides G, Marinello MJ, Stein AM, and Browman G Therapy of secondary acute nonlymphocytic leukemia with cytarabine. N Engl J Med 1983 308:21–23.

Pui C-H, Dahl GV, Melvin S, Williams DL, Peiper S, Mirro J, Murphy SB, and Stass S Acute leukemia with mixed lymphoid and myeloid phenotype. Br J Haematol 1984 56:121–130.

Pui C-H, Raimondi SC, Behm FG, Ochs J, Furman WL, Bunin NJ, Ribeiro RC, Tinsley PA, and Mirro J Shifts in blast cell phenotype and karyotype at relapse of childhood lymphoblastic leukemia. Blood 1986 68:1306–1310.

Pui C-H, Raimondi SC, Murphy SB, Ribeiro RC, Kalwinsky DK, Dahl GV, Crist WM, and Williams DL An analysis of leukemic cell chromosomal features in infants. Blood 1987 69:1289–1293.

Pui C-H, Behm FG, Raimondi SC, Dodge RK, George SL, Rivera GK, Mirro J Jr, Kalwinsky DK, Dahl GV, Murphy SB, Crist WM, and Williams DL Secondary acute myeloid leukemia in children treated for acute lymphoid leukemia. N Engl J Med 1989b 321:136–142.

Pui C-H, Raskind WH, Kitchingman GR, Raimondi SC, Behm FG, Murphy SB, Crist WM, Fialkow PJ, and Williams DL Clonal analyses of childhood acute lymphoblastic leukemia with "cytogenetically independent" cell populations. J Clin Invest 1989a 83:1971–1977.

Pui C-H, Hancock ML, Raimondi SC, Head D, Thompson E, Wilimas JK, Kun LE, Bowman LC, Crist WM, and Pratt CB Myeloid neoplasia in children treated for solid tumor. Lancet 1990 (in press).

Ratain MJ, Kaminer LS, Bitran JD, Larson RA, LeBeau MM, Skosey C, Purl S, Hoffman PC, Wade J, Vardiman JW, Daly K, Rowley JD, and Golomb HM Acute nonlymphocytic leukemia following etoposide and cisplatin combination chemotherapy for advanced non-small-cell carcinoma of the lung. Blood 1987 70:1412–1417.

Redman JR, Vugrin D, Arlin ZA, Gee TS, Kempin SJ, Godbold JH, Schuttenfeld D, and Clarkson DB Leukemia following treatment of germ cell tumors in men. J Clin Oncol 1984 2:1080–1087.

Reimer RR Risk of a second malignancy related to the use of cytotoxic chemotherapy. Cancer 1982 32: 287–292.

Reimer RR, Hoover R, Fraumeni JF Jr, and Young RC Acute leukemia after alkylating agent therapy of ovarian cancer. N Engl J Med 1977 297:177–181.

Rieche K Carcinogenicity of antineoplastic agents in man. Cancer Treat Rev 1984 11:39–67.

Ross W, Rowe T, Glisson B, Yalowich J, and Liu L Role of topoisomerase II in mediating epipodophyllotoxin-induced DNA cleavage. Cancer Res 1984 44:5857–5860.

Rowley JD, Golomb HM, and Vardiman JW Nonrandom chromosome abnormalities in acute leukemia and dysmyelopoietic syndromes in patients with previously treated malignant disease. Blood 1981 58:759–767.

Saffhill R, Margeson GP, and O'Connor PJ Mechanisms of carcinogenesis induced by alkylating agents. Biochem Biophys Acta 1985 823:111–145.

Sandberg AA, Abe S, Kowalczyk JR, Zedgenidze A, Takeuchi J, and Kakati S Chromosomes and causation of human cancer and leukemia. L. Cytogenetics of leukemias complicating other diseases. Cancer Genet Cytogenet 1982 7:95–136.

Scheneck SA and Penn I De novo brain tumors in renal transplant recipients. Lancet 1971 1:983–986.

Schmahl D, Habs M, Lorenz M, and Wagner I Occurrence of second tumors in man after anticancer drug. Cancer Treat Rev 1982 9:167–194.

Selby P and Horwich A Secondary leukemia in Hodgkin's disease. Lancet 1986 1:1027.

Singh B and Gupta RS Mutagenic responses of thirteen anticancer drugs on mutation induction at multiple genetic loci and on sister chromatoid exchanges in Chinese hamster ovary cells. Cancer Res 1983 43:577–584.

Spector G, Youness E, and Culbert SJ Acute lymphoblastic leukemia followed by acute granulocytic leukemia in a pediatric patient. Am J Clin Pathol 1979 72:242–245.

Stass S, Mirro J, Melvin S, Pui C-H, Murphy SB, and Williams D Lineage switch in acute leukemia. Blood 1984 64:701–706.

Stott H, Fox W, Girling DJ, Stephens RJ, and Galton DAG Acute leukaemia after busulphan. Br Med J 1977 2:1513–1517.

Strong LC, Herson J, Osborne BM, and Sutow WW risk of radiation-related subsequent malignant tumors in survivors of Ewing's sarcoma. JNCI 1979 62:1401–1406.

Strong LC, Stine M, and Norsted TL Cancer in survivors of childhood soft tissue sarcoma and their relatives. JNCI 1987 79:1213–1220.

Takaue T, Sullivan MP, Ramirez I, Cleary KR, and van Eys J Second malignant neoplasm in treated Hodgkin's disease: Report of a patient and scope of the problem. Am J Dis Child 1986 140:49–51.

Terracini B, Pastore G, Zurlo MG, Masera G, Fossati-Bellane F, Castello M, Tamaro P, Massolo F, Rosati D, Biddau PF, and Russo A Late deaths and second primary malignancies among long-term survivors of childhood cancer: An Italian multicentre study. Eur J Cancer Clin Oncol 1987 23:499–504.

Tester WJ, Kinsella TJ, Waller B, Makuch RW, Kelley PA, Glatstein E, and DeVita VT Second malignant neoplasms complicating Hodgkin's disease: The National Cancer Institute experience. J Clin Oncol 1984 2:762–769.

Tucker MA, Boice JD Jr, and Hoffman DC Second cancer following cutaneous melanoma and cancers of the brain, thyroid, connective tissue, bone, and eye in Connecticut, 1935–82. NCI Monogr 1985 68:161–189.

Tucker MA, Misfeldt D, Coleman CN, Clark WH Jr, and Rosenberg SA Cutaneous malignant melanoma after Hodgkin's disease. Ann Intern Med 1985 102:37–41.

Tucker MA, D'Angio GJ, Boice JD, Strong LC, Li FP, Stovall M, Stone BJ, Green DM, Lombardi F, Newton W, Hoover RN, and Fraumeni JF Jr Bone sarcomas linked to radiotherapy and chemotherapy in children. N Engl J Med 1987 317:588–593.

Tucker MA and Fraumeni JF Jr Treatment-related cancers after gynecologic malignancy. Cancer 1987 60:2117–2122.

Tucker MA, Meadows AT, Boice JD Jr, Stovall M, Oberlin O, Stone BJ, Birch J, Voûte PA, Hoover RN, and Fraumeni JF Jr, for the Late Effects Study Group. Leukemia after therapy with alkylating agents for childhood cancer. JNCI 1987 78:459–464.

Tucker MA, Coleman CN, Cos RS, Varghese A, and Rosenberg SA Risk of second cancers after treatment for Hodgkin's disease. N Engl J Med 1988 318:76–81.

Valagussa P, Santoro A, Fossati-Bellani F, Franchi F, Banfi A, and Bonadonna G Absence of treatment-induced second neoplasms after ABVD in Hodgkin's disease. Blood 1982 59:488–494.

Valagussa P, Santoto A, Fossati-Bellani F, Banfi A, and Bonadonna G Second acute leukemia and other malignancies following treatment for Hodgkin's disease. J Clin Oncol 1986 4:830–837.

Valagussa P, Tancini G, and Bonadonna G Second malignancies after CMF fòr resectable breast cancer. J Clin Oncol 1987 5:1138–1142.

Van Lierde S, Mecucci C, Casteels-Van Daele M, and Van den Berghe H Lineage switch and translocation t(9;11) in acute leukemia. Am J Pediatr Hematol Oncol 1989 11:20–22.

van der Velden JW, van Putten WLJ, Guinee VF, Pfeiffer R, van Leeuwen FE, van der Linden EAM, Vardomskaya I, Lane W, Durand M, Lagarde C, Hagemeister FB, Hagenbeek A, and Eghbali H Subsequent development of acute non-lymphocytic leukemia in patients treated for Hodgkin's disease. Int J Cancer 1988 42:252–255.

de Vathaire F, Schweisguth O, Rodary C, Francois P, Sarrazin D, Oberlin O, Hill C, Raquin MA, Dutreix A, and Flamant R Long-term risk of second malignant neoplasm after a cancer in childhood. Br J Cancer 1989 59:448–452.

Wacholder S and Boivin JF External comparisons with the case-cohort design. Am J Epidemiol 1987 126:1198–1209.

Wahlin A, Roos O, and Holm J Melphalan-related leukemia in multiple myeloma. Acta Med Scand 1982 21:203–208.

Weh HJ, Kabisch H, Landbeck G, and Hussfeld DK Translocation (9;11) (p21;q23) in a child with acute monoblastic leukemia following 2 1/2 years after successful chemotherapy for neuroblastoma. J Clin Oncol 1986 4:1518–1520.

Whang-Peng J, Young RC, Lee EC, Longo DL, Schechter GP, and DeVita VT Jr Cytogenetic studies in patients with secondary leukemia/dysmyelopoietic syndrome after different treatment modalities. Blood 1988 71:403–414.

White L, Ortega JA and Ying KL Acute non-lymphocytic leukemia following multimodality therapy for retinoblastoma. Cancer 1985 55:496–498.

Wozniak AJ, Glisson BS, Hande KR, and Ross WR Inhibition of etoposide-induced DNA damage and cytotoxicity in L1210 cells by dehydrogenase inhibitors and other agents. Cancer Res 1984 44:626–632.

Young JL Jr, Percy CL, and Asive AJ Eds SEER Program: Incidence and mortality, 1973–1977. National Cancer Institute Monograph 57, Washington, DC, U.S. Government Printing Office 1981.

Zarrabi MH, Rosner F, and Grunwald HW Second neoplasms in acute lymphoblastic leukemia. Cancer 1983 52:1712–1719.

CHAPTER 4

Toxicity of Alkylating Agents: Clinical Characteristics and Pharmacokinetic Determinants

David R. Newell, Ph.D. and Martin E. Gore, M.D.

INTRODUCTION

The alkylating agents were the first type of cytotoxic drug to be used in the chemotherapy of cancer. As will be apparent from even a cursory glance at their toxicities, these drugs are extremely toxic and it may come as no surprise that the alkylating agents were initially derived from a warfare agent, that is, sulphur mustard gas. Although less vesicant than sulphur mustard the lead compound, nitrogen mustard, retained many of the side effects of the parent molecule. Indeed, it is only due to skill and care of the medical and nursing staff who administer these agents that their routine use has become widespread. The desire to identify alkylating agents with more antitumor selectivity than nitrogen mustard led to the synthesis of many hundreds of compounds of which ten or so are still in clinical use. The common feature of the alkylating agents is that they are all antiproliferative drugs which produce hematological toxicity and gonadal dysfunction (see below). Other antiproliferative toxicities, that is, damage to the epithelium of the gastrointestinal tract and alopecia, are seen less frequently at standard doses although with the advent of high dose chemotherapy they are being reported more often. The introduction of high dose alkylating agent therapy has been stimulated by the observation that for many antitumor agents there is a clear dose–response relationship and that improved response rates can be achieved by the use of larger doses (Hryniuk, 1988). This approach has only been feasible, until recently, with the use of autologous bone marrow transplantation. However, with the availability of hematopoietic growth factors bone marrow transplantation may not be necessary. In either case, it is clear that the nonhematological toxicities of alkylating agents will assume more importance than they have previously assumed in the study of toxicity. This change in focus may create a need for the development of "cleaner" alkylating agents which display less in the way of nonhematological side effects.

Much of the early work on the molecular pharmacology of the alkylating agents implicated DNA as the locus of action for the group of compounds as a whole (Connors, 1975; Ludlum, 1975). This is still the prevalent view although it is now clear that the details of the interaction of alkylating agents with DNA are complex. For example, recent studies have shown that there may be some DNA sequence specificity (Kohn et al., 1987) with guanine situated within runs of guanine being the preferred site of alkylation. Furthermore, consideration of interpatient variability in the levels of DNA reaction for the alkylating agents may well be necessary to fully explain the toxicity and activity of these agents. In this respect, with the development of immunological methods for performing such studies on patient material (Tilby et al., 1987), it may soon be possible to do this on a routine basis. In addition, these methods have the advantage of allowing the measurement of specific types of DNA-alkylating agent adduct and as such they may indicate the nature of the DNA lesion responsible for antitumor activity in patients.

Although the mechanistic studies alluded to above are still at an early stage, there has been significant progress over the past decade in our understanding of the clinical pharmacokinetics of alkylating agents and it is now clear that these can be a major determinant of the toxicity of this class of drugs. In view of this progress, the aim of the current chapter is not only to review the clinical characteristics of the toxicities of alkylating agents but also to describe their clinical pharmacokinetics, particularly where these have been shown to relate to side effects. Despite being in clinical use for 50 years it seems likely that the full clinical potential of the alkylating agents has yet to be realized and that this article may play a role in that occurrence.

SPECIFIC AGENTS

Oxazaphosphorines—Cyclophosphamide and Ifosphamide

Clinical Toxicities

The oxazaphosphorine, cyclophosphamide, is the most widely used alkylating agent and possibly the most widely used anticancer drug. Unlike most of the other alkylating agents, such as melphalan, cyclophosphamide is not a hematopoietic stem cell poison and its effects on the bone marrow are less marked. Leucopenia is more of a feature than thrombocytopenia and the nadir blood count is reached on day 10. Nausea, vomiting, and alopecia only appear when higher doses are administered and cyclophosphamide is a nonvesicant. Prolonged oral doses may cause hemorrhagic cystitis because of the presence of the metabolite acrolein in the urine (see below); chronic bladder inflammation due to prolonged administration can lead to transitional cell neoplasms (Manohoran, 1984). Other toxicities that have been reported are interstitial pneumonitis (Hunt, 1972) and inappropriate antidiuretic hormone (ADH) secretion (DeFronzo et al., 1973). Cyclophosphamide in low dose is preferentially toxic to suppressor cells but it enhances natural killer cells, activates macrophages, and is synergistic to lymphokine activated killer cells (Hengst and Kempf, 1984). Like all alkylating agents it is carcinogenic and there is an increased risk of leukemia with prolonged use. In one study, patients with carcinoma of the ovary had a two- to threefold increased risk of acute leukemia (Green et al., 1986).

The toxicity of cyclophosphamide increases with dose so that above 50 mg/kg most patients suffer from nausea and vomiting and by 7 g/m^2 all patients suffer from this, although it is only severe (World Health Organization [WHO] grade 3–4) in 40% of patients and never lasts more than 72 hr (Fetting et al., 1982; Smith et al., 1985). The frequency of alopecia increases with dose, so that at 50 mg/kg, 2 gm/m^2, and 7 g/m^2, the incidence is 32, 77, and 100%, respectively (Araujo et al., 1979; Solidoro et al., 1981; Smith et al., 1985). Similarly, although the severity and duration of myelosuppression increases with increasing dose, it has been demonstrated that even at very high doses (7 g/m^2) the median time to bone marrow recovery is unaffected by autologous bone marrow rescue: the neutrophil count reaches 1×10^9 per liter in 18 days (Smith et al., 1985). Similar results have been obtained by others using 7 g/m^2 and 120 mg/kg (Souhami et al., 1983; Osbourne et al., 1987; Collins et al., 1989). Serious infection develops in 12 to 32% of patients receiving high dose cyclophosphamide but treatment related mortality is generally below 10% (Allen and Helson, 1981; Bell et al., 1982; Souhami et al., 1983; Lenhart et al., 1984; Smith et al., 1985; Osbourne et al., 1987; Collins et al., 1989). Severe gastrointestinal toxicity such as WHO grade 3 to 4 diarrhea is not common, although transient mild diarrhea occurs in about 28 to 40% of patients (Souhami et al., 1983; Smith et al., 1985). Similarly, severe hemorrhagic cystitis is rare provided bladder protection with intravenous (IV) hydration and mesna (sodium mercaptoethanesulphonate) are used although mild hematuria or dysuria has been reported in 9 to 35% of patients (Araujo et al., 1979; Solidoro et al., 1981; Bell et al., 1982; Souhami et al., 1983; Smith et al., 1985). A transient erythematous rash is often seen around the necklace area (Souhami et al., 1985; Smith et al., 1985; Osbourne et al., 1987).

High doses of cyclophosphamide are potentially cardiotoxic, the severity of which ranges from transient asymptomatic dysrhythmias to fatal myocardial necrosis. Doses of 120 mg/kg are associated with transient changes on ECG but as the dose rises to 150 mg/kg cardiac failure and myocarditis are encountered (Appelbaum et al., 1976; Mills and Roberts, 1979). The frequency of these complications is difficult to assess, but at 7 g/m^2 Smith and colleagues reported transient asymptomatic arrhythmias in 6/34 patients (Smith et al., 1985). Fatal cardiac complications occur in 19% of patients when high doses of cyclophosphamide (180 mg/kg) are given either together with noncardiotoxic cytotoxic drugs or alone but after the patient has been exposed to adriamycin (Gottdiener et al., 1981). However, at very high doses of 240 mg/kg the incidence is at least 25% (Santos et al., 1971; Buckner et al., 1972).

Ifosphamide in conventional dosage has a similar toxicity profile to cyclophosphamide, myelosuppression affects leucocytes and platelets alike but little cumulative toxicity occurs. Similarly nausea, vomiting, and alopecia start to appear at higher doses. Small divided doses result in subclinical nephrotoxicity (Van Dyke et al., 1972) but the dose limiting toxicity of early Phase I trials was hemorrhagic cystitis which occurred at 150 mg/kg (Bruhl et al., 1976). This urotoxicity is due to the oxazaphosphorine metabolite acrolein (Brock et al., 1979) and can be abrogated by a number of measures the most effective and convenient of which being the administration of mesna (Bryant et al., 1980).

Myelosuppression is dose limiting at 300 mg/kg with 41% of patients developing WHO grade 4 leucopenia but no nephro- or uro-toxicity is seen at this dose when mesna is used (Falkson et al., 1982). Others have however been able to escalate the dose further to 5 and 8 g/m^2 without bone marrow rescue (Stuart-Harris et al., 1983) with 4% and 54% of patients, respectively, developing WHO grade 4 leucopenia in this study. The mean leucocyte nadir was only 2.1×10^9 per liter and in only four patients did the platelet count drop below 100×10^9 per liter. However, at these high doses vomiting was severe in 45% of patients. Macroscopic hematuria occurred in 3% of the cases probably caused by insufficient mesna and in 24% of patients microscopic hematuria was detected. Seven out of 10 patients showed a deterioration of creatinine clearance and in two cases fatal renal failure developed. The authors concluded that the scheduling and the total dose of ifosphamide might be an important factor in the development of renal failure and because there was no apparent increase in response rate with the higher dose, 5 not 8 g/m^2 should be used (Stuart-Harris et al., 1983).

Encephalopathy is an important side effect of high dose ifosphamide and it has been noted that up to 9% of patients receiving 5 g/m^2 develop this side effect with a further 56% of patients exhibiting abnormalities on electroencephalogram (EEG) (Meanwell et al., 1986). These authors suggested a series of factors that could predict the development of encephalopathy: hypoalbuminemia, high serum creatinine, and the presence of pelvic disease. They constructed a nomogram using these parameters which could predict for this side effect. However, more recently it has been suggested that drug metabolism may plan an important role in the etiology of ifosphamide encephalopathy (see below).

Pharmacokinetics

The oxazaphosphorines represent classic examples of the importance of pharmacokinetics as a determinant of drug toxicity. Studies by a large number of groups have shown that both cyclophosphamide and ifosphamide require metabolic activation to display activity. However, metabolism is a double-edged sword in that it also leads to the formation of toxic metabolites and only with a full understanding of the metabolic pathways for the compounds has their optimal clinical use been made possible. The more important steps in the metabolism of cyclophosphamide are outlined in Fig. 4-1. Excellent reviews on the development and pharmacokinetics of the oxazaphosphorines are available and the reader is referred to these for many of the original references (Grochow and Colvin, 1983; Sladek, 1987; Brock, 1989).

The original aim in the development of the oxazaphosphorines was to produce cyclic N-phosphorylated prodrugs of nor-nitrogen mustard which upon phosphoramidase catalyzed hydrolysis would yield reactive bifunctional alkylating species (Arnold et al., 1958). In reality, it was soon found that drug activation was achieved by hepatic enzymes (Foley et al., 1961) and it was later shown that these were mixed function oxidases which catalyzed the formation of the 4-hydroxylated metabolite (Fig. 4-1B) (Connors et al., 1974; Sladek, 1973; Struck, 1974; Fenselau et al., 1977). The 4-hydroxy metabolite exists in equilibrium with the ring-opened aldehyde tautomer (Fig. 4-1C) which, following the beta-elimination of acrolein (Fig. 4-1F), gives rise to phosphoramide mustard (Fig. 4-1E) (Struck et al., 1975; Fenselau et al., 1975). Phosphoramide mustard is recognized by most authors as the species responsible for the cytotoxic activity of cyclophosphamide whereas acrolein is the entity which causes oxazaphosphorine-induced bladder toxicity (see above). Ifosphamide follows a similar pathway for metabolic activation although a different structural isomer of phosphoramide mustard is formed. The other major metabolic pathway for oxazaphosphorine metabolism is the oxidation of the aldehyde tautomer of the 4-hydroxy metabolite to the corresponding carboxylic acid (Fig. 4-1D) (Hill et al., 1972; Sladek, 1973; Connors et al., 1974). The carboxylic acid is unable to undergo beta-elimination and therefore is an inactive metabolite. The oxidation of the aldehyde to the carboxylic acid is probably catalyzed in vivo by aldehyde dehydrogenase (Domeyer and Sladek, 1980) and because this results in the formation of an inactive metabolite it has been argued that the selectivity of the oxazaphosphorines is caused by the action of this enzyme. Thus, both normal and certain resistant tumor cell lines have elevated levels of aldehyde dehydrogenase in comparison to sensitive tumor cells (Cox et al., 1975, 1976; Hilton, 1984; Sladek and Landkamer, 1985). It is therefore envisaged that normal tissues preferentially metabolize the 4-hydroxy/aldehyde compound to the inactive carboxyl species and it is this process which confers selectivity on the oxazaphosphorines. This is supported by the relatively poor therapeutic index of phosphoramide mustard in experimental systems (Brock and Hohorst, 1977). Also, following cyclophosphamide administration, there was preferential formation of DNA cross links in tumor as opposed to normal tissues in mice (Colvin and Hilton, 1981) which was not the case with phosphoramide mustard. Although the above data strongly suggests that the selectivity of the oxazaphosphorines is caused by their preferential inactivation in normal tissues the selective uptake of the 4-hydroxy/aldehyde metabolite or its conversion to phosphoramide mustard in tumor tissue cannot be excluded. However, there are no convincing data to support these latter possibilities (Sladek, 1987).

Interest in the selective inactivation of the oxazaphosphorines in normal tissues has been further stimulated by recent observations that there can be considerable interpatient variability in the urinary excretion of carboxycyclophosphamide following cyclophosphamide administration. Thus, it appears that patients can be divided into two groups dependant upon their carboxylator phenotype (Hadidi et al., 1988), a finding which strongly suggests pharmacogenetic variability in oxazaphosphorine metabolism. A number of lines of evidence point to acrolein as the species responsible for the bladder toxicity seen with oxazaphosphorines. Phosphoramide mustard is not toxic to the bladder (Phillips et al., 1961) when administered systemically to rats. Furthermore, phosphoramide mustard, nor-nitrogen mustard, and cyclophosphamide itself are also relatively nontoxic when instilled directly into the bladder which is not the case for 4-hydroxycyclophosphamide and acrolein (Brock et al., 1979; Sladek et al., 1982). In addition, the derivative of the cyclophosphamide in which the two chloroethyl groups have been replaced with ethyl substituents *was* toxic to the bladder when administered to experimental animals (Cox, 1979). These observations, and other data, strongly implicate acrolein as the causative agent in oxazaphosphorine-induced bladder toxic-

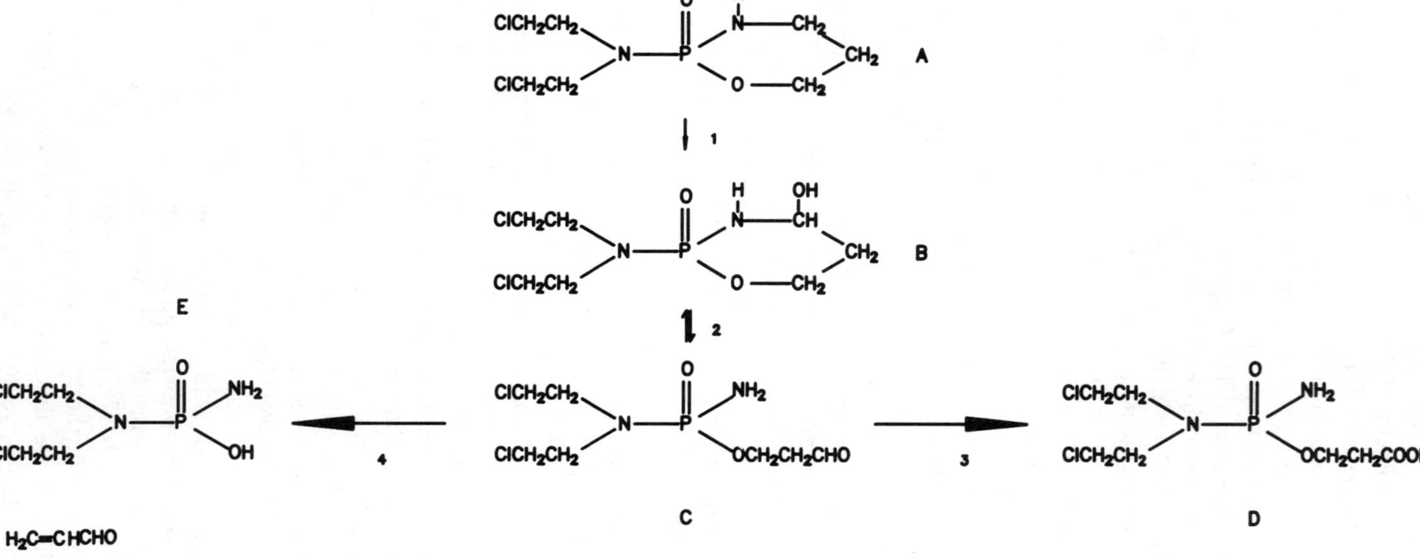

FIGURE 4-1. Pathways of biological significance in the metabolism of cyclophosphamide. Compounds: A–cyclophosphamide; B–4-hydroxycyclophosphamide; C–aldophosphamide; D–carboxyphosphamide; E–phosphoramide mustard; F–acrolein.
Pathways: 1–mixed function oxidase catalyzed 4-hydroxylation; 2–4-hydroxycyclophosphamide/aldophosphamide tautomerization; 3–aldehyde dehydrogenase catalyzed oxidation; 4–chemical beta-elimination of acrolein.

ity. An understanding of this mechanism led to the use of mesna which undergoes rapid renal elimination and is thus available for alkylation by acrolein which is thought to be formed from the decomposition of the 4-hydroxy/aldehyde metabolite in the urine. Therefore by the use of mesna the urothelium is spared and oxazaphosphorine bladder toxicity circumvented.

Although, as indicated above, the metabolic pathway of ifosphamide is similar to that of cyclophosphamide there is one important exception, namely, N-dechloroethylation. In the case of ifosphamide this can account for 25% of the metabolism of the drug (Norpoth, 1976) whereas for cyclophosphamide N-dechloroethylation is a minor pathway. In view of this metabolic difference it has been suggested that the central nervous system (CNS) toxicity seen with ifosphamide is caused by the release of chlorolacetaldehyde (Goren et al., 1986). CNS toxicity is a particular problem following oral ifosphamide therapy and this could occur because of the more extensive formation of chloroacetaldehyde during first pass metabolism.

With regard to intra and interindividual variation in oxazaphosphorine metabolism, it is now clear that both cyclophosphamide and ifosphamide cause induction of their own metabolism. On repeated administration the plasma half-life of the parent compound declines and the whole body clearance increases (D'Incalci et al., 1979; Graham et al., 1983; Lind et al., 1989a). This effect is presumably because of the induction of hepatic mixed-function oxidases and, following IV administration, this results in the production of elevated levels of alkylating species in plasma (Schuler et al., 1987; Lind et al., 1989a). One interpatient variable which has been identified is body weight with both cyclophosphamide and ifosphamide terminal half-life being increased in heavier patients however, since the active species were not measured in either study, the relevance to pharmacodynamics is not clear (Powis et al., 1987; Lind et al., 1989b). Recently a limited sampling method for cyclophosphamide has been described (Egorin et al., 1989) which should allow the more widespread description of the pharmacokinetics of the parent compound. However, in view of the large number of toxic and active metabolites, it is unlikely that on its own it will allow the optimization of the use of the drug. More probably this will require the application of methods which allow the measurement of the full range of oxazaphosphorine metabolites. Such methods are now available (Sladek et al., 1984; Struck et al., 1987; Hadidi and Idle, 1988) and their use should in theory improve the use of what is already an important class of drugs.

Although it is now 30 years since the introduction of oxazaphosphorines it will be clear from the above discussion that the complexities of their pharmacokinetics are only just becoming fully understood. With this understanding it should be possible, for the first time, to define relationships between pharmacokinetics and pharmacodynamics such that the care of individual patients is optimized. It is worth noting that, despite the complexity of their pharmacokinetics, the oxazaphosphorines are among the most selective and hence useful antitumor agents. The challenge now is to exploit the selectivity conferred by oxazaphosphorine pharmacokinetics and in so doing reveal their true therapeutic potential.

Melphalan

Clinical Toxicities

The principle side effect of melphalan is myelosuppression. Neutrophils and platelets are equally affected and when it is administered in conventional dosage the nadir occurs at 28 days. Nausea and vomiting are dose dependent as is the frequency of alopecia. Melphalan is nonirritant to subcutaneous tissues and peritoneal surfaces and is therefore not useful as a sclerosant for the treatment of pleural effusions. The dose of melphalan needs to be adjusted when renal function is impaired, otherwise severe bone marrow suppression results (see below). In addition, melphalan itself can be nephrotoxic, particularly in high doses. Melphalan is carcinogenic and long-term exposure is associated with an increased risk of acute leukemia. In one study patients with ovarian cancer who were treated with melphalan had a 93-fold increase in the incidence of leukemia (Green et al., 1986).

Melphalan is a bone marrow stem cell poison and cumulative myelotoxicity is a feature of prolonged dosing. The dose-limiting toxicity is myelosuppression and it appears that the maximum dose that can safely be given without autologous bone marrow rescue is 140 mg/m^2. At this dose it takes about 28 days for the leucocyte count to recover to 1×10^9 per liter and about 24 days for the platelet count to recover to 25×10^9 per liter (Maraninchi et al., 1986; Selby et al., 1987a). Autologous bone marrow transplantation reduces the neutropenia time by about 10 days but does not affect the time to platelet recovery (McElwain et al., 1979; Maraninchi et al., 1986; Gore et al., 1989). There seems to be a relationship, at least in children, between the nucleated cell count of the re-infused marrow and the time taken for the blood count to recover (Kingston et al., 1984). Doses above 140 mg/m^2 are invariably associated with alopecia and almost invariably associated with nausea and vomiting (Selby et al., 1987a), tiredness and anorexia are likewise very common. Stomatitis and diarrhea of WHO grade 2 or greater occurs in 70% and 61% of patients respectively (Gore et al., 1989).

The dose-limiting toxicities of high dose melphalan, when given in association with autologous bone marrow rescue, are stomatitis and diarrhea and doses above 200 mg/m^2 are associated with severe gastrointestinal side effects. It has been shown that pretreating or "priming" mice or sheep with a small dose of cyclophosphamide prior to a large dose of an alkylating agent such as melphalan, reduces gastrointestinal toxicity and increases the survival of these animals (Millar et al., 1978a and 1978b). In man, priming with cyclophosphamide enhances peripheral leucocyte recovery following high dose melphalan (Hedley et al., 1978) and reduces gut damage (Selby et al., 1987b). Diarrhea is dose limiting at 245 mg/m^2 in primed patients and 170 mg/m^2 in unprimed patients but in these situations the toxicity is severe (Cornbleet et al., 1983). However, not all groups have demonstrated that there is a clinical benefit from priming (Lazarus et al., 1983).

The severe infection rate in patients treated with high doses of melphalan ranges from 15 to 33% and accounts for most of the treatment-related deaths which range from 2.5 to 23% (Cornbleet et al., 1983; Corringham et al., 1983; Dewar et al., 1984; Graham-Pole et al., 1984; Maraninchi et al., 1984). Gram-negative organisms account for many of these infections and there is evidence that with increasing clinical experience, and the use of prophylactic antibiotics, the treatment-related death rate can be reduced (Selby et al., 1987a).

Less commonly recorded side effects include: transient rises in liver enzymes and blood urea, depression, early hypotension, inappropriate ADH secretion, palmar erythema, and the development of acute leukemia (Cornbleet et al., 1983; Lazarus et al., 1983; Maraninchi et al., 1984; Greenbaum-Lefkoe et al., 1985; Leff et al., 1986).

Pharmacokinetics

Although it was originally designed as a transport form of nitrogen mustard only recently have the transport characteristics of melphalan been elucidated in detail. It is now clear that melphalan can enter cells by amino acid transport systems and that levels of amino acids present in biological fluids can modulate the uptake of the drug (Vistica, 1983). In addition to tissue uptake, melphalan clearance involves both renal elimination (see below) and chemical hydrolysis. Metabolism is not thought to play an important role in determining the disposition of the drug.

With melphalan, there are two areas where relationships between pharmacokinetics and clinical pharmacodynamics have been studied. The first of these relates to the oral bioavailability of the compound where, following the advent of High Performance Liquid Chromatography (HPLC) methods for measuring the drug, it soon became clear that there was considerable inter- and intrapatient variability. In their early study Alberts et al. (1979) found a greater than 10-fold variation in melphalan area under the curve (AUC) following oral administration, a result which was in agreement with that of Brox et al. (1979) who were unable to detect any melphalan in the plasma of some patients. Studies by Woodhouse et al. (1983) and Bosanquet and Gilby (1982) further confirmed the variable and sometimes poor bioavailability of oral melphalan and these latter authors suggested that melphalan absorption could be improved if patients were fasted prior to and for four hours after melphalan administration (Bosanquet and Gilby, 1984). This result was confirmed by Reece et al. (1986) who went on to study the effect of co-administration of L-leucine (Reece et al., 1987) since it had been shown (Adair and McElnay, 1986) that melphalan uptake from the gastrointestinal tract was by an active process, that is, probably an amino acid transporter. In fact, L-leucine co-administration had little or no effect on the plasma levels of melphalan achieved following oral administration (Reece et al., 1987) and this is in accord with the data of Adair and McElnay (1987) who showed no marked effect of dietary amino acids on melphalan absorption. Following high dose oral melphalan there is also considerable intra- and interpatient variability and in the recent study by Choi et al. (1989) the trend towards lower melphalan AUC values on repeat administration may well have occurred because of concurrent damage to the gastrointestinal tract epithelium as a result of both the melphalan, and the cyclophosphamide and thiotepa the patients were also receiving. With regard to intrapatient variability in melphalan bioavailability, one small study suggests that the intrapatient variation is less than the interpatient variation (Taha et al., 1982), however further data on this subject would be useful. In general, it is clear that the oral bioavailability of melphalan cannot be considered satisfactory, either in extent or reproducibility.

The obvious solution to this problem is parenteral administration and there have been a number of studies performed addressing the pharmacokinetics of the IV drug, often when administered at high doses. A number of these studies have also encompassed the question of the relationship between melphalan pharmacokinetics and renal function, the second area where pharmacokinetic–toxicity relationships are apparent with melphalan. The first study to suggest a relationship between melphalan exposure in patients and renal function was that of Cornwell et al. (1982). These authors showed that patients with a blood urea nitrogen level of > 30 mg/100 mL were more likely to suffer severe leucopenia. The pharmacokinetic basis for this observation has been suggested by a number of studies which have shown a weak correlation between renal function and melphalan exposure (Bosanquet and Gilby, 1982; Adair et al., 1986; Zucchetti et al., 1988) which in one investigation was apparent even after oral administration (Osterborg et al., 1989). Although other studies have failed to show any such relationship (Ninane et al., 1985; Reece et al., 1988; Choi et al., 1989), note that in a number of cases renal function (glomerular filtration rate) was calculated from serum creatinine levels and therefore may not have been an accurate value (Daugaard et al., 1988). It has recently been argued that the ultimate solution to the problem of variability in melphalan pharmacokinetics is to resort to the use of a test dose (Tranchaud et al., 1989). Melphalan pharmacokinetics appear to be linear and therefore this approach is feasible, however, it would be far more satisfactory to accurately define the relationship between renal function and melphalan renal clearance such that a dose formula could be derived and applied. Once variation in melphalan exposure as a consequence of differences in renal function can be controlled, and the use of the IV route becomes routine, it should then be possible to derive the maximum benefit from the drug.

Chlorambucil

Clinical Toxicities

Chlorambucil has similar myelosuppressive affects on both leucocytes and platelets. The nadir of the myelosuppression is 14 days and like other stem cell poisons it exhibits cumulative myelotoxicity. It is very well-tolerated, only occasionally causing nausea and anorexia when it is used in conventional doses. Rarely patients may be allergic to the drug and develop bronchospasm, fever, and skin hypersensitivity (Sawitsky et al., 1971; Knisley et al., 1977) and interstitial pneumonitis is associated with prolonged exposure (Rubino, 1972; Refsum et al., 1977; Cole et al., 1978) or high dose therapy (Lane et al., 1981). Intermediate doses of 16 mg/m^2 daily for five days are associated with virtually no myelosuppression and only minor gastrointestinal upset, provided the treatment is given intermittently (Cadman et al., 1982; Portlock et al., 1987). However, when very high doses are used (2 mg/kg/d for 3 days) CNS toxicity occurs (Ciobanu et al., 1987) which has been our own experience at the Royal Marsden Hospital (unpublished data). As with other alkylating agents chlorambucil has been associated with the development of acute leukemia (Fiere et al., 1978).

Pharmacokinetics

The clinical pharmacokinetics of chlorambucil have been studied by a number of groups and on the basis of available data there are no clear instances of pharmacokinetic variables influencing toxicities of the compound. In routine clinical use chlorambucil is administered orally. Whereas there is considerable interpatient variability in the plasma levels of chlorambucil achieved the bioavailability is thought to be satisfactory (Farmer and Newell, 1983; Ehrsson et al., 1984; Adair and McElany, 1987; Oppitz et al., 1989). The major metabolic process for chlorambucil is beta-oxidation of the butyric side chain which results in the formation of phenyl acetic mustard. It is now clear that the levels of this metabolite formed in patients are such that it is likely to contribute to the biological actions of the drug. Although it has been argued, on the basis of data from preclinical models, that phenyl acetic mustard has less antitumor selectivity than chlorambucil (McLean et al., 1980; Godeneche et al., 1980; Lee et al., 1986) there are no clinical data to support this contention.

In addition to beta-oxidation, N-dechloroethylation is also an important step in the metabolism of chlorambucil (McLean et al., 1980). By analogy with ifosphamide (see above) this should lead to the release of chloroacetaldehyde which could give rise to CNS toxicity. Indeed, CNS toxicity is recognized as a complication of chlorambucil therapy (Ciobanu et al., 1987) although its symptoms (seizures) differ from those of ifosphamide (CNS depression) and therefore is unlikely to have the same etiology.

With the exception of CNS toxicity, chlorambucil remains a well-tolerated drug with satisfactory bioavailability following oral administration. Both chlorambucil and its major metabolite are active species and therefore dose modification in the case of metabolic insufficiency is not required.

Nitrosoureas

Clinical Toxicities

The nitrosoureas are again bone marrow stem cell poisons and their main toxicity is myelosuppression. Leucocytes and platelets are affected alike and the nadir of the counts is at 28 days and cumulative myelosuppression occurs with chronic dosing. The severity of nausea and vomiting is dose dependant as is the alopecia. The nitrosoureas are leukemogenic (Greene et al., 1985), and can occasionally be associated with renal failure (Harmon et al., 1979). Cumulative doses of 2733 mg/m^2 for methyl-CCNU (N-(z-chloroethyl)-N′-(trans-4-methylcyclohexyl)N-nitrosourea) and 100 mg/m^2 for BCNU (N, N′-bis(2-chloroethyl)-N-nitrosourea) cause pulmonary fibrosis (Hundley and Lukens, 1979).

High doses of BCNU require bone marrow rescue and when given IV, BCNU seems to be associated with mild flushing, tachycardia, and hypotension although these symptoms may be due to the alcohol vehicle (Takvorian et al., 1983; Mbidde et al., 1988). These latter authors found that bone marrow infusions should be delayed to 48 hr in patients receiving high dose BCNU otherwise there is a risk on nonengraftment. The most serious complications are clearly dose related thus, anorexia, nausea, and vomiting are severe above 900 mg/m^2, mucositis and diarrhea are severe above 2000 mg/m^2, and in addition at this dose fatal encephalomyelopathy can develop (Phillips et al., 1983). These authors found that sepsis occurred in 9/143 (6%) of patients and was fatal in five. The overall treatment related death rate was 20% and causes included pancytopenic complications, interstitial pneumonitis, and hepatotoxicity. Total alopecia occurs above doses of 1200 mg/m^2 and very occasionally maculopapular rashes and optic neuritis were seen. This latter complication together with CNS complications seems to be particularly common with intracarotid infusions of BCNU (Kapp et al., 1982).

Hepatotoxicity with high-dose nitrosoureas occurs in 26 to 46% of patients (DeVita et al., 1965; Phillips et al., 1983; Takvorian et al., 1987) and occurs in two patterns: the first is a nondose related mild transient asymptomatic rise in liver function tests. The second form of hepatotoxicity appears to be dose related, is delayed in onset (median 40 days), the liver function tests present a cholestatic picture, and often there is progression to liver failure. Phillips and colleagues (1983) found that 10 (11%) patients developed this type of hepatotoxicity, eight of whom died. This study demonstrated the dose relationship for its side effect: 6/17 evaluable patients who received > 1500 mg/m^2 of BCNU as compared to 4/76 evaluable patients who had received < 1500 mg/m^2 developed this side effect ($p = 0.01$). In contrast, interstitial pneumonitis was found not to be dose related in this same series. Overall this adverse effect occurred in 19% of the patients (16/83 evaluable patients) but only patients who received between 1050 to 1200 mg/m^2 developed this complication. The median time of onset of pneumonitis was 52 days, the presenting symptoms were usually cough and dyspnea and 6/16 patients (37.5%) died.

Pharmacokinetics

The chloroethylnitrosoureas are used primarily for the treatment for brain tumors. This use is a reflection of the lipophilicity of these compounds and hence, by virtue of their distribution into the CNS, this pharmacodynamic property can be seen as related to pharmacokinetics, that is, tissue distribution.

In comparison to preclinical models the clinical activity of the chloroethylnitrosoureas is, to say the least, disappointing. A large body of evidence now indicates that it is differences in DNA repair capacity which underlies the species differences in the activity of these compounds (D'Incalci et al., 1988); pharmacokinetics are not implicated to any great extent. Although chloroethylnitrosoureas can undergo metabolism, most notably the ring hydroxylation of CCNU, there is again no clear evidence of any relationship between this process and pharmacodynamics (Reed, 1987). Of the clinical toxicities seen with chloroethylnitrosoureas, particularly at high doses, lung damage is among the most problematic with serious toxicity being reported (Weiss et al., 1981). Studies by Smith and Boyd (1984) have shown that destruction of pulmonary glutathione reductase precedes the onset of lung damage in rats and that this destruction may be caused by reaction with the isocyanate released from BCNU and CCNU during their chemical decomposition. Because chloroethylnitrosoureas are now available that do not release carbamoylating species, the lung toxicity of this class of compounds should be overcome and again it could be argued that an understanding of the molecular pharmacology of the compounds as a class has led to improvements in their use.

Busulphan

Clinical Toxicities

The pattern of myelosuppression encountered with busulphan is similar to that seen with the nitrosoureas. Both leucocytes and platelets are equally affected, the nadir of the myelosuppression is 28 days and cumulative toxicity occurs. Weakness, gynecomastia, cataracts and pulmonary fibrosis are all seen and hyperpigmentation is the most common dermatological effect although a variety of skin rashes have been described including, bullous eruptions (Dosik et al., 1970) and porphyria cutanea tarda (Kyle and Dameshek, 1964).

At higher doses (16–20 mg/kg) almost all patients develop anorexia, mucositis, nausea and vomiting, diarrhea, stomatitis, and some degree of hepatotoxicity (Peters et al., 1987), furthermore at these doses patients require bone marrow rescue. Radiotherapy induced skin reactions seemed to be enhanced after high dose busulphan (Vassal et al., 1989b) and convulsions have been reported. It is therefore advisable that patients receiving high doses of busulphan be given prophylactic anticonvulsants.

Pharmacokinetics

Busulphan and treosulphan are the sole clinical representatives of the methanesulphonates and the former drug is deemed to be a useful compound in the treatment of chronic myelogenous leukemia. Early pharmacokinetic studies with both drugs were reviewed by Farmer and Newell (1983). More recently developed HPLC and gas chromatography-mass spectrometry (GC-MS) methods (Ehrsson and Hassan, 1983; Henner et al., 1987; Vassal and Gouyette, 1988) have allowed a more detailed description of the pharmacokinetics of busulphan both at conventional (Ehrsson et al., 1983) and high doses (Vassal et al., 1989a; Grochow et al., 1989). One interesting correlation which arose from the study of Grochow and co-workers was that the veno-occlusive disease of the liver which occurs in some 20% of patients treated with high dose busulphan may relate to an elevated busulphan AUC. Because there is a significant mortality rate associated with veno-occlusive disease, these authors went on to suggest that patients should be monitored and doses decreased so as to reduce the risk of this side effect. However note that, hepatic veno-occlusive disease can be seen at high doses with other agents (for example, nitrosoureas [see above] and mitomycin C) and thus the higher busulphan AUC seen in patients with the syndromes may simply be due to underlying hepatic dysfunction.

Thiotepa

Clinical Toxicities

Thiotepa is now only rarely used as a parenteral anticancer agent although it still has a place as a serosal surface sclerosant. Recent Phase I studies with bone marrow rescue indicated that severe toxicity occurred at doses of 810 to 1215 mg/m^2 with mucositis, hepatotoxicity, and CNS toxicity all being encountered (Lazarus et al., 1987).

Pharmacokinetics

Recent interest in thiotepa has extended to pharmacokinetic studies and this has again been stimulated by the development of more specific and sensitive assays (Egorin et al., 1985). Although it has been suggested that interindividual variations in thiotepa pharmacokinetics warrant dose adjustment on the basis of pharmacokinetic monitoring (Hagen et al., 1988), this suggestion has not been widely followed. Pharmacokinetic studies have shown that thiotepa efflux from the peritoneal cavity is rapid and therefore the drug is not a good candidate for intraperitoneal (IP) therapy (Wadler et al., 1989); in addition, metabolism is the major route of thiotepa elimination (Cohen et al., 1986). Major thiotepa metabolites include the oxygen derivative tepa whose formation in vitro can be catalyzed by cytochrome P450 (Waxman et al., 1989). Both thiotepa and tepa distribute well into the cerebrospinal fluid (CSF) and it has been suggested that this pharmacokinetic property makes the agent a good candidate for the treatment of central nervous system tumors (Heideman et al., 1989). It is clear from recent studies that our understanding of thiotepa is, despite over 30 years of clinical use, inadequate. Further studies with the agent are thus warranted particularly as the drug appears to lack significant toxicities other than hematological side effects at conventional doses. Thus, thiotepa may well be a useful agent in high dose studies with either bone marrow or growth factor support and initial experience in this area has been reported (Ackland et al., 1988). Because it has been indicated that the plasma clearance of thiotepa may be saturable (Heideman et al., 1989), pharmacokinetic monitoring in high dose studies is essential.

GONADAL DYSFUNCTION

All alkylating agents have similar effects on gonadal function. In men irreversible azoospermia can occur although it is difficult to give precise doses at which this will happen. It seems that cumulative doses of 400 mg of chlorambucil (Richter et al., 1970) or 6 to 10 g of cyclophosphamide (Fairley et al., 1972) will result in sterility. In prepubertal boys the cumulative dose of cyclophosphamide probably needs to be greater, possibly as much as before 20 g permanent azoospermia results (Rapola et al., 1973; Lentz et al., 1977). Studies at the Royal Marsden Hospital are currently addressing the question of male fertility after high dose of melphalan. In adult males the main pathological lesion is one of germinal aplasia, thus testosterone levels are usually normal and patients can be assured that libido and sexual performance will be unaffected. However, during puberty there is a risk of Leydig cell damage and this may result in lowered testosterone levels with all its concomitant problems such as gynecomastia.

In women treated with single alkylating agents about 50% develop permanent ovarian failure (Louis et al., 1956; Galton et al., 1958; Warne et al., 1973). The probability of infertility in women appears to be related to age. The nearer a woman is to menopause the more likely she is to be rendered infertile. In one study amenorrhea occurred after 5.2 g of cyclophosphamide in women over 40 but only after 9.3 g in those under 40. Furthermore, 50% of this latter group resumed normal mensuration within six months of discontinuing treatment (Koyama et al., 1977). A similar relationship between amenorrhea and age has been noted for patients treated with melphalan (Fisher et al., 1979). However, high dose melphalan given to adolescent girls may be associated in some cases with permanent ovarian failure (Kellie and Kingston, 1987).

The issue of sterility must be discussed with every patient, and males who wish to father children in the future should be offered sperm banking.

A number of measures have been attempted to try and protect patient's fertility; they have been based on the premise that future gonadal function can be protected by suppressing the gonads during treatment. Therefore men have been given testosterone, women have been given oral contraceptives and both men and women have been given gonadotrophin releasing hormones (Redman and Bajorunas, 1987).

Alkylating agents should be avoided during the first trimester of pregnancy because of their teratogenic potential but it is safe to administer them during the third trimester. Clearly however, there is a theoretical risk to the fetus of leukemia in later life but the actual risk, if there is one, is completely unknown.

CONCLUSIONS

From the extensive literature reviewed in this article it should be clear that the alkylating agents represent a class of compounds the toxicity of which dictates that they should be prescribed solely by experienced practitioners. However, in the right hands, they are compounds which can offer real therapeutic benefit to the cancer patient and they are indeed components of certain curative chemotherapeutic regimens, for example in the treatment of lymphomas. The major challenge for the future is to improve the activity of these drugs in the treatment of the common solid tumors and reduce the level of interpatient variability both in terms of toxicity and response. With regard to the former challenge, the most hopeful approach lies in the use of high dose alkylating agent therapy with hematological support. Such support may take the form of bone marrow transplantation or the administration of hematopoietic growth factors. Regardless of which is chosen, the dose of the alkylating agent should then be limited by nonhematological toxicity and, as indicated from the work covered in this chapter, the organ that becomes dose limiting will depend upon the drug used.

Turning to the question of interpatient variability in the toxicity of alkylating agents, it should again be clear from this chapter that pharmacokinetics are a significant causative factor. The exact role, if any, of therapeutic drug monitoring in alkylating agent therapy remains to be determined. However, it is already clear that in dose escalation studies pharmacokinetics should always be performed and that for most types of alkylating agent further studies are required to fully define the impact of pharmacokinetics on drug toxicity.

The alkylating agents are an extremely important class of antitumor agent and it is likely that they will remain so for the foreseeable future. Despite being highly toxic their safe clinical use is possible and the experienced clinician in a specialist center should not be deterred from using them.

REFERENCES

Ackland SP, Choi KE, Ratain MJ, Egorin MJ, Williams SF, Sinkule JA, and Bitran JD Human plasma pharmacokinetics of thiotepa following high dose administration of thiotepa and cyclophosphamide. J Clin Oncol 1988 6:1192–1196.

Adair CG, Bridges JM, and Desai ZR Renal function in the elimination of oral melphalan in patients with multiple myeloma. Cancer Chemother Pharmacol 1986 17:185–188.

Adair CG and McElnay JC Studies on the mechanism of gastrointestinal absorption of melphalan and chlorambucil. Cancer Chemother Pharmacol 1986 17:95–98.

Adair CG and McElnay JC The effect of dietary amino acids on the gastrointestinal absorption of melphalan and chlorambucil. Cancer Chemother Pharmacol 1987 20:343–346.

Alberts DS, Chang SY, Chen HS-G, Evans TL, and Moon TE Oral melphalan kinetics. Clin Pharm Ther 1979 26:737–745.

Allen JC and Helson L High-dose cyclophosphamide chemotherapy for recurrent CNS tumours in children. J Neurosurg 1981 55:749–756.

Appelbaum FR, Strauchen JA, and Gram RG Acute lethal carditis caused by high-dose combination chemotherapy. Lancet 1976 31:58–62.

Araujo CE, Barrague J, Tagle J, and Tessler J Lung cancer treatment with high cyclophosphamide doses versus high cyclophosphamide doses plus radiotherapy. Int J Radiat Oncol Biol Phys 1979 3:1449–1453.

Arnold H, Bourseaux F, and Brock N Chemotherapeutic action of a cyclic nitrogen mustard phosphamide ester (B 518-ASTA) in experimental tumours of the rat. Nature 1958 181:931.

Bell R, Gallangher CJ, Ford J, Malpas JS, and Lister TA Phase II study of a high-dose regimen of cyclophosphamide and prednisolone in advanced non-Hodgkin's lymphoma of favourable histologic type. Cancer Treat Rep 1982 66:377–380.

Bosanquet AG and Gilby ED Pharmacokinetics of oral and intravenous melphalan during routine treatment of multiple myeloma. Eur J Cancer Clin Oncol 1982 18:355–362.

Bosanquet AG and Gilby ED Comparison of the fed and fasting states on the absorption of melphalan in multiple myeloma. Cancer Chemother Pharmacol 1984 12:183–186.

Brock N Oxazaphosphorine cytostatics: Past-present-future. Cancer Res 1989 49:1–7.

Brock N and Hohorst HJ The problem of the specificity and selectivity of alkylating cytostatics: Studies on N-2-chloroethylamido-oxazaphosphorines. Z Krebsforsch 1977 88:185–215.

Brock N, Stekar J, Pohl J, Niemeyer U, and Scheffler G Acrolein, the causative factor of urotoxic side-effects of cyclophosphamide, ifosfamide, trofosfamide and sufosfamide. Arzneimittel-Forschung, Drug Research 1979 29:659–661.

Brox L, Birkett L, and Belch A Pharmacology of intravenous melphalan in patients with multiple myeloma. Cancer Treat Rev 1979 6:(Suppl) 27–32.

Bruhl P, Gunther U, Hoefer-Janker H, Huls W, Scheef W, and Vahlensieck W Results obtained with fractionated ifosphamide massive-dose treatment in generalized malignant tumours. Int J Clin Pharmacol 1976 14:29–39.

Bryant BM, Ford HT, Jarman M, and Smith IE Prevention of isophosphamide-induced urothelial toxicity with 2-mercaptoethane sulphonate sodium (Mesna) in patients with advanced carcinoma. Lancet 1980 27:657–659.

Buckner CD, Rudolph RH, Fefer A, Clift RA, Epstein RB, Funk DD, Neiman PE, Slighter SJ, Storb R, and Thomas ED High-dose cyclophosphamide therapy for malignant disease. Cancer 1972 29: 357–365.

Cadman ED, Drislane F, Waldron JA, Farber L, Prosnitz L, and Bertino JR High-dose pulse chlorambucil. Cancer 1982 50:1037–1041.

Choi KER, Ratain MJ, Williams SF, Golick JA, Beschorner JC, Fullem LJ, and Bitran JD Plasma pharmacokinetics of high-dose oral melphalan in patients treated with trialkylator chemotherapy and autologous bone marrow reinfusion. Cancer Res 1989 49:1318–1321.

Ciobanu N, Runowicz C, Gucalp R, Frank M, Charuvanki V, Kaufman D, and Wiernik PH Reversible central nervous system toxicity associated with high-dose chlorambucil in autologous bone marrow transplantation for ovarian carcinoma. Cancer Treat Rep 1987 71:1324–1325.

Cohen BE, Egorin MJ, Kohlhepp EA, Aisner J, and Gutierrez PL Human plasma pharmacokinetics and urinary excretion of thiotepa and its metabolites. Cancer Treat Rep 1986 70:859–864.

Cole SR, Myers TJ, and Klatsky AU Pulmonary disease with chlorambucil therapy. Cancer 1978 41: 455–459.

Collins C, Mortimer J, and Livingston RB High-dose cyclophosphamide in the treatment of refractory lymphomas and solid tumour malignancies. Cancer 1989 63:228–232.

Colvin M and Hilton J Pharmacology of cyclophosphamide and its metabolites. Cancer Treat Rep 1981 65:89–95.

Connors TA Mechanism of action of 2-chloroethylamine derivatives, sulphur mustards, epoxides, and aziridines. In: Antineoplastic and Immunosuppressive Agents, Pt II Sartorelli AC and Johns DG Eds Springer-Verlag, Berlin 1975 pp. 18–34.

Connors TA, Cox PJ, Farmer PB, Foster AB, and Jarman M Some studies on the active intermediates formed in the microsomal metabolism of cyclophosphamide and isophosphamide. Biochem Pharmacol 1974 23:115–129.

Cornbleet MA, McElwain TJ, Kumar PJ, Filshie J, Selby P, Carter RL, Hedley DW, Clark ML, and Millar JL Treatment of advanced malignant melanoma with high-dose melphalan and autologous bone marrow transplantation. Br J Cancer 1983 48:329–334.

Cornwell III GG, Pajak TF, McIntyre OR, Kochwa S, and Dosik H Influence of renal failure on myelosuppressive effects of melphalan: Cancer and acute leukaemia group B experience. Cancer Treat Rep 1982 66:473–481.

Corringham R, Gilmore M, Prentice HG, and Boesen E High-dose melphalan with autologous bone marrow transplant. Cancer 1983 52:1783–1787.

Cox PJ Cyclophosphamide cystitus—identification of acrolein as the causative agent. Biochem Pharmacol 1979 28:2045–2049.

Cox PJ, Phillips BJ, and Thomas P The enzymatic basis for the selective action of cyclophosphamide. Cancer Res 1975 35:3755–3761.

Cox PJ, Phillips BJ, and Thomas P Studies on the selective action of cyclophosphamide (NSC-26271): Inactivation of the hydroxylated metabolite by tissue soluble enzymes. Cancer Treat Rep 1976 60: 321–326.

Daugaard G, Rossing N, and Rorth M Effects of cisplatin on different measures of glomerular function in the human kidney with special emphasis on high-dose. Cancer Chemother Pharmacol 1988 21: 163–167.

DeFronzo RA, Braine H, and Colvin M Water intoxication in men after cyclophosphamide therapy: Time course and relation to drug activation. Ann Intern Med 1973 78:861–869.

DeVita VT, Carbone PP, and Owens Jr AH Clinical trials with 1,3-bis-(2-chloroethyl)-1-nitrosourea. Cancer Res 1965 25:1876–1881.

Dewar JM, Forgeson GV, and Dady PJ High-dose melphalan with autologous marrow rescue in cancer treatment. N Z Med J 1984 97:816–818.

D'Incalci M, Bolis G, Facchinetti T, Mangioni C, Morasc L, Morazoni P, and Salmona M Decreased half life of cyclophosphamide in patients under continual treatment. Eur J Cancer 1979 15:7–10.

D'Incalci M, Citti L, Taverna P, and Catapano CV Importance of the DNA repair enzyme O^6-alkyl guanine alkyltransferase (AT) in cancer chemotherapy. Cancer Treat Rev 1988 15:279–292.

Domeyer BE and Sladek NE Metabolism of 4-hydroxycyclophosphamide/aldophosphamide in vitro. Biochem Pharmacol 1980 29:2903–2912.

Dosik H, Hurewitz DJ, Rosner F, and Schwartz JM Bullous eruption and elevated leukocyte alkaline phosphatase in the course of busulfan-treated chronic granulocytic leukaemia. Blood 1970 35:543–548.

Egorin MJ, Cohen BE, Kohlhepp EA, and Gutierrez PL Gas-liquid chromatographic analysis of

N,N′,N″-triethylenethiophosphoramide and N,N′,N″-triethylenephosphoramide in biological samples. J Chromatog Biomed Appl 1985 343:196–202.

Egorin MJ, Forrest A, Belani CP, Ratain MJ, Abrams JS, and Van Echo DA A limited sampling strategy for cyclophosphamide pharmacokinetics. Cancer Res 1989 49:3129–3133.

Ehrsson H, Hassan M, Ehrnebo M, and Beran M Busulphan kinetics. Clin Pharmacol Ther 1983 34: 86–89.

Ehrsson H and Hassan M Determination of busulphan in plasma by GC-MS with selected-ion monitoring. J Pharm Sci 1983 72:1203–1205.

Ehrsson H, Wallin I, Simonsson B, Hartvig P, and Oberg G Effect of food on pharmacokinetics of chlorambucil and its main metabolite, phenyl acetic mustard. Eur J Clin Pharmacol 1984 27:111–114.

Fairly KF, Barrie JU, and Johnson W Sterility and testicular atrophy related to cyclophosphamide therapy. Lancet 1972 1:568–569.

Falkson G, Van Dyke JJ, Stapelberg R, and Falkson HC Mesna as a protector against kidney and bladder toxicity with high-dose ifosphamide treatment. Cancer Chemother Pharmacol 1982 9:81–84.

Farmer PB and Newell DR Alkylating agents. In: Pharmacokinetics of Anticancer Drugs in Humans MM Ames, G Powis, and JS Kovach Eds Elsevier, Amsterdam 1983 pp. 77–111.

Fenselau C, Kan M-NN, Billets S, and Colvin M Identification of phosphorodiamidic acid mustard as a human metabolite of cyclophosphamide. Cancer Res 1975 35:1453–1457.

Fenselau C, Kan M-NN, Rao SS, Myles A, Friedman OM, and Colvin M Identification of aldophosphamide as a metabolite of cyclophosphamide in vitro and in vivo in humans. Cancer Res 1977 37: 2538–2543.

Fetting JH, Grochow LB, Folstein MF, Ettinger DS, and Colvin M The course of nausea and vomiting after high-dose cyclophosphamide. Cancer Treat Rep 1982 66:1487–1493.

Fiere D, Felman P, and Vivian H Acute myeloid leukaemia following the administration of chlorambucil: Two cases. Nouv Presse Med 1978 7:756.

Fisher B, Sherman B, and Rockette H L-Phenylalanine mustard in the management of premenopausal patients with primary breast cancer. Cancer 1979 44:847–857.

Foley GE, Friedman OM, and Drolet BP Studies on the mechanism of activation of cytoxan-evidence of activation in vivo and in vitro. Cancer Res 1961 21:57–63.

Galton DAG, Till M, and Wiltshaw E Busulfan: Summary of clinical results. Ann NY Acad Sci 1958 68: 967–973.

Godeneche D, Madelmont JC, Moreau MF, Plagne R, and Meyneil G Comparative physico-chemical properties, biological effects and disposition in mice of four nitrogen mustards. Cancer Chemother Pharmacol 1980 5:1–9.

Gore ME, Viner C, Meldrum M, Bell J, Milan S, Zuiable A, Slevin M, Selby PJ, Clark PI, Millar B, Maitland JA, Judson IR, Tillyer C, Malpas JS, and McElwain TJ Intensive treatment of multiple myeloma and criteria for complete remission. Lancet 1989 ii:879–889.

Goren MP, Wright RK, Pratt CB, and Pell FE Dechlorethylation of ifosfamide and neurotoxicity. Lancet 1986 ii:1219–1220.

Gottdiener JS, Appelbaum FR, Ferrans VJ, Deisseroth A, and Ziegler J Cardiotoxicity associated with high-dose cyclophosphamide therapy. Arch Intern Med 1981 141:758–763.

Graham MI, Shaw IC, Souhami RL, Sidau B, Harper PG, and McLean AEM Decreased plasma half life of cyclophosphamide during repeated high dose administration. Cancer Chemother Pharmacol 1983 10:192–193.

Graham-Pole J, Lazarus HM, Herzig RH, Cross S, Coccia P, Weiner R, and Strandjord S High-dose melphalan therapy for the treatment of children with refractory neuroblastoma and Ewing's sarcoma. Am J Paediat Haemato/Oncol 1984 6:17–26.

Green MH, Harris EL, and Gershenson DM Melphalan may be a more potent leukaemogen than cyclophosphamide. Ann Intern Med 1986 105:360–367.

Greene MH, Boile JD, and Strike TA Carmustine as a cause of acute nonlymphocytic leukaemia. N Engl J Med 1985 313:579.

Greenbaum-Lefkoe B, Rosenstock JG, Belasco JB, Rohrbaugh TM, and Meadows AT Syndrome of inappropriate antidiuretic hormone secretion. Cancer 1985 55:44–46.

Grochow LB and Colvin M Clinical pharmacokinetics of cyclophosphamide. In: Pharmacokinetics of Anticancer Drugs in Humans MM Ames, G Powis, and JS Kovach Eds Elsevier, Amsterdam 1983 pp. 135–154.

Grochow LB, Jones RJ, Brundrett RB, Braine HG, Chen T-L, Saral R, Santos GW, and Colvin MO Pharmacokinetics of busulphan: Correlation with veno-occlusive disease in patients undergoing bone marrow transplantation. Cancer Chemother Pharmacol 1989 25:55–61.

Hadidi A-HFA, Coulter CEA, and Idle JR Phenotypically deficient urinary elimination of carboxyphosphamide after cyclophosphamide administration to cancer patients. Cancer Res 1988 48:5167–5171.

Hadidi A-HFA and Idle JR Combined thin-layer chromatography-photography-densitometry for the quantitation of cyclophosphamide and its four principle urinary metabolites. J Chromatog Biomed Appl 1988 427:121–130.

Hagen B, Walstad RA, and Nilsen OG Pharmacokinetics of thio-tepa at two different doses. Cancer Chemother Pharmacol 1988 22:356–358.

Harmon WE, Cohen HJ, and Schneeberger EE Chronic renal failure in children treated with methyl CCNU. N Engl J Med 1979 300:1200–1203.

Hedley DW, McElwain TJ, Millar JE, and Gordon MY Acceleration of bone marrow recovery by pretreatment with cyclophosphamide in patients receiving high-dose melphalan. Lancet 1978 ii:966–967.

Heideman RL, Cole DE, Balis F, Sato J, Reaman GH, Packer RJ, Singher LJ, Ettinger LJ, Gillespie A, Sam J, and Poplack DG Phase I and pharmacokinetic evaluation of thiotepa in the cerebrospinal fluid and plasma of pediatric patients: Evidence for dose-dependent plasma clearance of thiotepa. Cancer Res 1989 49:736–741.

Hengst JCD and Kempf RA Immunomodulation by cyclophosphamide. Clin Immunol Allergy 1984 4: 199–216.

Henner WD, Furlong EA, Flaherty MD, and Shea TC Measurement of busulphan in plasma by high-performance liquid chromatography. J Chromatog Biomedical Appl 1987 416:426–432.

Hill DL, Laster WR, and Struck RF Enzymatic metabolism of cyclophosphamide and nicotine and production of a toxic cyclophosphamide metabolite. Cancer Res 1972 32:658–665.

Hilton J Role of aldehyde dehydrogenase in cyclophosphamide-resistant L1210 leukemia. Cancer Res 1984 44:5156–5160.

Hundley R and Lukens JN Nitrosourea-associated pulmonary fibrosis. Cancer Treat Rep 1979 63:2128–2130.

Hunt KK Post cyclophosphamide pneumonitis. N Engl J Med 1972 287:668–669.

Hryniuk WM The importance of dose intensity in the outcome of cancer chemotherapy. In: Important Advances in Oncology 1988 VT Devita, SM Hellman, and SA Rosenburg Eds JB Lippincott Co., Philadelphia 1988 pp. 121–141.

Kapp J, Vance R, Parker JL, and Smith RR Limitations of high-dose intra-arterial 1,3-Bis(2-chloroethyl)-1-nitrosourea (BCNU) chemotherapy for malignant gliomas. Neurosurgery 1982 10:715–719.

Kellie SJ and Kingston JE Ovarian failure after high-dose melphalan in adolescents. Lancet 1987 i: 1425.

Kingston JE, Malpas JS, Stiller Ca, Pritchard J, and McElwain TJ Autologous bone marrow transplantation contributes to haemopoietic recovery in children with solid tumours treated with high-dose melphalan. Brit J Haematol 1984 58:589–595.

Knisley RE, Settipane GA, and Albala MM Unusual reaction to chlorambucil in a patient with chronic lymphocytic leukaemia. Arch Dermatol 1977 104:77.

Kohn KW, Hartley JA, and Mattes WB Mechanisms of DNA sequence selective alkylation of guanine-N7 positions by nitrogen mustards. Nucleic Acid Res 1987 24:10531–10549.

Koyama H, Wada T, and Nishizawa Y Cyclophosphamide-induced ovarian failure and its therapeutic significance in patients with breast cancer. Cancer 1977 39:1403–1409.

Kyle RA and Dameshek W Porphyria cutanea tarda associated with chronic granulocytic leukemia treated with busulfan (Myleran). Blood 1964 23:776–785.

Lane SD, Besa EC, Justh G, and Joseph RR Fatal interstitial pneumonitis following high-dose intermittent chlorambucil therapy for chronic lymphocytic leukaemia. Cancer 1981 47:32–36.

Lazarus HM, Herzig RH, Graham-Pole J, Wolff SN, Phillips GL, Strandjord S, Hurd D, Forman W, Gordon EM, Coccia P, Gross S, and Herzig GP Intensive melphalan chemotherapy and cryopreserved autologous bone marrow transplantation for the treatment of refractory cancer. J Clin Oncol 1983 1:359–367.

Lazarus HM, Reed MD, Spitzer TR, Rabaa MS, and Blumer JL High-dose IV thiotepa and cryopreserved autologous bone marrow transplantation for therapy of refractory cancer. Cancer Treat Rep 1987 71:689–695.

Lee FYF, Coe P, and Workman P Pharmacokinetic basis for the comparative antitumour activity and toxicity of chlorambucil, phenyl acetic mustard and β,β-difluorochlorambucil (CB7103) in mice. Cancer Chemother Pharmacol 1986 17:21–29.

Leff RS, Thompson JM, Johnson DB, Mosley KR, Daly MB, Knight III WA, Ruxer Jr RL and Messerschmidt GL Phase II trial of high-dose melphalan and autologous bone marrow transplantation for metastatic colon carcinoma. J Clin Oncol 1986 4:1586–1591.

Lenhard Jr RE, Oken MM, Barnes JM, Humphrey RL, Glick JH, and Silverstein MN High-dose cyclophosphamide. An effective treatment for advanced refractory multiple myeloma. Cancer 1984 53:1456–1460.

Lentz RD, Bergstein J, and Steffes MW Post-pubertal evaluation of gonadal function following cyclophosphamide therapy before and during puberty. J Pediatr 1977 91:385–394.

Lind MJ, Margison JM, Cerny T, Thatcher N, and Wilkinson PM Comparative pharmacokinetics and alkylating activity of fractionated intravenous and oral ifosfamide in patients with bronchogenic carcinoma. Cancer Res 1989a 49:753–757.

Lind MJ, Margison JM, Cerny T, Thatcher N, and Wilkinson PM Prolongation of ifosphamide elimination half-life in obese patients due to altered drug distribution. Cancer Chemother Pharmacol 1989b 25:139–142.

Louis J, Limarzi LR, and Best WR Treatment of chronic granulocytic leukaemia with myleran. Arch Intern Med 1956 97:299–308.

Ludlum DB Molecular biology of alkylation: An overview. In: Antineoplastic and Immunosuppressive Agents, Pt II Sartorelli AC and Johns DG Eds Springer-Verlag, Berlin 1975 pp. 6–17.

Manohoran A Carcinoma of the urinary bladder in patients receiving cyclophosphamide. Aust NZ J Med 1984 14:507–512.

Maraninchi D, Abecasis M, Gastaut JA, Herve P, Sebahoun G, Flesch M, Blanc AP, and Carcassonne Y High-dose melphalan with autologous bone marrow rescue for the treatment of advanced adult solid tumours. Cancer Treat Rep 1984 68:471–474.

Maraninchi D, Pico JL, Hartmann O, Gastaut JA, Kamioner D, Hayat M, Mascret B, Beaujean F, Sebahoun G, Novakovitch G, Lemerle J, and Carcassonne Y High-dose melphalan with or without marrow transplantation: A study of dose-effect in patients with refractory and/or relapsed acute leukaemias. Cancer Treat Rep 1986 70:445–448.

Mbidde EK, Selby PJ, Perren TJ, Dearnaley DP, Whitton A, Ashley S, Workman P, Bloom HJG, and McElwain TJ High dose BCNU chemotherapy with autologous bone marrow transplantation and full dose radiotherapy for grade IV astrocytoma. Br J Cancer 1988 58:779–782.

McLean A, Newell D, Baker G, and Connors T The metabolism of chlorambucil. Biochem Pharmacol 1980 29:2039–2047.

McElwain TJ, Hedley DW, Burton G, Clink HM, Gordon MY, Jarman M, Juttner CA, Millar JL, Milsted RAV, Prentice G, Smith IE, Spence D, and Woods M Marrow autotransplantation accelerates haematological recovery in patients with malignant melanoma treated with high-dose melphalan. Br J Cancer 1979 40:72–80.

Meanwell CA, Blake AE, Kelly KA, Honigsberger L, and Blackledge G Prediction of ifosphamide/mesna associated encephalopathy. Eur J Cancer Clin Oncol 1986 22:815–819.

Millar JL, Hudspith BN, McElwain TJ, and Phelps TA Effect of high-dose melphalan on marrow and intestinal epithelium in mice pretreated with cyclophosphamide. Br J Cancer 1978a 38:137–142.

Millar JL, Phelps TA, Carter RL, and McElwain TJ Cyclophosphamide pre-treatment reduces the toxic effect of high-dose melphalan on intestinal epithelium in sheep. Eur J Cancer 1978b 11:1283.

Mills BA and Roberts RW Cyclophosphamide-induced cardiomyopathy: A report of two cases and review of the English literature. Cancer 1979 43:2223–2226.

Ninane J, Baurain R, de Selys A, Trouet A, and Cornu G High dose melphalan in children with advanced malignant disease. Cancer Chemother Pharmacol 1985 15:263–267.

Norpoth K Studies on the metabolism of isophosphamide (NSC-109724) in man. Cancer Treat Rep 1976 60:437–443.

Osbourne R, Evans B, Gallagher C, Wood C, Slevin M, Shepherd J, and Wiltshaw E High-dose cyclophosphamide followed by cisplatin in the treatment of ovarian cancer. Cancer Chemother Pharmacol 1987 20:48–52.

Oppitz MM, Musch E, Malek M, Rug HP, von Unruh GE, Loos U, and Muhlenbruch B Studies on the pharmacokinetics of chlorambucil and prednimustine in patients using a new high-performance liquid chromatography assay. Cancer Chemother Pharmacol 1989 23:208–212.

Osterborg A, Ehrsson H, Eksborg S, Wallin I, and Mellstedt H Pharmacokinetics of oral melphalan in relation to renal function in multiple myeloma patients. Eur J Cancer Clin Oncol 1989 25:899–903.

Peters WP, Henner WD, Grochow LB, Olsen G, Edwards S, Stanbuck H, Stuart A, Gockerman J, Moore J, Bast Jr RC, Seigler HF, and Colvin OM Clinical and pharmacologic effects of high-dose single agent busulfan with autologous bone marrow support in the treatment of solid tumours. Cancer Res 1987 47:6402–6406.

Philips FS, Sternberg SS, Cronin AP, and Vidal PM Cyclophosphamide and urinary bladder toxicity. Cancer Res 1961 21:1577–1589.

Phillips GL, Fay JW, Herzig GP, Herzig RH, Weiner RS, Wolff SN, Lazarus HM, Karanes C, Ross WE and Kramer BS Intensive 1,3-Bis(2-chloroethyl)-1-nitrosourea (BCNU), NSC #4366650 and cryopreserved autologous marrow transplantation for refractory cancer. Cancer 1983 52:1792–1802.

Portlock CS, Fischer DS, Cadman E, Lundberg B, Levy A, Bobrow S, Bertino JR, and Farber L High-dose pulse chlorambucil in advanced, low-grade non-Hodgkin's lymphoma. Cancer Treat Rep 1987 71:1029–1031.

Powis G, Reece P, Ahmann DL, and Ingle JN Effect of body weight on the pharmacokinetics of cyclophosphamide in breast cancer patients. Cancer Chemother Pharmacol 1987 20:219–222.

Rapola J, Koskimies O, and Huttanen NP Cyclophosphamide and the pubertal testis. Lancet 1973 i:98–99.

Redman JR and Bajorunas DR Suppression of germ cell proliferation to prevent gonadal toxicity associated with cancer treatment. Proceedings of the workshop on psychosexual and reproductive issues effecting patients with cancer. 1987:90–94.

Reece PA, Kotasek D, Morris RG, Dale BM, and Sage RE The effect of food on melphalan oral absorption. Cancer Chemother Pharmacol 1986 16:194–197.

Reece PA, Dale BM, Morris RG, Kotasek D, Gee D, Rogerson S, and Sage RE Effect of L-leucine on oral melphalan kinetics in patients. Cancer Chemother Pharmacol 1987 20:256–258.

Reece PA, Hill HS, Green RM, Morris RG, Dale BM, Kotasek D, and Sage RE Renal clearance and protein binding of melphalan in patients with cancer. Cancer Chemother Pharmacol 1988 22:348–352.

Reed DJ 2-Chloroethylnitrosoureas. In: Metabolism and Action of Anticancer Drugs G Powis and RA Prough Eds Taylor and Francis London 1987 pp. 1–28.

Refsum O Fatal intraalveolar and interstitial lung fibrosis in chlorambucil-treated chronic lymphocytic leukaemia. Mount Sinai J Med 1977 44:847.

Richter P, Calamera JC, and Morgenfeld MD Effect of chlorambucil on spermatogenesis in the human with malignant lymphoma. Cancer 1970 25:1026–1030.

Rubino FA Possible pulmonary effects of alkylating agents. N Engl J Med 1972 287:1150.

Santos GW, Sensenburger LL, and Burke P Marrow transplantation in man following cyclophosphamide. Transplant Proc 1971 3:400–404.

Sawitsky A, Boklan BR, and Benjamin Z Drug fever produced by chlorambucil. NY J Med 1971 71: 2434.

Schuler U, Ehninger G, and Wagner T Repeated high-dose cyclophosphamide administration in bone marrow transplantation: Exposure to activated metabolites. Cancer Chemother Pharmacol 1987 20: 248–252.

Selby PJ, McElwain TJ, Nandi AC, Perron TJ, Powles RL, Tillyer CR, Osborne RJ, Slevin ML, and Malpas JS Multiple myeloma treated with high-dose intravenous melphalan. Brit J Haematol 1987a 66:55–62.

Selby PJ, Lopes N, Mundy J, Crofts M, Millar JL, and McElwain TJ Cyclophosphamide priming reduces intestinal damage in man following high-dose melphalan chemotherapy. Br J Cancer 1987b 55:531–533.

Sladek NE Evidence for an aldehyde possessing alkylating activity as the primary metabolite of cyclophosphamide. Cancer Res 1973 33:651–658.

Sladek NE, Smith PC, Bratt PM, Low JE, Powers JF, Borch RF, and Coveney JR Influence of diuretics on urinary general base catalytic activity and cyclophosphamide-induced bladder toxicity. Cancer Treat Rep 1982 66:1889–1900.

Sladek NE, Doeden D, Powers JF, and Krivit W Plasma concentrations of 4-hydroxycyclophosphamide and phosphoramide mustard in patients repeatedly given high doses of cyclophosphamide in preparation for bone marrow transplantation. Cancer Treat Rep 1984 68:1247–1254.

Sladek NE and Landkamer GL Restoration of sensitivity to oxazaphosphorines by inhibitors of aldehyde dehydrogenase activity in cultured oxazaphosphorine-resistant L1210 and cross-linking agent-resistant P388 cell lines. Cancer Res 1985 45:1549–1555.

Sladek NE Oxazaphosphorines. In: Metabolism and Action of Anticancer Drugs G Powis and RA Prough Eds Taylor and Francis, London 1987 pp. 48–90.

Smith AC and Boyd MR Preferential effects of 1,3-bis-(2-chloroethyl)-1-nitrosourea (BCNU) on pulmonary glutathione reductase and glutathione/glutathione disulfide ratios: Possible implications for lung toxicity. J Pharmacol Exp Ther 1984 229:658–663.

Smith IE, Evans BD, Hartland SJ, Robinson BA, Yarnold JR, Glees JG, and Ford HT High-dose cyclophosphamide with autologous bone marrow rescue after conventional chemotherapy in the treatment of small cell lung carcinoma. Cancer Chemother Pharmacol 1985 14:120–124.

Solidoro A, Otero J, Vallejos C, Casanova L, Salas F, Pasco T, Quiroz L, Orlandini O, and Marcial J Intermittent continuous IV infusion of high-dose cyclophosphamide for remission injection in acute lymphocytic leukaemia. Cancer Treat Rep 1981 65:213–218.

Souhami RL, Harper PG, Linch D, Trask C, Goldstone AH, Tobias JS, Spiro SG, Geddes DM, and Richards DM High-dose cyclophosphamide with autologous marrow transplantation for small cell carcinoma of the bronchus. Cancer Chemother Pharmacol 1983 10:205–207.

Souhami RL, Finn G, Gregory WM, Birkhead BG, Buckman R, Edwards D, Goldstone AH, Harper PG, Spiro SG, Tobias JS, and Geddes D High-dose cyclophosphamide in small cell carcinoma of the lung. J Clin Oncol 1985 3:958–963.

Struck RF Isolation and identification of a stabilized derivative of aldophosphamide, a major metabolite of cyclophosphamide. Cancer Res 1974 34:2933–2935.

Struck RF, Kirk MC, Witt MH, and Laster WR Isolation and mass spectral identification of blood metabolites of cyclophosphamide: Evidence for phosphoramide mustard as the biologically active metabolite. Biomed Mass Spec 1975 2:46–52.

Struck RF, Alberts DS, Horne K, Phillips JG, Peng Y-M, and Roe DJ Plasma pharmacokinetics of cyclophosphamide and its cytotoxic metabolites after intravenous versus oral administration in a randomized crossover trial. Cancer Res 1987 47:2723–2726.

Stuart-Harris RC, Harper PG, Parsons CA, Kaye SB, Mooney CA, Gowing NF, and Wiltshaw E High-dose alkylation therapy using ifosphamide infusion with mesna in the treatment of adult advanced soft-tissue sarcoma. Cancer Chemother Pharmacol 1983 11:69–72.

Taha IA-K, Ahmed RA, Gray H, Roberts CI, and Rogers HJ Plasma melphalan and prednisone concentrations during oral therapy for multiple myeloma. Cancer Chemother Pharmacol 1982 9:57–60.

Takvorian T, Parker LM, Hochberg FH, and Canellos GP Autologous bone marrow transplantation: Host effects of high-dose BCNU. J Clin Oncol 1983 1:610–620.

Tilby MJ, Styles JM, and Dean CJ Immunological detection of DNA damage caused by melphalan using monoclonal antibodies. Cancer Res 1987 47:1542–1546.

Tranchand B, Ploin Y-D, Minuit M-P, Sapet C, Biron P, Philip T, and Ardiet C High dose melphalan dosage adjustment: Possibility of using a test dose. Cancer Chemother Pharmacol 1989 23:95–100.

Van Dyke JJ, Falkson HC, and Van Der Merwe AM Unexpected toxicity in patients treated with iphosphamide. Cancer Res 1972 32:921–924.

Vassal MRE and Gouyette A Gas-chromatographic-mass spectrophotometric assay for busulphan in biological fluids using a deuterated internal standard. J Chromatog Biomedical Appl 1988 428:357–361.

Vassal G, Gouyette A, Hartmann O, Pico JL, and Lemerle J Pharmacokinetics of high-dose bulsulphan in children. Cancer Chemother Pharmacol 1989a 24:386–390.

Vassal G, Hartmann O, Habrand JL, Pico HL, and Lemerle J Enhanced cutaneous radiation effects following high-dose busulfan therapy. Cancer Chemother Pharmacol 1989b 23:117–118.

Vistica DT Cellular pharmacokinetics of phenylalanine mustards. Pharmacol Ther 1983 22:379–405.

Wadler S, Egorin MJ, Zuhowski EG, Tortorello L, Salva K, Runowicz CD, and Wiernik P Phase 1 clinical and pharmacokinetic study of thiotepa administered intraperitoneally in patients with advanced malignancies. J Clin Oncol 1989 7:132–139.

Warne GL, Fairley KF, and Hobbs JB Cyclophosphamide-induced ovarian failure. N Engl J Med 1973 289:1159–1162.

Waxman DJ, Clarke L, and Ng S-F Oxidative metabolism of thio-TEPA: Role of hepatic cytochrome P-450. Proc Am Assoc Cancer Res 1989 30:463.

Weiss RB, Posada DS, and Penta JS The nitrosoureas and pulmonary toxicity. Cancer Treat Rev 1981 8: 111–125.

Woodhouse KW, Hamilton P, Lennard A, and Rawlins MD The pharmacokinetics of melphalan in patients with multiple myeloma: An intravenous/oral study using a conventional dose regimen. Eur J Clin Pharmacol 1983 24:283–285.

Zucchetti M, D'Incalci M, Willems Y, Cavalli F, and Sessa C Lack of effect of cisplatin on iv L-PAM plasma pharmacokinetics in ovarian cancer patients. Cancer Chemother Pharmacol 1988 22:87–89.

CHAPTER 5

Toxicity of Antimetabolites

David J. Sweeny, Ph.D. and Robert B. Diasio, M.D.

INTRODUCTION

Antimetabolites are chemically similar to endogenous cofactors and metabolic precursors that have an important function in the biosynthesis of nucleic acids. Antimetabolites use similar cellular uptake processes and metabolic pathways as these endogenous metabolites. However, because of small but significant structural differences, use of antimetabolites results in disruption of nucleic acid synthesis either by inhibiting key enzymes in this process or by altering cellular function following incorporation into RNA or DNA. Because antimetabolites produce their pharmacological action by disrupting nucleic acid synthesis, these agents typically have a major effect on cells in S-phase. Host cells (e.g., bone marrow precursors and gastrointestinal cells) which actively divide, requiring increased DNA synthesis, will also use antimetabolites and are therefore often major sites of toxicities. However, some therapeutic advantage results because tumor cells (particularly more rapidly growing tumors, e.g., leukemia) use antimetabolites to a greater extent than these host cells.

The present chapter presents our current knowledge on the toxicities associated with the use of the three classes of antimetabolites: (a) antifolates, (b) pyrimidine analogues, and (c) purine analogues. Because the most common toxicities produced by antimetabolites often result from a mechanism similar to that responsible for their antitumor activity, the pharmacology of these agents is presented prior to discussion of their toxicities. This will allow for an understanding of the mechanism by which antimetabolites produce these toxicities and also, for some of these drugs, provide a rationale by which the severity of these toxicities can be reduced.

ANTIFOLATES

Methotrexate

Pharmacology

Antifolates were developed for use as chemotherapeutic agents following recognition of the importance of reduced folates in the biosynthesis of nucleic acid precursors. These agents are used in the treatment of a variety of cancers (e.g., leukemia, breast cancer) as well as in the management of psoriasis and rheumatoid arthritis. Aminopterin, the 4-NH_2 analogue of folic acid (Fig. 5-1), was the first antifolate introduced clinically (Farber et al., 1948). This compound was later replaced by its N^{10}-methyl derivative methotrexate (MTX) which, despite the introduction of newer antifolates, continues to be the most widely used antifolate.

The biochemical action responsible for the chemotherapeutic action of MTX is inhibition of dihydrofolate reductase (DHFR) (Futterman and Silverman, 1957). Dihydrofolate reductase functions in maintaining a cellular pool of reduced folate (tetrahydrofolate, FH_4), which serves as a cofactor in the de novo synthesis of purine nucleotides and thymidylate (dTMP). In the thymidylate synthetase (TS) reaction (Fig. 5-2), 5,10-methylene tetrahydrofolate

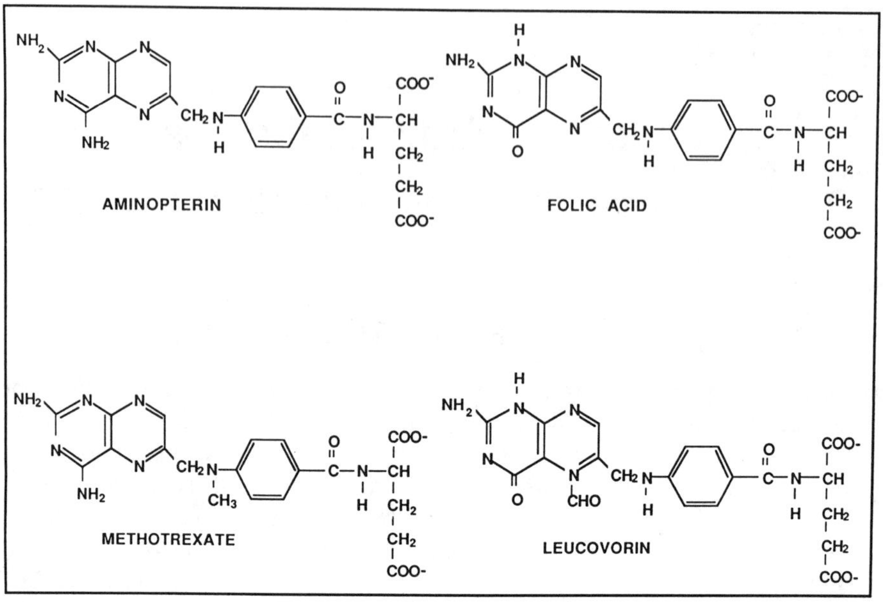

FIGURE 5-1. Structures of folic acid, the folate antimetabolites aminopterin and methotrexate, and the rescue agent leucovorin.

(CH_2–FH_4) is oxidized to inactive dihydrofolate (FH_2) during the reductive methylation of 2′-deoxyuridylate (dUMP). Dihydrofolate is usually reduced back to tetrahydrofolate by DHFR. Inhibition of DHFR by MTX, however, prevents the reduction of dihydrofolate, leading to a depletion of reduced folate and an impairment of dTMP synthesis. The inhibition of thymidylate formation appears to be the important mechanism of tumor cell toxicity (Rueckert and Mueller, 1960), however an effect on de novo purine nucleotide biosynthesis may also contribute to the chemotherapeutic action of MTX (Taylor and Tattersall, 1981).

Methotrexate is a competitive inhibitor of DHFR, with an estimated Ki of 5×10^{-12} M and 7×10^{-12} M in mouse L1210 and human lymphoblast cells, respectively (Jackson et al., 1976). Methotrexate binds very tightly to DHFR, but this interaction is reversible and therefore an amount of MTX in excess of the cellular concentration of DHFR is required for complete inhibition of this enzyme (Goldman, 1974).

Methotrexate is administered clinically by a number of routes, including oral, intravenous (IV), and intrathecal. Low dose (2.5–25 mg) MTX that is commonly used in the management of psoriasis and rheumatoid arthritis is administered orally. However, with oral doses above 80 mg/m^2 absorption is often incomplete and therefore with high dose MTX therapy (as is used in some cancer chemotherapy regimens) the IV route is usually used.

The plasma pharmacokinetics of MTX following IV administration is characterized by three phases with the terminal half-life being approximately 8 to 10 hr (Wilkinson et al., 1978). Greater than 90% of the administered MTX dose is eliminated unchanged through the kidney (Henderson et al., 1965). However, a fraction of the dose undergoes polyglutamylation in both normal and malignant tissue. The MTX-polyglutamates are active in inhibiting DHFR and the intracellular persistence of these polyglutamates may account for the long duration of DHFR inhibition (Rosenblatt et al., 1978). Methotrexate can also be metabolized in the liver by aldehyde oxidase to its 7-hydroxy derivative, and plasma concentrations of 7-hydroxy-MTX usually exceed those of the parent compound 24 hr after the administration of a moderate (>378 mg/24 hr) dose of MTX (Lankelma et al., 1980). The 7-hydroxy-MTX, however, is a poor inhibitor of DHFR (Jacobs et al., 1977).

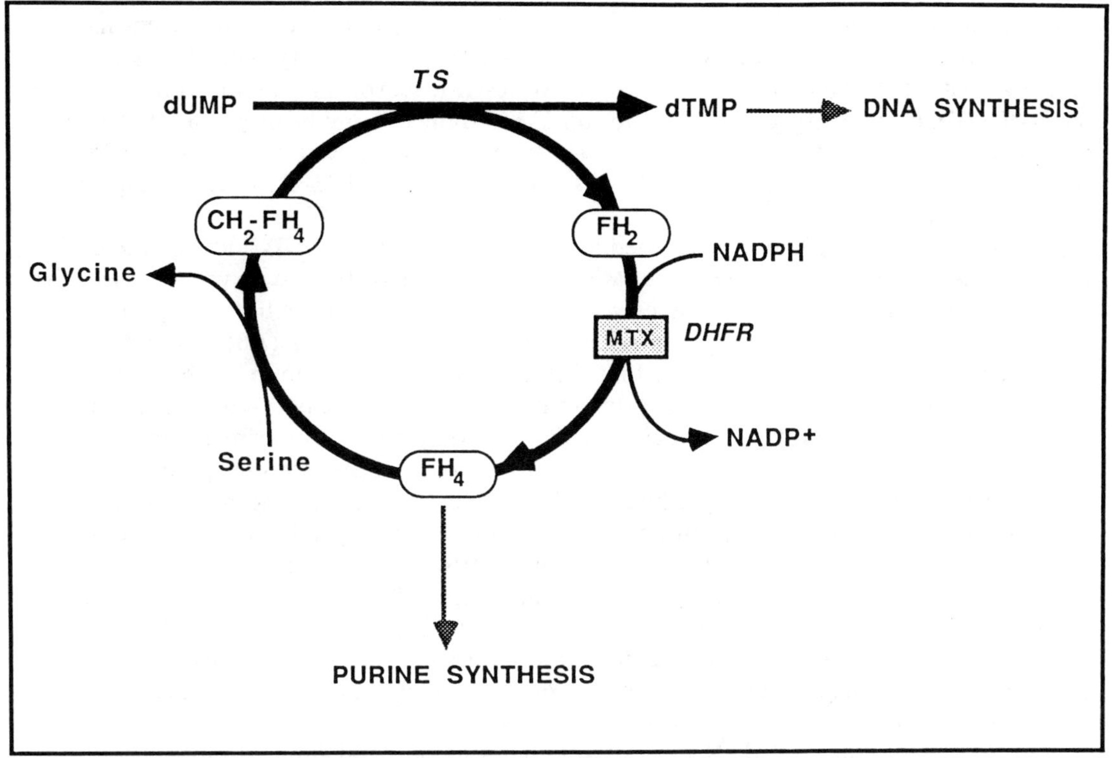

FIGURE 5-2. Schematic of folate use in synthesis of thymidylate. Reduced folates (FH_4) serve as methyl donors (CH_2–FH_4) in the reductive methylation of 2′-deoxyuridylate (dUMP) to thymidylate (dTMP), a reaction catalyzed by thymidylate synthase (TS). Use of CH_2-FH_4 leads to the formation of the inactive dihydrofolate (FH_2), which is normally reduced back to FH_4 by dihydrofolate reductase (DHFR). Inhibition of DHFR by MTX prevents the reduction fo FH_2, leading to the depletion of FH_4 and the inhibition of dTMP and DNA synthesis.

Toxicology

The most frequent toxicities associated with MTX are observed in normal tissues that undergo rapid cell division (e.g., gastrointestinal mucosa and bone marrow). These toxicities are due to inhibition of DNA synthesis as a consequence of DHFR inhibition. The production of these toxicities does not result solely from the total dose of MTX administered, but results as a consequence of the persistence (>48 hr) of MTX in plasma above a threshold level (1×10^{-8} M. Therefore, whereas a dose of 7 gm infused over 48 hr was found to produce severe gastrointestinal and hematological toxicity, a dose of 20 gm infused over 24 hr produced no toxicity (Goldie et al., 1972). Furthermore, in patients receiving MTX (50–250 mg/kg) over a six-hour period, toxicity was only observed in patients whose plasma levels of MTX were elevated ($>9 \times 10^{-7}$ M) 48 hr following administration of MTX (Stoller et al., 1977).

Gastrointestinal toxicity typically presents as nausea and vomiting, and usually begins on the day of treatment and lasts an average of two days. Mucositis usually begins 3 to 5 days following MTX administration and lasts on the average four days. Myelosuppression becomes evident between 4 and 7 days following administration of MTX and is characterized by a decrease in white blood cell count (500–2300 cells/m^2) and platelet count (500–60,000 cell/m^2) that may persist from 6 to 13 days (Reggev and Djerassi, 1988).

Because the gastrointestinal and bone marrow toxicities result from MTX's inhibition of DHFR, compounds that can bypass the cellular effects resulting from this inhibition have been used as a means of reducing the severity of these toxicities. Leucovorin, 5-formyltetrahydrofolate (Fig. 5-1), was first used clinically in combination with high dose-MTX in the 1960s (Bertino, 1977) and remains the most effective agent for reducing the gastrointestinal and bone marrow toxicity associated with MTX therapy. The most important mechanism by which leucovorin reduces these toxicities is by replenishing the cellular pool of reduced folates (Jackson and Grindey, 1984). However, leucovorin also reduces intracellular levels of MTX by competing with MTX for uptake into the cell and by displaying MTX from intracellular binding sites. Moreover, leucovorin increases intracellular levels of dihydrofolate, which compete with and thereby displace MTX from DHFR, thus leading to the reactivation of DHFR.

Thymidine "rescue" has also been used as a means of reducing MTX-induced bone marrow and gastrointestinal toxicities. The rationale for the use of thymidine was that selective rescue of nontumor cells could be achieved because tumor cells have been suggested to be more sensitive to the antipurine effect of MTX than nontumor cells (Abelson and Gorka, 1983). The basis for this rationale was that certain tumor cells were found to be deficient in the salvage pathways for purine nucleotide synthesis. These salvage pathways use free purine bases (i.e., from the hydrolysis of nucleic acids) for the synthesis of purine nucleotides and thus are insensitive to MTX. Therefore, tumor cells deficient in these salvage pathways would be more sensitive to the toxicity produced by MTX because they are dependent on de novo pathways (MTX-sensitive) for purine nucleotide synthesis. Thymidine has been shown to reduce the severity of the gastrointestinal and bone marrow toxicities in experimental animals (Tattersall et al., 1981) and humans (Ensminger and Frei, 1977). However, thymidine does not appear to provide any greater clinical benefits over leucovorin and therefore the extended hospital stay required for thymidine administration does not rationalize the use of this agent as a means of reducing the MTX-induced gastrointestinal and bone marrow toxicities (Meyer et al., 1987).

Because the clearance of MTX from plasma depends on renal elimination, the concomitant use of drugs that interfere with renal excretion of MTX may result in an increased incidence of MTX-induced gastrointestinal and bone marrow toxicities. Drug interactions with ketoprofen (Thyss et al., 1980), aminoglycosides (Freeman-Narrod et al., 1982), and probenecid (Aherne et al., 1978) have all been reported to increase the incidence and severity of MTX-induced gastrointestinal and bone marrow toxicities. Therefore, the use of these drugs in patients receiving MTX should be avoided. However, if these drugs must be used in conjunction with MTX, plasma levels of MTX should be monitored closely and the leucovorin schedule adjusted appropriately.

Following introduction of regimens of high dose MTX with leucovorin, renal toxicity was found to be a frequent complication of MTX therapy. This toxicity was characterized by increased serum creatinine and BUN levels, and a decreased urine output. Because of high urinary concentrations of MTX (1.7 to 11.0 $\times$ 10^{-3} M) that result during high dose MTX therapy (Stoller et al., 1975) and the limited solubility of MTX and 7-hydroxy MTX at acidic pH (Bratlid and Moe, 1978), the renal toxicity has been suggested to result from mechanical obstruction of the kidney tubules as a result of precipitation of MTX or its 7-hydroxy metabolite. In support of this proposed mechanism, an amorphous yellow material (i.e., precipitated MTX) has been demonstrated in kidneys of patients who died as a result of the MTX-induced renal toxicity (Pitman et al., 1975). Alkalinization of urine by administration of bicarbonate and vigorous hydration (3 L/m^2/24 hr, beginning 12 hr prior to MTX administration) have led to a decrease in the incidence of renal toxicity. However, renal toxicity may still occur despite these measures. This has led to the suggestion that a mechanism(s) other than physical precipitation of MTX in the renal tubule (e.g., prolonged exposure to MTX) may contribute to the renal toxicity of MTX (Freeman-Nanod et al., 1982). In support of this contention, aminopterin was found to produce renal toxicity at a dose 50-fold lower than MTX, where precipitation of aminopterin in the tubule would not occur (Glade et al., 1979).

High dose intermittent MTX administration has been shown to produce significant abnormalities in liver function tests, with an increase in SGPT being the most noticeable sign of hepatotoxicity observed during MTX therapy (Weber et al., 1987). The abnormalities in liver function tests are usually transient and serum enzymes return to normal during the 2 to 3 week period following discontinuation of therapy. Liver biopsies obtained during intermittent MTX therapy may occasionally demonstrate moderate portal inflammatory reaction without signs of liver necrosis (Hersh et al., 1966). Furthermore, no long-term histological changes result from short-term high dose MTX.

Progressive hepatotoxicity, characterized by hepatic steatosis, hepatic fibrosis, and hepatocellular necrosis, is a common problem associated with long-term low dose (7.5–15 mg/wk) MTX therapy that is routinely used in the management of psoriasis. These hepatic changes are not typically detected by monitoring standard liver function tests nor noninvasive tests of hepatic function (e.g., ultrasound) and at present the most reliable means of assessing hepatotoxicity is by routine liver biopsy (Reynolds and Lee, 1986). Patients receiving MTX continuously for six months usually show some sign (e.g., mild fatty infiltration) of hepatotoxicity. These histological changes usually progress during the course of therapy, with the most severe changes being observed following five years of therapy and after a cumulative dose of 2 g MTX (Lewis and Schiff, 1988). It is recommended therefore that patients have yearly liver biopsies after five years on MTX. Methotrexate should be discontinued when liver toxicity is grade III (i.e., marked fibrosis, fatty infiltration, and prominent nuclear vacuoles) or IV (i.e., fully developed cirrhosis). Hepatotoxicity does not progress following the discontinuation of MTX.

The mechanism by which MTX produces hepatotoxicity isn't known. However, it has been suggested that hepatic changes may result as a consequence of depletion in hepatic levels of reduced folates, since similar hepatic changes are observed in folate depleted rats (Barek et al., 1984). Moreover, hepatic changes in humans have been shown to correlate with decreased reduced folate levels in reticulocytes and liver (Kamen et al., 1981). Moderate alcohol consumption and additional factors (e.g., previous arsenic therapy) have been implicated as predisposing factors for development of this toxicity (Lewis and Schiff, 1988). Reduction of MTX dose may be a means of delaying or even preventing the hepatotoxicity, since doses (< 15 mg/weekly) used in the management of rheumatoid arthritis rarely produces hepatotoxicity (Tolman et al., 1985).

Neurotoxicity is observed in approximately 5 to 15% of patients receiving high dose intravenous MTX (Jaffe et al., 1985). In addition, neurotoxicity may be observed in patients receiving intrathecal MTX (Kay et al., 1972). The onset of neurotoxicity is usually abrupt and symptoms may develop from several hours to 20 days following the start of therapy. In some instances, symptoms of neurotoxicity may be preceded by severe headaches. Neurotoxicity is manifest by apathy, confusion, slurred speech, and ataxia, which progresses to total neuromuscular paralysis. Severe grand mal convulsions are also observed in some patients. Computerized tomographic scans have demonstrated demyelenation of white matter, especially in the anterior and frontal lobes (Allen et al., 1980). Administration of leucovorin in most cases fails to prevent or reverse symptoms of neurotoxicity, but most deficits reverse following discontinuation of MTX. However, in patients receiving multiple cycles of MTX therapy some symptoms (e.g., ataxia) may remain. In patients receiving MTX who died as a result of their metastatic disease, microscopic analysis of brain tissue revealed congruent foci of white matter necrosis which was characterized by myelin loss, clusters of macrophages, and dystrophic axons (Allen et al., 1980).

A direct effect of MTX on neurotissues may be responsible for the neurotoxicity, since high levels of MTX have been detected in cerebrospinal fluid (CSF) of patients (receiving IV MTX) who developed neurotoxicity (Allen et al., 1980). However, the mechanism by which MTX produces neurotoxicity has not been established. Although neurons do not replicate, glial and endothelial cells do undergo cell division. Therefore, one possible mechanism may be that the MTX-induced neurotoxicity results from toxicity to neuronal glial and endothelial cells as a consequence inhibition of DNA synthesis by MTX. Alternatively, it has been suggested that neurotoxicity may result from a decreased synthesis of neurotransmitters (e.g., serotonin) (Abelson, 1978). The decreased neurotransmitter synthesis resulting from the reduced levels of tetrahydrobiopterin, a required cofactor for this synthesis, that occurs as a consequence of the inhibition of DHFR by MTX.

MTX-induced pneumonitis usually occurs in 5 to 7% of patients receiving MTX (Sostman et al., 1976), although an incidence as high as 40% has been reported in children receiving MTX for the treatment of acute lymphocytic leukemia (Acute leukemia group B, 1969). The development of pneumonitis does not appear to correlate with dose, since patients receiving intermittent high dose MTX or long-term low dose MTX are at risk to develop pulmonary complications (Everts et al., 1973; Goldman and Moschella, 1973). Furthermore, the development of MTX-induced lung toxicity is not related to duration of therapy, since pneumonitis has been reported in patients receiving MTX for as little as 12 days or as long as 17 years (Sostman et al., 1976; Lewis and Walter, 1979). MTX-induced pneumonitis usually presents with a nonproductive cough, dyspnea, and fever. Tachypnea and crepitant rales are also usually present. Although the peripheral blood profiles are at times within normal limits, the majority of affected patients have an increased eosinophil count. Blood, sputum, and lung biopsy cultures are almost always negative for bacterial, fungal, and viral infections. Pulmonary function tests demonstrate a marked reduction in gas transfer function. Chest X rays may be normal, but in a majority of cases linear and reticulonodular inflitrates are observed in the base and mid-lung zones (Sostman et al., 1976). Upon histological examination, lung biopsies demonstrate diffuse alveolar damage and interstitial infiltrates of predominantly mononuclear cells (Sostman et al., 1976). Administration of corticosteroids may provide some relief, but most symptoms resolve following discontinuation of MTX.

The MTX-induced pneumonitis has been suggested to have an immunological basis because of the increased eosinophil count observed in many of the affected patients and by the lack of correlation of toxicity with dose or duration of therapy (Searles and McKendry, 1987). Supportive of this hypothesis, peripheral lymphocytes isolated from patients displaying MTX-induced pneumonitis were found to produce a lymphokine (leukocyte inhibitory factor) following incubation with MTX in the direct leukocyte migration inhibition test (Akoun et al., 1987). No lymphokine was found to be produced in lymphocytes from patients receiving MTX, but not displaying pneumonitis, or controls who had never received MTX.

PYRIMIDINE ANALOGS

Fluoropyrimidines

Pharmacology

Fluoropyrimidines (Fig. 5-3) are widely used in the palliative treatment of solid tumors of the breast, gastrointestinal tract and ovaries, and in the curative treatment of noninvasive basal cell carcinoma. 5-fluorouracil (5FU) is the most commonly used fluoropyrimidine. This agent was rationally synthesized in 1957 by Durchinsky, following the observation that certain tumors (e.g., rat hepatoma) used uracil to a greater extent than normal hepatic tissue (Rutman et al., 1954). The antitumor properties of 5FU depend on the anabolism of this agent to cytotoxic nucleotides (Diasio and Harris, 1989). Three pathways of anabolism have been identified: (a) conversion to 5-fluorouridine-5′-monphosphate (FUMP) by the sequential action of uridine phosphorylase and uridine kinase, (b) direct conversion of 5FU to FUMP by uracil phosphoribosyltransferase, and (c) conversion to the deoxyribonucleotide 5-fluoro-2′-deoxyuridine-5′-monophosphate (FdUMP) by thymidine phosphorylase and thymidine kinase.

Following anabolism of FUra to nucleotides, cytotoxicity may result at three intracellular sites (Diasio and Harris, 1989). First, the fluoropyrimidine nucleotide FdUMP has been shown to inhibit thymidylate synthase, leading to impaired synthesis of thymidylate and cell

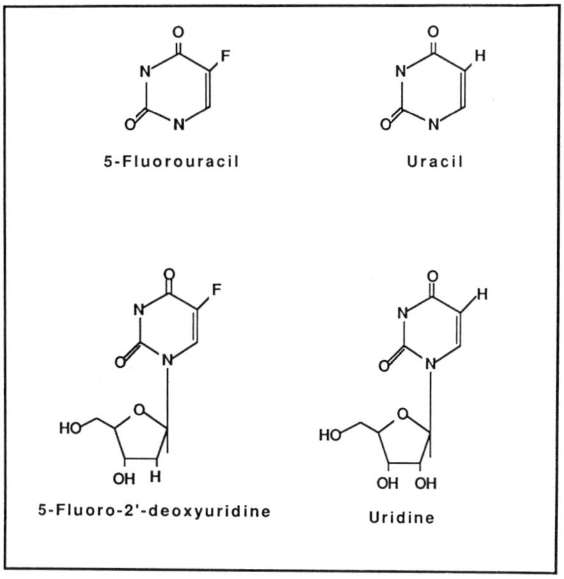

5-Fluorouracil

Uracil

5-Fluoro-2'-deoxyuridine

Uridine

FIGURE 5-3. Structures of fluorouracil and uracil bases and nucleosides.

death as a result of a "thymineless state". Second, 5-fluorouridine-5′-triphosphate (FUTP) can be incorporated into RNA preventing further processing of newly synthesized RNA. This may in turn result in RNA dysfunction that may affect control activities in the cell leading to cytotoxicity. Finally, 5-fluoro-2′-deoxyuridine-5′-triphosphate (FdUTP), particularly in the presence of decreased 2′-deoxythmidine-5′-triphosphate (dTTP) (resulting from thymidylate synthetase inhibition) can be incorporated into DNA. Subsequent removal of the 5FU from DNA by repair enzymes may fragment newly formed DNA resulting in toxicity (Schuetz et al., 1984; 1988). The pathway that is primarily responsible for fluoropyrimidine cytotoxicity, however, has not been determined.

Whereas anabolism of fluoropyrimidines is responsible for the chemotherapeutic action of these agents, the availability of fluoropyrimidines for anabolism appears to be controlled by the rate of catabolism of these agents (Diasio and Harris, 1989). Catabolism (Fig. 5-4) occurs primarily in the liver. It has been shown that greater than 85% of the dose administered to cancer patients is catabolized (Heggie et al., 1987). The conversion of 5FU to dihydro5FU (FUH_2) by dihydropyrimidine dehydrogenase (DPD) is the initial step in 5FU catabolism and activity of this enzyme may therefore control the availability of 5FU for anabolism. FUH_2 is further converted to α-fluoro-ureidopropionic acid (FUPA), which is subsequently metabolized to 2-fluoro-β-alanine (FBAL), CO_2 and NH_4. FBAL is eliminated by the kidney and urinary FBAL accounts for up to 63% of the administered dose excreted within 24 hr (Heggie et al, 1987). In the liver FBAL is also conjugated with bile acids by the enzyme N-acyltransferase. These FBAL-bile acid conjugates are eliminated exclusively into bile where they account for greater than 90% of biliary fluoropyrimidine metabolites (Sweeny et al., 1987).

Oral administration of 5FU is erratic, possibly because the first pass effect in the liver. Therefore, 5FU is usually administered IV either as a bolus or by continuous infusion. Following IV bolus, 5FU is rapidly catabolized as indicated by its short plasma half-life ($T^{1/2} \sim 13$ min) and the concomitant increase in plasma FBAL levels (Heggie et al., 1987). Whereas 5FU is most frequently administered systemically, in recent years continuous regional infusion (e.g., hepatic arterial infusion) of the nucleoside of 5FU (fluorodeoxyuridine) has proven useful in increasing the response rate of hepatic metastases (Balch and Levin, 1987).

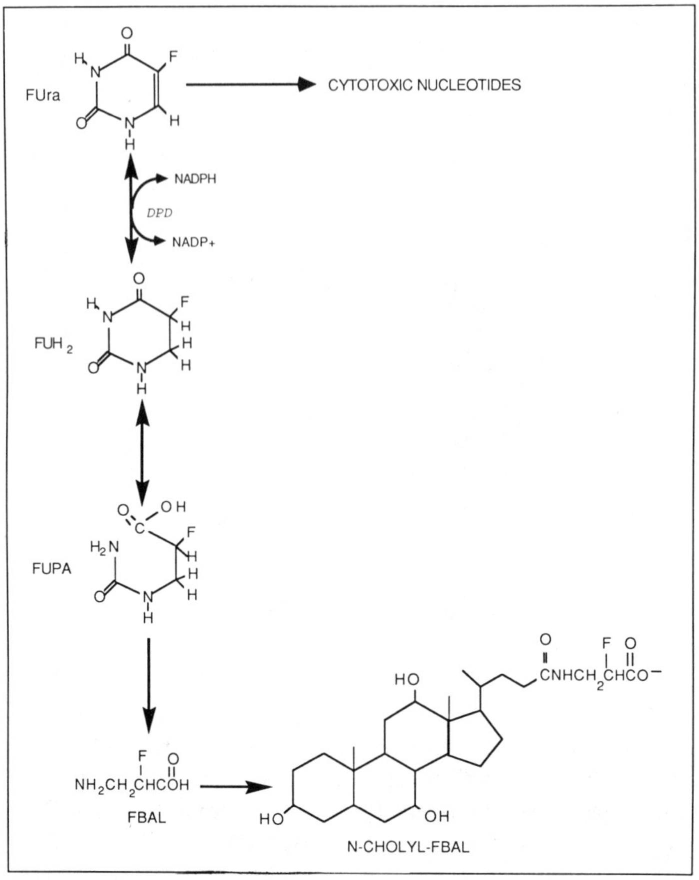

FIGURE 5-4. Pathway of 5-fluorouracil catabolism. 5-fluorouracil (FUra) is catabolized by dihydropyrimidine dehydrogenase (DPD) to dihydroFUra (FUH_2). FUH_2 is subsequently metabolized to α-fluoro-ureidoproionic acid (FUPA), which is further metabolized to α-fluoro-β-alanine (FBAL). FBAL is primarily eliminated into the urine. However, FBAL may also be conjugated with bile acids (e.g., N-cholyl-FBAL) which represent greater than 90% of the biliary metabolites of FUra.

Toxicology

Gastrointestinal toxicity and myelosuppression are the most frequent toxicities observed with 5FU. However, the pattern of these toxicities is dependent on whether 5FU is administered by rapid or continuous infusion. Thus, administration of 5FU (12.0 mg/kg × 5 days) by IV bolus produces a relatively high incidence of leukopenia (<4000 cells/m^3), whereas severe gastrointestinal toxicity (e.g., stomatitis) occurs infrequently (Seifert et al., 1975). On the other hand, continuous IV 5FU administration (30 mg/kg/d × 5d) produces a high incidence of stomatitis, but less leukopenia. The differential incidence of bone marrow toxicity following continuous and bolus IV 5FU administration appears to result from the higher levels of 5FU that are achieved in bone marrow following bolus administration than are produced during continuous infusion of this agent (Fraile et al., 1980).

Neurotoxicity is an infrequent toxicity associated with 5FU therapy, occurring in approximately 2 to 5% of patients receiving 5FU (Moertel et al., 1964; Lynch et al., 1981). Early symptoms of neurotoxicity include coarse nystagmus, dizziness, slurred speech, and severe ataxia of gait (Riehl and Brown, 1964). Following development of symptoms, neurotoxicity usually progresses rapidly over the next five to ten days to a point where many patients are unable to walk or feed themselves. The neurological syndrome results from primary disruption of cerebellar pathways, and to a lesser degree disruption of vestibular and corticospinal tracts. Symptoms disappear following discontinuation of 5FU. Readministration of 5FU (at a similar dose) may result in reoccurrence of neurotoxicity, but a subsequent reduction in dose may be well-tolerated (Riehl and Brown, 1964).

The underlying mechanism of the 5FU-induced neurotoxicity is still not known. Koenig and Patel (1970) have suggested that 5FU-induced neurotoxicity may result from catabolism of 5FU to fluorocitrate, a known neurotoxin which blocks the tricarboxlylic acid cycle by inhibiting the enzyme aconitase. The formation of fluoroacetate or fluorocitrate from FUra has never been documented. However, it has been suggested that only a small percentage (< 2%) of the 5FU dose needs to be converted to fluorocitrate to produce symptoms of neurotoxicity (Koening and Patel, 1970).

In support of "fluorocitrate" hypothesis, severe ataxia can be produced in cats following IV administration of either 5FU (15–30 mg/kg), FBAL (5 mg/kg), or fluoroacetate (0.1–0.4 mg/kg) (Koenig and Patel, 1970; Riehl and Brown, 1964). However, ataxia in cats usually occurred after a period of neuromuscular excitement and severe convulsions, symptoms that have not been reported to occur in patients displaying 5FU-induced neurotoxicity. Furthermore, neurotoxicity usually becomes apparent within 24 hr following the administration of 5FU, a period of time much shorter than is required to produce symptoms of neurotoxicity in patients receiving 5FU. The differences in the time course and symptoms displayed in the cat, however, may not discount the "fluorocitrate" hypothesis, because these dissimilarities could be due to the greater sensitivity of the cat to the neurotoxicity produced by 5FU (fluorocitrate).

Alternatively, there is evidence to suggest that the neurotoxicity may be due to anabolism of 5FU to cytotoxic nucleotides, since intracisternal injection of the fluorinated pyrimidine 5-fluororotic acid (3–10 mg) was found to produce symptoms of neurotoxicity (e.g., sluggish activity) in cats after five to 10 symptom free days (Koenig, 1958). Over the next few days symptoms of neurotoxicity progress to where cats exhibited severe ataxia and were so incapacitated that they were unable to feed themselves. The development of these symptoms of neurotoxicity was correlated with anabolism of 5-fluororotic acid to its nucleotide derivatives and subsequent incorporation into RNA of neuronal tissue (Koenig, 1967). Similar behavioral changes could be produced by intrathecal administration of the nucleoside derivative of 5FU (5-fluoro-deoxyuridine). FUra, on the other hand, produced only minor symptoms of neurotoxicity when administered intrathecally, possibly because of poor anabolic conversion of 5FU to cytotoxic nucleotides in the feline nervous system (Adams, 1965).

A role for anabolism in producing 5FU-induced neurotoxicity was further suggested by findings in two patients who developed neurotoxicity after they received IV 5FU (see Tuchman et al., 1985; Diasio et al., 1988). Both patients became sluggish and developed ataxia two to three weeks after administration of 5FU, with neurotoxicity progressing to where patients became semicomatose. Both patients were found to have increased plasma and urinary pyrimidine levels, suggesting an abnormality in pyrimidine catabolism. In one patient, the lack of 5FU catabolism was demonstrated by the absence of 5FU catabolites in plasma and urine (Diasio et al., 1988). Moreover, this inability to catabolize 5FU was suggested to result from the absence of dihydropyrimidine dehydrogenase activity, because activity of this enzyme was completely deficient in blood mononuclear cells isolated from this patient. Whereas the development of neurotoxicity in patients with a deficiency in 5FU catabolism strongly suggests a role for anabolism in the etiology of 5FU-induced neurotoxicity, it remains to be determined whether other patients developing neurotoxicity demonstrate a similar reduced capacity for 5FU catabolism.

Overt cardiotoxicity is an infrequent (1–2%), yet often severe toxicity associated with 5FU therapy (Collins and Weiden, 1987; Gamucci and Zampa, 1980). Patients may complain of severe substernal chest pain, accompanied with nausea and vomiting two to three days following the start of FUra administration. ECG obtained during an episode of cardiotoxicity may show ST segment changes consistent with cardiac ischemia. Changes in serum cardiac enzymes (e.g., lactate dehydrogenase) in most cases have not been noted, however in a few patients a rise in serum levels of cardiac enzymes have been observed (Pottage et al., 1978; Stevenson et al., 1977). Symptoms of cardiotoxicity are usually relieved by administration of vasodilators (e.g., nitrates), and in most cases all symptoms and ECG changes disappeared following discontinuation of FUra. Patients with a prior history of heart disease appear to be at a greater risk to develop FUra-induced cardiotoxicity. Moreover, the consequences of the cardiotoxicity may be more severe, as patients with a prior history of infarction have died as a consequence of the FUra-induced cardiotoxicity (Collins and Weiden, 1987).

Whereas the incidence of overt cardiotoxicity may be low, a high incidence of ECG changes have been noted in patients receiving 5FU who were asymptomatic for cardiac distress (Rezkalla et al., 1988). In this study, all patients (7/7) with known coronary artery disease demonstrated ST segment changes on ECG (suggestive of cardiac ischemia) following FUra administration, whereas 56% (10/18) of patients with no history of coronary artery disease demonstrated similar ECG changes.

ECG changes similar to those observed in humans have been produced in the guinea pig following an IV administration of 5FU (see Matsubara et al., 1980). This effect was dose related and no cardiac changes were noted following administration of 10 to 20 mg/kg 5FU, whereas 100% (7/7) of the guinea pigs demonstrated ECG changes suggestive of ischemia within three hr after receiving 60 mg/kg 5FU. Biochemical analysis of heart tissue from animals receiving 60 mg/kg 5FU demonstrated a significant decrease in intracellular levels of high energy phosphates (adenosine triphosphate [ATP] and creatine phosphate) and a slight increase in adenosine 5′-diphosphate (ADP), adenosine monophosphate (AMP), and inorganic phosphate. Intracellular citrate levels were increased, leading the investigators to suggest that cardiac changes may have resulted from an inhibition of the tricarboxylic acid cycle enzyme aconitase by fluorocitrate. These studies, however, did not document the presence of fluorocitrate or demonstrate that fluorocitrate can produce similar cardiac changes in these animals.

Hepatotoxicity is not a problem typically associated with systemic IV administration of fluoropyrimidines. However, hepatotoxicity occurs frequently (>75%) when 5-fluorodeoxyuridine (FUDR) is administered by hepatic arterial infusion (Balch and Levin, 1987; Venook et al., 1988). This toxicity usually develops between one and six courses of chemotherapy (0.3 mg/kg/d, 14 days on/14 days off) and is characterized by abnormalities in liver function tests and elevated serum bilirubin levels. Furthermore, in many patients cholangiographic changes similar to those seen with primary biliary sclerosis have been observed in both intrahepatic and extrahepatic bile ducts (Botet et al., 1985).

Initially, it was thought that the FUDR-induced toxicity was primarily hepatocellular in nature. However, more recent studies have suggested that biliary toxicity (without primary hepatocellular injury) is more typical (Hohn et al., 1985). At present the mechanism for this toxicity is not known. Our laboratory has recently identified conjugates of FBAL and bile acids as the major biliary metabolites of fluoropyrimidines in humans (Sweeny et al., 1987; Sweeny et al., 1988a). We have suggested a possible role for these metabolites in the biliary toxicity produced by fluoropyrimidines, since the FBAL conjugate of chenodeoxycholic acid has been shown to produce a marked cholestasis in the isolated perfused rate liver (Sweeny et al., 1988b). However, administration of FBAL-bile acid conjugates to a dog model for the toxicity (Andrews et al., 1989) failed to produce any of the changes (e.g., bile duct) that are characteristic of the FUDR-induced hepatotoxicity, indicating that these FBAL-bile acid conjugates may not have a role in the development of this hepatotoxicity.

Because the bile duct cells receive their blood supply primarily from the hepatic artery (Northover and Terblanche, 1979), these cells would be exposed to high concentrations of FUDR for an extended period of time. Therefore, it is possible that the biliary toxicity may result as a consequence of the anabolism of FUDR to cytotoxic nucleotides, which results in the inhibition of DNA or RNA synthesis in the cells lining the bile duct.

Cytosine Arabinoside (ARA-C)

Pharmacology

Cytosine arabinoside (ARA-C) is an analogue of the pyrimidine nucleoside deoxycytidine, differing only in that the 2′ hydroxyl group of the sugar residue is in the beta configuration (Fig. 5-5). Cytosine arabinoside is effective either alone or in combination with other agents (e.g., anthracyclines) in the treatment of leukemias. It has minimal activity against solid tumors. The cytotoxic action of ARA-C depends on anabolism to ARA-CTP and subsequent incorporation into DNA (Kufe et al., 1980). The exact mechanism by which ARA-C produces cytotoxicity is not known. However, cytotoxicity may result as a consequence of DNA chain termination or from the formation of abnormal DNA (Momparler, 1974).

Cytosine arabinoside is usually administered IV as a single high dose (3 gm/m^2) infused over one to two hr and repeated every 12 hr for 4–12 doses. The terminal plasma half-life following IV administration is 111 min, due to rapid deamination to pharmacologically inactive ARA-uridine. Greater than 70% of the administered dose is excreted in the urine within 24 hr, primarily as ARA-uridine (Ho and Frei, 1971). Low levels of ARA-C are detected in CSF following IV injection. However, levels of ARA-C in the CSF approach 40% of those in plasma following continuous IV infusion of this agent (Ho and Frei, 1971). Levels of ARA-C persist in CSF following continuous IV infusion or intrathecal administration as a result of the absence of deaminase enzymes in the CSF and CNS.

Toxicology

The most frequent toxicities associated with ARA-C occur in the gastrointestinal tract and bone marrow (Frei et al., 1969; Goodell et al., 1970). Gastrointestinal toxicity is generally mild, presenting as nausea, vomiting, diarrhea, abdominal pain, and upper gastrointestinal bleeding. Symptoms subside during the course of ARA-C administration and resolve completely following termination of therapy. Bone marrow depression is very common and often severe. The severity of bone marrow suppression is related to dose and duration of ARA-C infusion (Frei et al., 1969). The most marked effects are seen in reticulocytes and granulocytes, but a reduction in megakaryocytes can also be observed. Lymphocytes are typically not affected. The nadir for granulocytopenia and thrombocytopenia usually range from three to 16 days, whereas the nadir for reticulocytopenia is typically three to nine days (Frei et al., 1969). During this time, patients may present with fever and positive blood cultures, and may develop fatal sepsis. The use of broad spectrum antibiotics and antifungals in these patients appears beneficial in reducing the incidence of fatal infections.

Neurotoxicity is frequently observed during intravenous high dose ARA-C therapy. The development of neurotoxicity appears dose related since patients treated with consecutive doses of 4.5 gm/m^2 had a higher incidence (67% vs 15%) of neurotoxicity than those receiving consecutive doses of 3 gm/m^2 (Lazarus et al., 1981). Furthermore, development of neurotox-

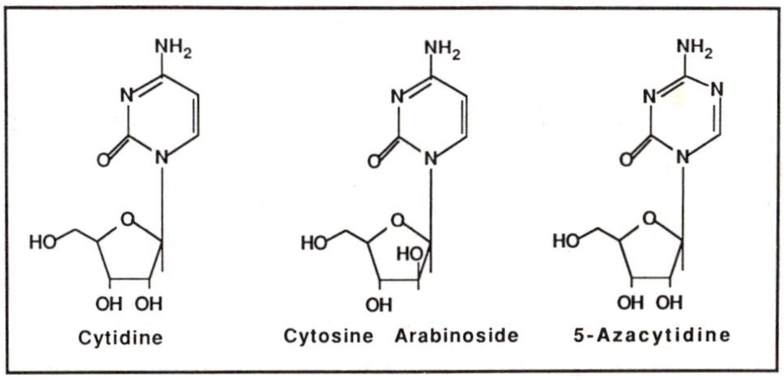

FIGURE 5-5. Structures of cytidine, cytosine arabinoside, and 5-azacytidine.

icity has been suggested to be age related since a higher incidence of neurotoxicity was observed in older patients (>55 years) (Gootlieb et al., 1987). Symptoms of neurotoxicity usually develop between three and four days after initiation of therapy but resolve following discontinuation of therapy. Toxicity is primarily cerebellar in nature, although some alterations in cerebral function (i.e., somnolence, confusion) may occur. Slurred speech and horizontal nystagmus are typically the first noticeable signs and toxicity usually progresses to include marked truncal and extremity ataxia. Computerized tomography scans may demonstrate moderate to severe focal or diffuse atrophy of posterior fossa structures (Grossman et al., 1983). On autopsy, histological examination reveals marked changes in the Purkinjie cell population throughout both cerebellar hemispheres (Salinsky et al., 1983). Purkinjie cells may be reduced in number, but the most common changes are condensation and clumping of nuclear chromatin, with loss of Purkinjie cell processes. At present, the mechanism responsible for this toxicity is not known. However, because Purkinjie cells are not actively dividing cells, this effect may be mediated through an effect of ARA-C on the neuronal glia cells, which are capable of cell division.

Abnormalities in liver function tests and elevation of serum bilirubin levels may be observed during ARA-C administration (Barrios et al., 1987). However, signs of hepatotoxicity usually resolve following discontinuation of therapy. Other common toxicities include conjunctivitis and skin rash. The mechanisms responsible for these different toxicities are unknown.

5-Azacytidine

Pharmacology

5-azacytidine (5-AZC) is an analog of cytidine, differing only in that the fifth carbon of the pyrimidine ring has been replaced with nitrogen (Fig. 5-5). 5-azacytidine is effective in the treatment of leukemias, but has little activity against solid tumors. The cytotoxic action of 5-AZC requires anabolism to its corresponding ribonucleotide and deoxribonucleotide triphosphates and the subsequent incorporation of these triphosphates into RNA and DNA. Incorporation of 5-AZC into RNA results in a number of effects including; decreased acceptor activity of tRNA (Kalousek et al., 1966), breakdown of polyribosomes (Levitan and Webb, 1969), and an inhibition of protein synthesis (Raska et al., 1966), whereas incorporation into DNA results in the inhibition of DNA synthesis (Li et al., 1970).

5-azacytidine is administered IV (150–200 $mg/m^2/d \times$ 5–7 days) either by rapid (over 5–10 min) or continuous (over 30 hr, repeated every 6 hr) infusion. Despite the extensive clinical use of 5-AZC, little information is available on the pharmacokinetics and metabolism of this agent in humans. 5-azacytidine was found to be rapidly metabolized in humans following IV bolus administration, with most of the dose being eliminated in the urine within 24 hr (Israili et al., 1976). However, a detailed analysis of the pharmacokinetics of 5-AZC and its metabolites has not been performed.

Toxicology

Gastrointestinal and bone marrow toxicities are the most frequent complications associated with 5-AZC therapy. Gastrointestinal toxicity, manifest as severe nausea, vomiting, and diarrhea, is frequently observed when 5-AZC is administered by rapid infusion (Levi and Weirnik, 1976). However, gastrointestinal toxicity is usually less severe and more easily controlled (i.e., with antiemetics) when 5-AZC is administered by continuous infusion (Vogler et al., 1976). With both rapid and continuous infusions, symptoms of gastrointestinal toxicity usually develop within 12 hr of initiation of therapy and persist until after the discontinuation of therapy.

Leukopenia, specifically granulocytopenia, is the most frequent hematological toxicity observed in patients receiving 5-AZC. The development of leukopenia with both rapid and continuous IV administration is dose related (Lomen et al., 1975; Vogler et al., 1974). With continuous infusion the frequency of 5-AZC courses also has a pronounced effect on the development of leukopenia. Thus, when 5-AZC was administered by continuous infusion (100 mg/m^2/d $\times$ 5 days) on a 14 day cycle all patients developed leukopenia (Vogler et al., 1976). However, when the 5-AZC was administered on a 21 day schedule only 50% of the patients developed leukopenia.

Renal tubular dysfunction characterized by polyuria, glucosuria, and transient changes in serum concentrations of bicarbonate and phosphorus is frequently seen in patients receiving 5-AZC (Peterson et al., 1981; Greenberg, 1979; Ho et al., 1976). Polyuria usually develops four days after the start of therapy and daily urinary output of between 4.2 and 16.5 liters is not uncommon. Urine output usually returns to normal following termination of therapy. However, polyuria may continue despite discontinuation of 5-AZC and may ultimately contribute to the death of patients receiving 5-AZC. Glucosuria, with daily urinary excretion of glucose up to 8 g, is often observed in patients receiving 5-AZC even though serum glucose levels are found to be normal (below 135 mg/mL). An increase (two- to tenfold) in the urinary excretion of amino acids also may be observed in patients receiving 5-AZC. The 5-AZC-induced renal dysfunction also results in a marked reduction in serum phosphate (59%) and bicarbonate (35%) levels, and an increase (125%) in serum creatine levels (Peterson et al., 1981).

The symptoms of renal tubular function suggest an effect of 5-AZC on both the proximal renal tubule (e.g., glucosuria), and the distal tubule and collecting duct (e.g., polyuria). Preclinical trials of 5-AZC in rhesus monkeys demonstrated that 5-AZC could produce swelling and focal necrosis of renal tubules (Palm et al., 1973). However, the precise mechanism by which 5-AZC produces renal toxicity is not known.

Generalized muscular pain and tenderness are often common complaints from patients receiving 5-AZC (Ho et al., 1976; Levi and Wiernik, 1976). The development of muscle pain has been associated with a reduction in serum phosphate levels. This finding has led to the suggestion that muscle pain and tenderness may result from depletion of high energy phosphate compounds (e.g., ATP) in muscle (Ho et al., 1976). However, a decrease in high energy phosphates in patients displaying 5-AZC-induced muscle pain has yet to be documented.

Hepatotoxicity was documented in 35% (7/20) of patients receiving 5-AZC (0.8 to 2.20 mg/kg/d for 10 days) by subcutaneous administration (Bellet et al., 1973). However, hepatotoxicity has not been reported in patients receiving 5-AZC IV (Vogler et al., 1974; Lomen et al., 1975). The 5-AZC-induced hepatotoxicity was characterized by a threefold increase in serum bilirubin levels and SGOT activity, but liver biopsies demonstrated no hepatocellular changes (Bellet et al., 1973). Four of these patients developed hepatic coma and died within 29 days following the start of 5-AZC therapy. No differences were noted in age, extent of hepatic tumor burden, prior therapy or dose of 5-AZC between patients who developed hepatotoxicity and those who did not. However, all patients who developed 5-AZC-induced hepatotoxicity had baseline serum albumin levels below 2.8 g%. All other patients had serum albumin levels above 3.0 g%. At present, the relationship between serum albumin levels and the development of 5-AZC-induced hepatotoxicity is not known.

PURINE ANALOGS

6-Mercaptopurine and 6-Thioguanine

Pharmacology

6-mercaptopurine (6-MP) and 6-thioguanine (6-TG), analogs of naturally occurring purines (Fig. 5-6), were introduced clinically in 1951 (Hitchings and Elion, 1954) and are still widely used today in the treatment of leukemia. The chemotherapeutic action of 6-MP and 6-TG

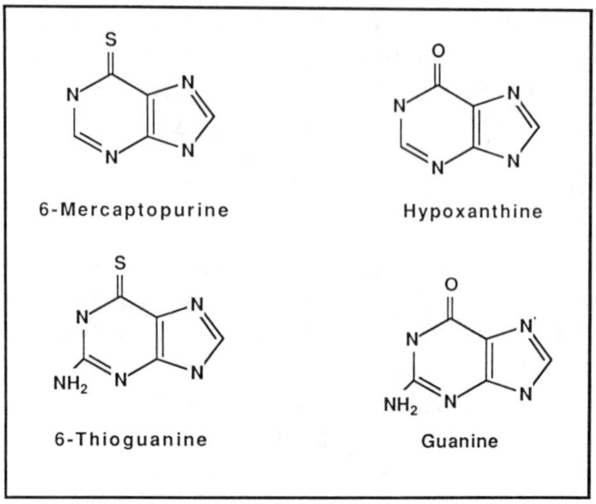

FIGURE 5-6. Structures of 6-mercaptopurine, 6-thioguanine, and corresponding purine bases.

depends on anabolism of these compounds to their respective nucleoside derivatives by the enzyme hypoxantine: guanine phosphoribosyltransferase (HGPRTase). The exact mechanism by which the nucleoside derivatives of 6-MP produces cytotoxicity is not completely understood, but it is thought to result from inhibition of purine biosynthesis or purine interconversion (Elion, 1967). On the other hand, cytotoxicity of 6-TG appears to result as a consequence of its incorporation into DNA (Nelson et al., 1975).

Both of these agents are administered orally, despite poor bioavailability and highly variable plasma levels achieved following this route of administration. Recent studies with both of these agents have employed IV administration and demonstrated that the plasma half-lives following this route of administration were 54 min and 20 min for 6-MP and 6-TG, respectively (Zimm et al., 1988; Kovach et al., 1986).

6-mercaptopurine undergoes metabolism (oxidation) by xanthine oxidase to the pharmacologically inactive thiouric acid, which is subsequently eliminated by the kidney. After low dose (25–100 mg) oral administration, less than 3% of the dose of 6-MP is excreted unchanged in the urine (Vogler et al., 1966). However, after continuous IV (Zimm et al., 1985) infusion or high dose IV (900–1000 mg) administration (Coffey et al., 1972) unchanged 6-MP may represent as much as 40% of the dose eliminated in urine. Co-administration of allopurinol, an inhibitor of xanthine oxidase, also results in an increased amount of unchanged 6-MP eliminated in the urine. The concomitant use of allopurinol may result in increased toxic manifestations and therefore when used together it is recommended that the 6-MP dose be reduced by 25%.

6-thioguanine can undergo degradation to inactive metabolite by two distinct pathways. First, the sulfur group can be methylated to form 6-methylthioguanine, which can subsequently be oxidized to inorganic sulfate and guanine. Alternatively, 6-TG can be deaminated in the liver to 6-thioxanthine, which is subsequently metabolized by xanthine oxidase to 6-thiouric acid. Essentially no unchanged 6-TG is eliminated in urine. After oral administration, approximately equal amounts of 6-methylthioguanine and 6-thiouric acid are found as urinary metabolites, whereas after IV administration 6-thiouric acid is the predominant urinary metabolite (Lepage and Whitecar, 1971).

Toxicology

Myelosuppression and gastrointestinal toxicities are the most common toxicities observed following administration of 6-MP and 6-TG. Daily oral doses of 2.5 mg/kg 6-MP rarely causes myelosuppression and gastrointestinal toxicity in children, but similar dose in adults or a higher dose in children often produces myelosuppression (e.g., leukopenia, anemia, thrombocytopenia) and gastrointestinal toxicity (e.g., nausea and vomiting) (Burchenal et al., 1953). Leukopenia and thrombocytopenia occurs in all patients receiving high dose intravenous 6-MP (100 mg/m^2/d $\times$ 5 days), with the leukopenia ($<$1000 cells/mm^3) and thrombocytopenia ($<$20,000 cells/m^3) often being severe (Esterhay et al., 1978). With continuous infusion of 6-MP (50 mg/m^2/h) bone marrow suppression is rarely seen with infusions less than 36 hr, whereas for infusions greater than 48 hr a variable, transient decrease in platelet, white blood and granulocyte count is observed (Zimm et al., 1985). Mucositis is dose limiting for continuous 6-MP infusion, with severe mucositis often being observed after 48 hr of continuous infusion.

Oral administration of 6-TG produces a qualitatively similar gastrointestinal toxicity and bone marrow depression as is seen with 6-MP, although the gastrointestinal toxicity is usually less severe. Intravenous administration of 6-TG (55–65 mg/m^2/d $\times$ 5 days) produces severe myelosuppression, without the development of any other significant toxicities (Kovach et al., 1986). Intraperitoneal administration of 6-TG (120–900 mg/m^2 over 48 hr) produced a dose related myelosuppression, with granulocytopenia being especially severe at the higher doses (Zimm et al., 1988). No peritonitis or other severe toxicities were seen with this route of administration.

Hepatotoxicity is frequently (34–42%) observed in patients receiving 6-MP (Einhorn and Davidsohn, 1964; Shorey et al., 1968), but is rarely encountered during therapy with 6-TG. Symptoms of hepatotoxicity may become apparent as early as six days after the start of continuous oral (5 mg/kg/d) administration or as long as 2 years after the start of intermittent 6-MP administration. Patients are usually anorexic, and complain of malaise. Stools may be light-colored and urine dark. Patients may be jaundiced (e.g., icteric sclera). Serum bilirubin levels ($>$3mg/100 mL) and transaminase levels (SGOT and SGPT) are elevated, peaking three to five days following completion of a course of 6-MP. In one patient displaying symptoms of hepatotoxicity, histological examination (hepatic biopsy) demonstrated centrilobular cholestasis with intracanalicular bile thrombi and bile lakes (Shorey et al., 1968). However, no significant inflammatory infiltration or hepatocellular necrosis was observed. Symptoms usually resolve following termination of 6-MP. However in some instances jaundice may persist or even worsen following discontinuation of 6-MP. Examination of livers from autopsied patients dying following 6-MP therapy may demonstrate intrahepatic cholestasis, but hepatocellular necrosis is not always evident (Shorey et al., 1968).

At present the mechanism by which 6-MP produces hepatotoxicity is not known. However, the toxicity appears to result from a direct effect of 6-MP, since systemic indicators of hypersensitivity (e.g., eosinophilia) are not observed., Furthermore, symptoms of hepatotoxicity normally resolve following the discontinuation of therapy and may reappear after the restarting of 6-MP.

SUMMARY

Because antimetabolites produce their chemotherapeutic action by primarily disrupting DNA or RNA synthesis, host tissues that undergo rapid cell turnover (e.g., bone marrow and gastrointestinal tract) are frequent sites of toxicity. In general, the development of the gastrointestinal and bone marrow toxicities is related to the dose and duration of antimetabolite administration. However, the rate at which antimetabolites are administered (i.e., rapid vs continuous infusion) can also influence the severity and pattern of gastrointestinal and bone marrow toxicities. With the exception of the use of leucovorin with MTX, there are no other pharmacological means of preventing or reducing these toxicities.

Antimetabolites also produce a variety of other toxicities (e.g., neurotoxicity, hepatotoxicity), although occurring less frequently than gastrointestinal and bone marrow toxicities. Whereas the mechanism by which some of these toxicities are produced is known, the basis for the majority of these toxicities is not fully understood. Despite the production of these often severe toxicities, antimetabolites remain a widely used and effective class of anticancer agents.

REFERENCES

Abelson HT Methotrexate and central nervous system toxicity. Cancer Treat Rep 1978 62:1999–2001.

Abelson HT and Gorka C Absence of Hypoxanthine quanine phosphoribosyltransferase activity in murine dunn osteosarcoma. Cancer Res 1983 43:4098–4101.

Acute Leukemia Group B. Acute lymphocytic leukemia in children: Maintenance therapy with methotrexate administered intermittently. JAMA 1969 207:923–928.

Adams DH Some observation in the incorporation of precursors into ribonucleic acid of rat brain. J Neurochem 1965 12:783–790.

Aherne GW, Piall E, Marks V, Mould G, and White WS Prolongation and enhancement of serum methotrexate concentrations by probenecid. Br Med J 1978 1:1097–99.

Akoun GM, Gauthier-Rahman S, Mayaud CM, Touboul JL, and Denis MF Leukocyte migration inhibition in methotrexate-induced pneumonitis. Chest 1987 91:96–99.

Allen JC, Rosen G, Mehta BM, and Horten B Leukoencephalopathy following high dose IV methotrexate chemotherapy with leucovorin rescue. Cancer Treat Rep 1980 64:1261–1273.

Andrews JC, Knol J, Wollner I, Knutsen C, Smith P, Prieskorn D, and Ensminger W Floxuridine-associated sclerosing cholangitis: A dog model. Invest Radiol 1989 24:47–51.

Balch CM and Levin B Regional and systemic chemotherapy for colorectal metastases to the liver. World J Surg 1987 11:521–526.

Barak AJ, Tuma DJ, and Beckenhauer HC Methotrexate hepatotoxicity. J Am Coll Nutr 1984 3:93–96.

Barrios NJ, Tebbi CK, Freeman AI, and Brecher ML Toxicity of high dose ARA-C in children and adolescents. Cancer 1987 60:165–169.

Bellet RE, Mastrangelo MJ, Engstrom PF and Custer RP Hepatotoxicity of 5-azacytidine (NSC-102816) (a clinical and pathologic study). Neoplasma 1973 20:303–309.

Bertino JR "Rescue" techniques in cancer chemotherapy use of leucovorin and other rescue agents after methotrexate treatment. Seminars Oncol 1977 4:203–216.

Botet JF, Watson RC, Kemeny N, Daley JM, and Yeh S Cholangitis complicating intraarterial chemotherapy in liver metastasis. Radiology 1985 156:335–337.

Bratlid D and Moe PJ Pharmacokinetics of high-dose methotrexate in children. Eur J Clin Pharmacol 1978 14:143–147.

Burchenal JH, Murphy ML, Ellison RR, Sykes MP, Tan TC, Leone LA, Karnofsky DA, Craver LF, Dargeon HW, and Rhoads CP Clinical evaluations of a new antimetabolite, 6-mercaptopurine, in the treatment of leukemia and allied diseases. Blood 1953 8:965–987.

Coffey JJ, White CA, Lesk AB, Rogers WI, and Serpick AA Effect of allopurnol on the pharmacokinetics of 6-mercaptopurine (NSC 755) in cancer patients. Cancer Res 1972 32:1283–1289.

Collins C and Weiden PL Cardiotoxicity of 5-fluorouracil. Cancer Treat Rep 1987 71:733–836.

Diasio RB, Beavers TL, and Carpenter JT Familial deficiency of dihydropyrimidine dehydrogenase. J Clin Invest 1988 81:47–51.

Diasio RB and Harris BE Clinical pharmacology of 5-fluorouracil. Clin. Pharmacokin 1989 16:215–237.

Einhorn M and Davidsohn I Hepatotoxicity of mercaptopurine. JAMA 1964 188:102–106.

Elion GB Biochemistry and pharmacology of purine analogues. Fed Proc 1967 26:898–903.

Ensminger WD and Frei E III The prevention of methotrexate toxicity by thymidine infusions in humans. Cancer Res 1977 37:1857–1863.

Esterhay RJ, Aisner J, Levi JA, and Wiernik PH High-dose 6-mercaptopurine in advanced refractory cancer. Cancer Treat Rep 1978 62:1229–1231.

Everts CS, Westcott JL, and Bragg DG Methotrexate therapy and pulmonary disease. Radiology 1973 107:539–543.

Farber S, Diamond LK, Mercer RD, Sylvester RF, and Wolff JA Temporary remissions in acute leukemia in children produced by folic antagonist 4-amethopteroylglutamic acid (aminopterin). N Eng J Med 1948 238:787–793.

Fraile RJ, Baker LH, Buroker TR, Horwitz J, and Vaitkevicius VK Pharmacokinetics of 5-fluorouracil administered orally, by rapid intravenous and by slow infusion. Cancer Res 1980 40:2223–2228.

Freeman-Narrod M, Kim JS, Ohanissian H, Mills K, Smiley JW and Djerassi I The effect of high-dose methotrexate on renal tubules as indicated by urinary lysozyme concentration. Cancer 1982 50:2775–2779.

Frei E, Bickers JN, Hewlett JS, Lane M, Leary WV, and Talley RW Dose schedule and antitumor studies of arabinosyl cytosine (NSC 63878). Cancer Res 1969 29:1325–1332.

Futterman S and Silverman M The "inactivation" of folic acid by liver. J Biol Chem 1957 224:31–40.

Gamucci T and Zampa G Cardiotoxicity of 5-fluorouracil. Tumori 1980 66:635–636.

Glade LM, Pitman SW, Ensminger WD, Rosowsky A, Papathanasopoulos N, and Frei E III A phase I study of high doses of aminopterin with leucovorin rescue in patients with advanced metastatic tumors. Cancer Res 1979 39:3707–3714.

Goldie JH, Price LA, and Harrap KR Methotrexate toxicity: Correlation with duration of administration, plasma levels, dose and excretion pattern. Eur J Cancer 1972 8:409–414.

Goldman GC and Moschella SL Severe pneumonitis occurring during methotrexate therapy. Arch Dermatol 1973 103:194–197.

Goldman ID The mechanism of action of methotrexate. I. Interaction with a low-affinity intracellular site required for maximum inhibition of deoxyribonucleic acid synthesis in L-cell mouse fibroblasts. Mol Pharmacol 1974 10:257–274.

Goodell B, Leventhal B, and Henderson E Cytosine arabinoside in acute granulocytic leukemia. Clin Pharmacol Ther 1970 12:599–606.

Gootlieb D, Bradstock K, Koutts J, Robertson T, Lee C, and Castaldi P The neurotoxicity of high-dose cytosine arabinoside is age-related. Cancer 1987 60:1439–1441.

Greenberg MS Reversible renal dysfunction due to 5-azacytidine. Cancer Treat Rep 1979 63:806.

Grossman L, Baker MA, Sutton DMC, and Deck JHN Central nervous system toxicity of high-dose cytosine arabinoside. Med Pediatr Oncol 1983 11:246–250.

Heggie GD, Sommadossi J-P, Cross DS, Huster WJ, and Diasio RB Clinical pharmacokinetics of 5-fluorouracil and its metabolites in plasma, urine, and bile. Cancer Res 1987 47:2203–2206.

Henderson ES, Adamson RH, and Oliverio VD The metabolic fate of tritiated methotrexate. II. Absorption and excretion in man. Cancer Res 1965 25:1018–1024.

Hersh EM, Wong VG, Henderson ES, and Freireich EJ Hepatotoxic effects of methotrexate. Cancer 1966 19:600–606.

Hitchings GH and Elion GB The chemistry and biology of purine analogs. Ann NY Acad Sci 1954 60: 195–199.

Ho DHW and Frei E Clinical pharmacology of 1-β-D-arabinofuranosyl cytosine. Clin Pharmacol Ther 1971 12:944–954.

Ho M, Bear RA, and Garvey MD Symptomatic hypophosphatemia secondary to 5-azacytidine therapy of acute nonlymphocytic leukemia. Cancer Treat Rep 1976 60:1400–1402.

Hohn D, Melnick J, Stagg R, Altman D, Friedman M, Ignoffo R, Ferrell L, and Lewis B Biliary sclerosis in patients receiving hepatic arterial infusions of floxuridine. J Clin Oncol 1985 3:98–102.

Israili ZH, Vogler WR, Mingioli ES, Pirkle JL, Smithwick RW, and Goldstein JH The disposition and pharmacokinetics in humans of 5-azacytidine administered intravenously as bolus or by continuous infusion. Cancer Res 1976 36:1453–1461.

Jackson RC, Hart LI, and Harrap KR Intrinsic resistance to methotrexate of cultured mammalian cells in relation to the inhibition kinetics of their dihydrofolate reductases. Cancer Res 1976 36:1991–1997.

Jackson RC and Grindey GB The biochemical basis for methotrexate cytotoxicity. In: Folate Antagonists as Therapeutic Agents, Vol. 1, Academic Press, Inc., 1984 pp. 289–315.

Jacobs SA, Stoller RG, Chabner BA, and Johns DG Dose-dependent metabolism of methotrexate in man and rhesus monkey. Cancer Treat Rep 1977 61:651–656.

Jaffe N, Takaue Y, Anzai T, and Robertson R Transient neurologic disturbances induced by high-dose methotrexate treatment. Cancer 1985 56:1356–1360.

Kalousek J, Raska K Jr, Jurovcik M, and Sorm F Effect of 5-azacytidine in the acceptor activity of s-RNA. Collection Czech Chem Commun 1966 31:1421–1424.

Kamen BA, Nylen PA, Camitta BM, and Bertino JR Methotrexate accumulation and folate depletion in cells as a possible mechanism of chronic toxicity to the drug. Br J Haematol 1981 49:355–360.

Kay HEM, Knapton PJ, O'Sullivan JP, Wells DG, Harris RF, Innes EM, Stuart J, Schwartz FCM, and Thompson EN Encephalopathy in acute leukemia associated with methotrexate therapy. Archiv Dis Child 1972 47:344–354.

Koenig H Production of injury to feline central nervous system with nucleic acid antimetabolite. Science 1958 127:1238–1239.

Koenig H Neurobiological action of some pyrimidine analogs. In: International Review of Neurobiology Pfeffer CC and Smythies JR Eds Academic Press, Inc., New York 1967 vol 10 pp. 199–233.

Koenig H and Patel A Biochemical basis for fluorouracil neurotoxicity. Arch Neurol 1970 23:155–160.

Kovach JS, Rubin J, Creagan ET, Schutt AJ, Kvols LK, Svingen PA, and Hu TC Phase I trial of parenteral 6-thioquanine given on 5-consecutive days. Cancer Res 1986 46:5959–5962.

Kufe WE, Major PP, Eagan EM, and Beardsley GP Correlation of cytotoxicity with incorporation of ARA-C into DNA. J Biol Chem 1980 255:8997–9000.

Lankelma J, van der Kleijn E, and Ramaekers F The role of 7-hydroxymethotrexate during methotrexate anticancer therapy. Cancer Lett 1980 9:133–142.

Lazarus HM, Herzig RH, Herzig GP, Phillips GL, Roessmann M, and Fishman DJ Central nervous system toxicity of high-dose systemic cytosine arabinoside. Cancer 1981 48:2577–2582.

LePage GA and Whitecar JP Pharmacology of 6-thioguanine in man. Cancer Res 1971 31:1627–1631.

Levi JA and Wiernik PH A comparative clinical trial of 5-azacytidine and guanazole in previously treated adults with acute nonlymphocytic leukemia. Cancer 1976 38:36–41.

Levitan IB and Webb TE EFfect of 5-azacytidine on polyribosomes and on the control of tysosine transaminase activity in rat liver. Biochim Biophys Acta 1969 182:491–500.

Lewis JH and Schiff E Methotrexate-induced chronic liver injury: Guidelines for detection and prevention. Am J Gastroenterol 1988 88:1337–1345.

Lewis WJ and Walter JF Methotrexate-induced pulmonary fibrosis. Arch Dermatol 1979 115:1169–1170.

Li LH, Olin EJ, Buskirk HH, and Reineke LM Cytotoxicity and mode of action of 5-azacytidine on L1210 leukemia. Cancer Res 1970 30:2760–2769.

Lomen PL, Baker LH, Neil GL, and Samson MK Phase I study of 5-azacytidine (NSC-102816) using 24-hour continuous infusion for 5 days. Cancer Chemother Rep 1975 59:1123–1126.

Lynch HT, Droszcz CP, Albano WA, and Lynch JF "Organic brain syndrome" secondary to 5-fluorouracil toxicity. Dis Colon Rectum 1981 24:130–131.

Matsubara I, Kamiya J, and Imai S Cardiotoxic effects of 5-fluorouracil in the guinea pig. Japan J Pharmacol 1980 30:871–879.

Meyer WH, Houghton JA, and Houghton PJ Hypoxanthine: guanine phosphoribosyltransferase activity in primary human osteosarcomas. A rationale for therapy with methotrexate-thymidine rescue? J Clin Oncol 1987 5:657–661.

Moertel CG, Reitemeier RJ, Bolton CF, and Shorter RG Cerebellar ataxia associated with fluorinated pyrimidine therapy. Cancer Chemother Rep 1964 41:15–18.

Mompaler R A model for the chemotherapy of acute leukemia with 1-β-D-arabinofuranosylcytosine. Cancer Res 1974 34:1775–1787.

Nelson JA, Carpenter JW, Rose LM, and Adamson DJ Mechanism of action of 6-thioquanine, 6-mercaptopurine and 8-azaquanine. Cancer Res 1975 35:2872–2878.

Northover JM and Terblanche J A new look at the arterial supply of the bile duct in man and its surgical implications. Br J Surg 1979 66:379–384.

Palm PE, Arnold EP, Rachwall PC, and Nick MS Repeated-dose toxicity of a new antimetabolite, 5-triazin-2(IH)-1,4-amino-1-B-D-ribofuranosyl-5-azacytidine in the rhesus monkey. Toxicol Appl Pharmacol 1973 25:492.

Peterson BA, Collins AJ, Vogelzang NJ, and Bloomfield CD 5-Azacytidine and renal tubular dysfunction. Blood 1981 57:182–185.

Pitman SW, Parker LM, Tattersall MHN, Jaffe N, and Frei E III Clinical trial of high-dose methotrexate (NSC-740) with citrovarum factor (NSC-3590)—toxicological and therapeutic observations. Cancer Chemother Rep 1975 6:43–49.

Pottage A, Holt S, Ludgate S, and Langlands AO Fluorouracil cardiotoxicity. Brit Med J 1978 1: 547.

Raska K Jr, Jurovcik M, Fucik J, Tykva R, Sormova L, and Sorm F Metabolic effects of 5-azacytidine in isolated nuclei of calf-thymus cells. Collection Czech Chem Commun 1966 31:2809–2815.

Reggev A and Djerassi I The safety of administration of massive doses of methotrexate (50 g) with equimolar citrovorum factor rescue in adult patients. Cancer 1988 61:2423–2428.

Reynolds FS and Lee WM Hepatotoxicity after long-term methotrexate therapy. South Med J 1986 79: 536–539.

Rezkalla S, Kloner RA, Sarraf MA, Bhasin S, Revels S, Ensley J, Kerpel-Fronius S, Olivenstein A, and Turi ZG Continuous ambulatory electrocardiographic monitoring during 5-fluorouracil therapy: A prospective study. (Abstract) Clin Res 1988 36:499.

Riehl J-L and Brown WJ Acute cerebellar syndrome secondary to 5-fluorouracil therapy. Neurology 1964 14:961–967.

Rosenblatt DS, Whitehead VM, Vera N, Pottier A, Dupont M, and Vuchich MJ Prolonged inhibition of DNA synthesis associated with the accumulation of methotrexate polyglutamates by cultured human cells. Mol Pharmacol 1978 14:1143–1147.

Rueckert RR and Mueller GC Studies on unbalanced growth in tissue culture. I. Induction and consequence of thymidine deficiency. Cancer Res 1960 20:1584–1590.

Rutman RJ, Cantarow A, and Paschkis KE Studies in 2-acetylfluorene carcinogenesis III. The utilization of uracil-2-^{14}C by prenoplastic rat liver and rat hepatone. Cancer Res 1954 14:119–134.

Salinsky MC, Levine RL, Aubuchon JP, and Schutta HS Acute cerebellar dysfunction with high-dose ARA-C therapy. Cancer 1983 51:426–429.

Schuetz JD, Wallace HJ, and Diasio RB 5-Fluorouracil incorporation into DNA of CF-1 mouse bone marrow cells as a possible mechanism of toxicity. Cancer Res 1984 44:1358–1363.

Schuetz JD, Wallace HJ, and Diasio RB DNA repair following incorporation of 5-fluorouracil into DNA of mouse bone marrow cells. Cancer Chemother Pharmacol 1988 21:208–210.

Searles G and McKendry RJR Methotrexate pneumonitis in rheumatoid arthritis: Potential risk factors. Four case reports and review of literature. J Rheumatol 1987 14:1164–1171.

Seifert P, Baker LH, Reed MD, and Vaitkevicius VI Comparison of continuously infused 5-fluorouracil with bolus injection in treatment of patients with colorectal adenocarcinoma. Cancer 1975 36:123–128.

Shorey J, Schenker S, Suki WN, and Combes B Hepatotoxicity of mercaptopurine. Arch Intern Med 1968 122:54–58.

Sostman HD, Matthay RA, Putman CE, and Smith GJW Methotrexate-induced pneumonitis. Medicine 1976 55:371–388.

Stevenson DL, Mikhailidis DP, and Gillet DS Cardiotoxicity of 5-fluorouracil. Lancet 1977 2:406–407.

Stoller RG, Jacobs SA, Drake JC, Lutz RJ, and Chabner BA Pharmacokinetics of high-dose methotrexate (NSC-740). Cancer Chemother Rep 1975 6:19–24.

Stoller RG, Hande KR, Jacobs SA, Rosenberg SA, and Chabner BA Use of plasma pharmacokinetics to predict and prevent methotrexate toxicity. N Engl J Med 1977 297:630–633.

Sweeny DJ, Barnes S, Heggie GD, and Diasio RB Metabolism of 5-fluorouracil to an N-cholyl-2-fluoro-β-alanine conjugate: Previously unrecognized role for bile acids in drug conjugation. Proc Natl Acad Sci USA 1987 84:5439–5443.

Sweeny DJ, Martin M, and Diasio RB N-chenodeoxycholyl-2-fluoro-β-alanine: A biliary metabolite of 5-fluorouracil in humans. Drug Metab Dispos 1988a 16:892–894.

Sweeny DJ, Daher G, Martin M, Barnes S, and Diasio RB Production of cholestasis by 2-fluoro-β-alanine-chenodeoxycholic acid. Possible role of this metabolite in the cholestasis associated with hepatic arterial infusion (HAI) of fluoropyrimidines (FPs) (abstract). Proc Am Assoc Cancer Res 1988b 29:486.

Tattersall MHN, Brown B, and Frei E III The reversal of methotrexate toxicity by thymidine with maintenance of antitumor effects. Nature 1981 253:198–200.

Taylor IW and Tattersall MHN Methotrexate cytotoxicity in cultured human leukemic cells studied by flow cytometry. Cancer Res 1981 41:1549–1558.

Thyss A, Milano G, Kubar J, Namer M, and Schneider M Clinical and pharmacokinetic evidence of a life-threatening interaction between methotrexate and ketoprofen. Lancet 1980 1:256–258.

Tolman KG, Clegg DO, Lee RG, and Ward JR Methotrexate and the liver. J Rheumatol 1985 12:29–34.

Tuchman M, Stoeckeler JS, Kiang DT, O'Dea RF, Ramnaraine ML, and Mirkin BL Familial pyrimidinemia and pyrimidinuria associated with severe fluorouracil toxicity. N Engl J Med 1985 313:245–249.

Venook AP, Stagg RJ, and Lewis BJ Regional chemotherapy for colorectal cancer metastatic to the liver. Oncol 1988 2:19–26.

Vogler WR, Arkun S, and Velez-Garcia E Phase I study of twice weekly 5-azacytidine (NSC-102816). Cancer Chemother Rep 1974 58:895–899.

Vogler WR, Bain JA, Huguley CM, Palmer HG Jr, and Lowrey ME Metabolic and therapeutic effects of allopurinol in patients with leukemia and gout. Am J Med 1966 40:548–559.

Vogler WR, Miller DS, and Keller JW 5-Azacytidine (NSC 102816): A new drug for the treatment of myeloblastic leukemia. Blood 1976 48:331–337.

Weber BL, Tanyer G, Poplack DG, Reaman GH, Feusner JH, Miser JS, and Bleyer WA Transient acute hepatotoxicity of high-dose methotrexate therapy during childhood. NCI Monogr 1987 5:207–212.

Wilkinson PM, Morice ER, and Lucas SB Chemical and kinetic parameters that influence the response and toxicity to methotrexate. In: Clinical Pharmacology of Antineoplastic Drugs Pinedo HM Ed. Elsevier/North Holland Biomedical Press, Amsterdam 1978 pp. 29–38.

Zimm S, Ettinger LJ, Holcenberg JS, Kamen BA, Vietti TJ, Belasco J, Cogliano-Shutta N, Balis F, Lavi LE, Collins JM, and Poplack DG Phase I clinical pharmacological study of mercaptopurine administered as a prolonged intravenous infusion. Cancer Res 1985 45:1869–1873.

Zimm S, Cleary SM, Horton CN, and Howell SB Phase I/pharmacokinetic study of thioguanine administered as a 48-hour continuous intraperitoneal infusion. J Clin Oncol 1988 6:696–700.

CHAPTER 6

Toxicity of Platinum-Based Anticancer Drugs

Miles P. Hacker, Ph.D.

HISTORICAL PERSPECTIVE

The search for effective drugs in the treatment of human cancer has resulted in the development of a wide variety of anticancer drugs. One class of compounds that has received a great deal of attention is the metal-based oncolytics which includes arsenic, mercury, gold, and platinum. Whereas several different metal-based complexes have demonstrated cell killing activity, only platinum-containing complexes have met with unqualified success.

The actual development of the prototypical drug, *cis*-diamminedichloroplatinum (II) (DDP), is an excellent example of serendipity in a inproper setting resulting important scientific advances and is worthy of a brief review. While investigating the effect of electric current on the mobility of bacteria, Dr. Barnett Rosenberg, a biophysicist by formal training, noted that motility not only ceased but the bacteria formed filamentous chains (Rosenberg et al., 1965). Because this type of bacterial structure is observed in nondividing cells, Dr. Rosenberg undertook an investigation to identify the cause of the growth inhibition.

After a series of elegant studies the agent responsible for growth inhibition was established as DDP, known in the chemical literature since the 1860s as Peyrode's salt (Fig. 6-1). Recognizing that any complex so effective in altering bacterial growth may also have important antitumor activity, Dr. Rosenberg and the National Cancer Institute initiated studies to assess this property of DDP (Rosenberg et al., 1969). By 1969, the activity of DDP in experimental tumor systems provided the impetus for limited human studies. Shortly thereafter, DDP was shown to be curative against metastatic testicular carcinoma when combined with other established oncolytics (Einhorn and Furnas, 1976; Rozencweig et al., 1977). By 1983, DDP had become one of the most widely used anticancer drugs having proven efficacy against testicular, ovarian, and head and neck cancers. In addition, DDP has important adjunct activity in cancers of the cervix, bladder, and lung (Yagoda et al., 1976).

MECHANISM OF ACTION

In spite of its relatively simple chemical structure, the elucidation of the mechanism of DDP activity has proven difficult. To date, it has been demonstrated that DDP remains chlorinated while in the plasma but after diffusion through the plasma membrane DDP encounters an environment of relatively low chloride concentration and undergoes aquation (Fig. 6-2) (Rosenberg, 1979). Once hydrated the platinum complex becomes highly reactive and has been shown to interact with a variety of cellular substituents. Of these, DNA appears to be the most likely candidate for the site of cytotoxic lesion formation (Erickson et al., 1981; Roberts et al., 1988).

The exact cytotoxic adduct has not yet been established but the preponderance of experi-

A)

NH_3 — Pt — Cl
NH_3 — — Cl

B)

NH_3 — Pt — OOC
NH_3 — — OOC

C)

OH
$(CH_3)_2CHNH_2$ — Pt — Cl
$(CH_3)_2CHNH_2$ — — Cl
OH

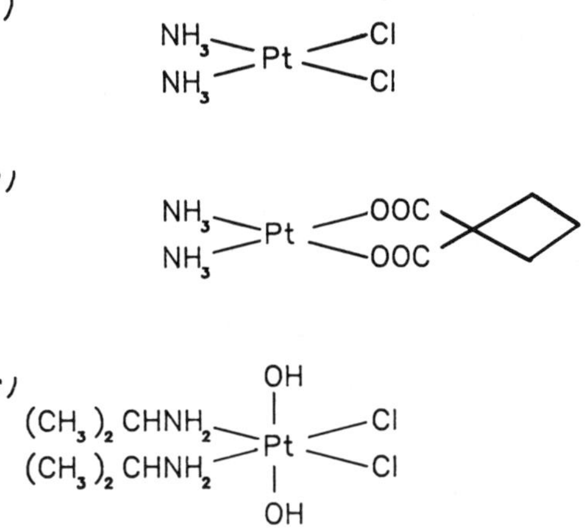

FIGURE 6-1. The chemical structures of: a.) *cis*-diamminedichloroplatinum (DDP); b.) carboplatin (CBDCA); and c.) iproplatin (CHIP).

mental data thus far accrued indicates that an intrastrand cross-link is the most likely candidate (Fig. 6-3). Data supporting this supposition include: (a) trans-diamminedichloroplatinum II, a congener of DDP lacking cytotoxic potential, cannot form intrastrand cross-links, (b) the vast majority of DNA-platinum adducts are intrastrand cross-links, and (c) the intrastrand cross-links appear to be more difficult to remove than the interstrand cross-links.

There is an apparent base selectivity for platinum adduct formation with the N7 position of guanosine nucleotides being the most frequent site of platination. The bifunctional lesion usually consists of adjacent guanosines, a guanosine-adenosine or two guanosines separated by an intervening base. Why such a lesion is cytotoxic is not known but it is hypothesized that the intrastrand cross-link causes a perurbation of the tertiary DNA structure and thereby inhibiting necessary DNA functions.

TOXICITIES

Myelosuppression

DDP

As with most anticancer drugs, DDP has myelosuppressive activity. Although significant in certain protocols or patient populations, DDP-induced hematologic toxicities are not often

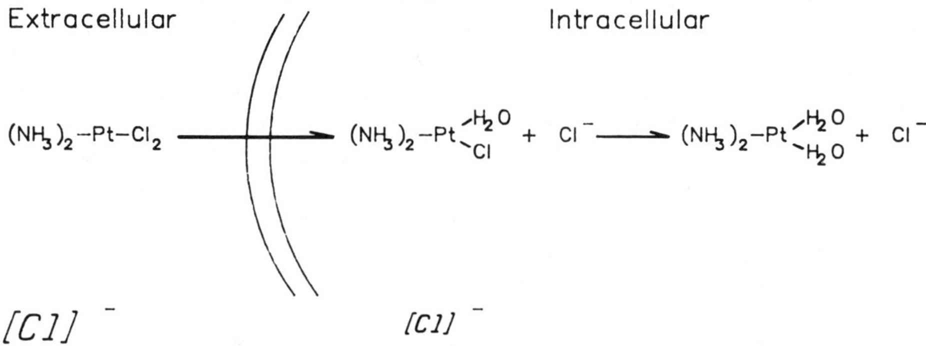

FIGURE 6-2. Proposed aquation of DDP following diffusion into the target cell.

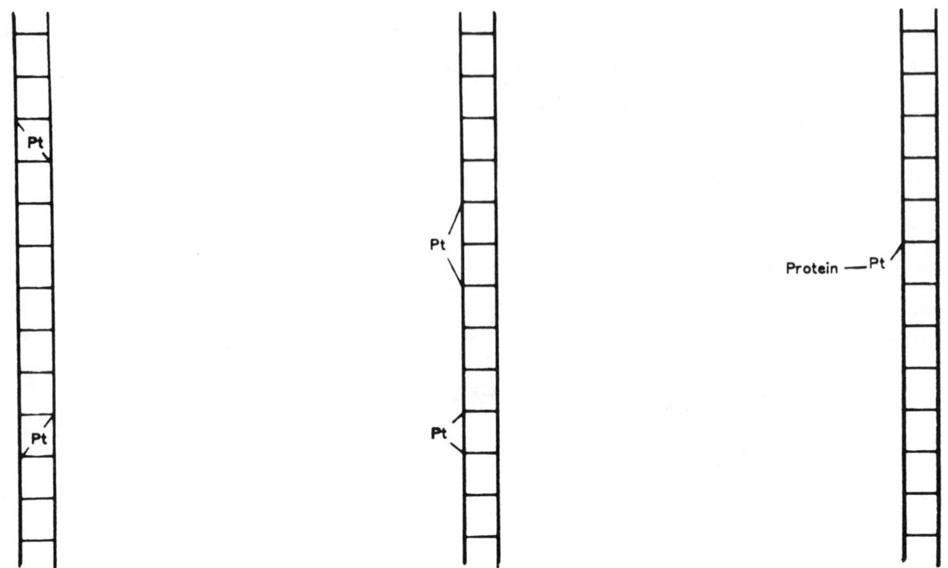

FIGURE 6-3. Potential sites of DNA interaction by fully aquated DDP including interstrand cross-link, intrastrand cross-link and DNA-protein crosslink.

considered to be dose limiting. Furthermore, each affected cell population, which includes leukocytes, platelets, and erythrocytes, recover following completion of the treatment protocol.

Leukocytopenia is a common occurrence in DDP treated patients but is seldom of sufficient severity to result in treatment related infections. The severity and incidence of this toxicity is related to the dose administered and the treatment schedule used. Prolonged infusions or multiple divided doses of DDP seem to yield equivalent oncolytic activity with much less myelosuppression than encountered with bolus injections of the drug. An exception to this is the recent report in which patients receiving DDP on a twice daily basis, developed an alarmingly high incidence of aplastic anemia 20 to 30 days after initiation of therapy. The nadir of leukocytopenia is somewhat delayed occurring as much as several weeks after the initiation of therapy. Even with high dose DDP, made possible with the advent of successful nephroprotection, leukocytopenia is infrequently the cause of cessation of treatment.

Bleeding from DDP-induced thrombocytopenia can be a significant, but readily manageable, problem for the patient (Hall et al., 1981; Talley et al., 1973). As above, the degree of thrombocytopenia is related to the total dose of DDP administered and treatment schedule used. With conventional doses of DDP, bleeding problems are rarely encountered and are easily managed with platelet transfusions. High dose DDP appears to cause greater thrombocytopenia as the nephroprotective regimens have little effect on DDP induced myelosuppression (Gandara et al., 1986; Holleran and deGregorio, 1988). Platelet decreases are reported to be severe enough to warrant interruption of treatment. Another circumstance that has been problematic when encountered is the combination of thrombocytopenia and gastrointestinal bleeding, observed in a few patients receiving DDP. For the most part this can be managed with platelet replacement without compromising the protocol.

DDP induced anemia is frequently seen in patients but is only rarely a significant clinical problem (Wiltshaw and Kroner, 1976; Von Hoff, et al., 1979). The mechanism of this toxicity has been a point of controversy. Obviously, the effect of DDP on dividing cells could explain some of the anemia seen in patients but oftentimes the onset is too rapid to be explained by interference of red blood cell production. Others have suggested a direct effect of DDP on the red blood cell through an interaction with red blood cell glutathione metabolism (Litterst, 1981; Milano et al., 1988).

An immune mediated mechanism similar to that seen with penicillin, has been suggested in which antibodies directed against DDP are adsorbed onto the surface of the red blood cell and hemolysis ensues (Cinollo et al., 1988). Reports of positive Coomb's tests in several patients have added credence to this hypothesis (Getaz et al., 1980; Van Nguyen et al., 1981). However, Zeger et al. have recently shown that the nonspecific direct antibody adsorption (DAT), and complement fixation can occur with red blood cells taken from DDP treated patients (Zeger et al., 1988). They suggest that unless specific DDP antibodies can be detected in the sera of patients, a positive DAT should not be considered proof of DDP-induced immune hemolytic anemia. In addition, the development of acute hemolytic anemia in a patient does not preclude this patient from further DDP therapy as most will not experience this toxicity in subsequent courses of treatment. However, further episodes of more severe nature must be considered a potential risk.

Platinum Analogues

Both carboplatin (CBDCA) and iproplatin (CHIP) have myelosuppression as their primary dose-limiting toxicities (Gaynon et al., 1987; Eisenberger et al., 1986; Al-Sarraf et al., 1987; Anderson et al., 1988). A number of Phase I and II studies have been completed on these two complexes and both have clearly proved to cause a dose and schedule dependent decrease in platelets and leukocytes.

Many treatment schedules have been examined for CBDCA, including single intravenous (IV) bolus (Motzer et al., 1987), single monthly IV 60 min infusions (Gaynon et al., 1987), and five daily IV bolus injections repeated every four to six weeks (Rozencweig et al., 1983; Van Echo et al., 1984; Eisenberger et al., 1986). In each of these studies, significant leukocytopenia, primarily of granulocytes, and thrombocytopenia were the dose-limiting toxicities. For each protocol tested these toxicities were delayed in onset with the nadir occurring three to five weeks after initiation of the study. When administered as a single injection in Phase I studies the recommended starting dose was determined to be 350 to 400 mg CBDCA/m^2 in nonpretreated patients and somewhat decreased in pretreated patients. When administered as five daily injections, the recommended starting doses for CBDCA were approximately 100 mg/m^2 in nonpretreated patients and 70 to 80 mg/m^2 in pretreated patients. Ozols et al. have reported that dose-limiting myelosuppression was encountered in at least 25% of patients receiving high dose CBDCA (800 mg/m^2 per cycle) when the drug was administered as a 48 hr infusion (Ozols et al., 1987). An encouraging observation made by these investigators was that few other toxicities were noted even at this relatively high dose of CBDCA. Phase II studies have subsequently verified these recommended doses and the relative myelotoxicity of CBCDA.

CHIP has received less extensive clinical evaluation than CBDCA but the reports to date indicate that CHIP has similar spectrum of myelotoxicity with thrombocytopenia and leukopenia being the primary dose-limiting toxicities. For the most part CHIP has been administered as a 30 to 60 min infusion at doses of 180 to 370 mg/m^2 (Al-Sarraf et al., 1987; Anderson et al., 1988; Clavel et al., 1988; Sessa et al., 1988) with nadir in platelet and leukocyte counts occurring seven to 35 days later. The extent of thrombocytopenia appears to be greater for CHIP than CBDCA because sporadic deaths have been reported for with this drug (Clavel et al., 1988). Further, nonmyelotoxic complications for CHIP were more frequent and severe than those observed with CBDCA.

Nephrotoxicity

Undoubtedly the most commonly cited toxicity associated with cisplatin administration is kidney damage. Early preclinical studies reported that cisplatin was highly nephrotoxic in rats, dogs and monkeys (Kociba and Sleight, 1971; Schaeppi et al., 1973; Ward and Fauvie, 1976). Degenerative renal lesions were mainly limited to the proximal tubules and were characterized by hydropic degeneration, necrosis, and occasional tubular atrophy. The severity of this toxicity was greatest between three to six days following drug administration and regenerative processes were noted within 10 days.

The nephrotoxic potential in humans was soon substantiated in clinical trials in which 20 to 30% of patients treated with single doses of 50 mg/m^2 developed impaired kidney function (Rossof et al., 1972; Kovach et al., 1973; Rozencweig et al., 1977). In most early studies this renal damage was mild and reversible. As clinical studies continued and a clear-cut dose response relationship between dose administered and effectiveness of cisplatin was established, patients received increasing doses of the drug. At doses of 100 mg/m^2 or more, it soon became apparent that nephrotoxicity was the major dose-limiting toxicity and that this toxicity was cumulative, dose dependent, and irreversible (Rossof et al., 1972; Schilsky, 1982).

Histological examination of kidney tissue revealed focal necrosis of the distal convoluted tubules and collecting ducts, dilation of convoluted tubules and the formation of casts (Gonzalez-Vitale et al., 1977; Dentino et al., 1978). In contrast to the lesions seen in experimental animals the proximal tubules of humans were far less affected by cisplatin than the distal convoluted tubules. The onset of renal damage appears during the second week after initiation of therapy and is manifested by a rise in blood urea nitrogen (BUN) and serum creatinine levels and a concomitant fall in creatinine clearance.

An area of controversy has centered around the appropriate marker(s) for monitoring the development of nephrotoxicity. Although BUN, serum creatinine, and creatinine clearance have been traditionally used for the measurement of renal damage, studies have indicated that changes in certain urinary enzymes may be more sensitive indicators of renal tubular toxicity of cisplatin. Urinary alanine aminopeptidase and N-acetyl-beta-D-glucosamidase, two high molecular weight proteins located within the microvilli and lysosomes of renal tubular cells, respectively, are released into the urine of patients following cisplatin-induced renal damage (Diener et al., 1981; Goren et al., 1986; Daugaard et al., 1988). Other indices of renal damage include beta-glucuronidase and beta-2-microglobulin (Kuhn et al., 1980; Cohen et al., 1981). Although several investigators have used the appearance of these urinary enzymes as indices of nephrotoxicity, no clear-cut advantage for the use of the markers as opposed to the more established indicators has been provided.

Another approach taken to monitor cisplatin-induced kidney damage has been to evaluate renal function of patients receiving cisplatin. The parameters followed have varied but have included glomerular filtration (GFR), filtration fraction (FF), urine output, and effective renal plasma flow (ERPF) (Meijer et al., 1983b; Offerman et al., 1984; Groth et al., 1986). Meijer et al. (1983a) demonstrated a significant fall in GFR without a corresponding rise in serum creatinine. Further, Safirstein et al. (1988) have reported that polyuria and decreased GFR persist long after BUN levels return to pretreatment values. Finally, altered renal function has been observed in patients receiving high dose cisplatin with hypersalination in spite of the absence of altered BUN or creatinine values. The data obtained from such studies suggest that patients may suffer subclinical renal damage that is not detected using the standard markers of kidney damage but the patient is at increased risk for kidney toxicity because of the subtle changes in kidney function.

The mechanism of this toxicity is not understood. A number of plausible hypotheses have been put forth but as yet none of these has proved to be the primary explanation. Several heavy metals are known to be nephrotoxic and appear to damage the kidney through interactions with sulfhydryl groups (Cafruny et al., 1955). This adduct formation results in the inactivation of enzymes, increased membrane fragility and depletion of intracellular glutathione. Studies with cisplatin have shown that renal sulfhydryl concentrations decrease prior to changes in BUN or serum creatinine (Levi et al., 1980). Others have reported that cisplatin can inhibit the Na-K-ATPase of renal tubular cells (Gaurino et al., 1979) which could account for the electrolyte imbalances seen in patients receiving cisplatin. Data have been presented suggesting that much of the damage induced in the kidney can be attributed to free radicals (Hannemann and Baumann, 1988; Sugihara et al., 1987a; 1987b) and that the kidney could be protected by the administration of free radical scavengers (Dobyan et al., 1986; Hannemann and Baumann, 1988; Sugihara et al., 1987b). Cisplatin is concentrated in the kidney to much higher degree than in other tissues including tumor (Dentino et al., 1978; Jacobs et al., 1980). The platinum is stored for long periods as DNA adducts but the importance of these adducts is unknown since the kidney has a relatively small growth fraction (Reed et al., 1988). Although it is not a biochemical mechanism, Macquet and Botour have suggested that the renal toxicity of platinum complexes is inversely related to the stability of the complex in solution (Maquet and Botour, 1983). The data seem to be supported by the clinical data accrued thus far with CBDCA, a far more stable and less nephrotoxic complex than cisplatin.

Given the clinical importance of this toxicity, a great deal of effort has gone into developing methods to eliminate or at least minimize the nephrotoxicity of cisplatin. Approaches taken include alteration of treatment schedule, administration of renal protectants and the development of nonnephrotoxic platinum analogs. This effort has resulted in some remarkable successes in controlling cisplatin-induced renal toxicity. Examples of each of these approaches will be discussed below.

Alteration of Treatment Schedule

In the initial clinical studies cisplatin was administered as a bolus injection in 10 to 15 min. As nephrotoxicity became evident alternative treatment schedules including divided doses, infusion times of two to six hr and continuous infusions over five day periods were evaluated. Ascribing decreased nephrotoxicity directly to these altered treatment schedules is complicated because most of these protocols also included vigorous hydration and diuretics. There are specific studies, however, in which the patients received only drug and mild prehydration. Salem et al. reported that in 96 patients who were hydrated 12 hr prior to cisplatin administration but received no diuretics during a five day continuous infusion of drug (20 mg/m^2/d) only four developed nephrotoxicity (Salem et al., 1984). Bozinno et al. administered 60 mg/m^2 cisplatin as a continuous 24 hr infusion and found no decrease in kidney function (Bozinno et al., 1980). In a pilot study Gandara et al. found that 200 mg/m^2 of cisplatin could be administered with significantly less kidney damage if given as two 3-hr infusions on days 1 and 8 compared to five daily infusions (Gandara et al., 1986).

This approach has assisted in decreasing the nephrotoxicity of cisplatin with no noticeable effect on the efficacy of the drug. Given the success of other nephroprotective interventions, however, the alteration of treatment schedule can be considered, at best, an adjunct procedure.

Hydration and Diuresis

Shortly after nephrotoxicity was identified as a clinical problem with cisplatin several of studies demonstrated that vigorous hydration in combination with an osmotic diuretic such as mannitol could significantly decrease the nephrotoxic potential of cisplatin (Hayes et al., 1977; Krakoff, 1979; Al-Sarraf et al., 1982). The mechanism of nephroprotection without loss of antitumor activity is not known. It has been proposed that hydration and diuresis may decrease the platinum concentration in the urine and perhaps decrease the exposure of the tubules to free platinum species (Vogl et al., 1980).

Currently, most protocols include some form of hydration and diuresis. When cisplatin is administered in conventional doses of <100 mg/m^2 patients are typically prehydrated with saline, dextrose and mannitol for 6 to 24 hr prior to administration of cisplatin. The drug is then given, either as a bolus or infusion, and hydration with diuresis continued for an additional 6 to 24 hr period. Variations of this basic approach can be found throughout the literature.

Whereas these types of interventions significantly decrease the incidence and severity of kidney damage, this complication continues to be a major hindrance in high-dose cisplatin therapy. Indeed, incidences as high as 50% have been reported in patients receiving 130 to 140 mg/m^2 (Ostrow et al., 1981; Baum et al., 1981; Bhuchar and Lanzotti, 1982).

It has been proposed that a vehicle of high NaCl concentration could inhibit the aquation of cisplatin and thereby diminish the reactivity of the drug. Litterst demonstrated that mice could be administered an LD_{50} dose of cisplatin (calculated from data obtained when cisplatin was dissolved in water) with no toxic deaths when the drug was administered in a 4.5% NaCl solution (Litterst, 1981). Following this experimental observation, Ozols et al. evaluated the effectiveness of hypersalination (40 mg/m^2 cisplatin in 250 mL of 3% NaCl daily for five days) in patients with poor prognosis nonseminomatous testicular cancer (Ozols et al., 1984). No evidence of renal damage was noted in patients after three to four courses of therapy. Note that all patients also received hydration and forced diuresis which may have also played a role in protecting the kidneys.

As a result of this initial observation a number of clinical studies have substantiated the fact that hypersalination allows much greater doses of cisplatin to be administered without causing nephrotoxicity (Gandara et al., 1986; Goren et al., 1987; Fuks et al., 1987). However, there is controversy concerning this intervention (Legha et al., 1984). Several groups have observed changes in renal function assays such as GFR, FF, and ERPF without concomitant changes in BUN or creatinine values (Daugaard et al., 1988; Safirstein et al., 1988). These investigators suggest that renal damage does occur but that for the most part these changes are subclinical. As discussed above, whether such changes predispose the patient to future kidney problems has yet to be determined.

Renal Protectants

A number of chemoprotectants have been evaluated for possible renal protection. Of these, sodium thiosulfate (ST), WR2721, and diethyldithiocarbamate (DDTC) have received the greatest clinical attention. More recently, clinical trials in Italy indicate that gluthathione may also function as an effective nephroprotectant. All four of these sulfur containing compounds appear to bind cisplatin through the S-moiety, thereby inactivating the drug (Borch et al., 1988).

Sodium thiosulfate protected mice from the nephrotoxicity of cisplatin when ST was administered from 60 min before to 30 min after cisplatin (Howell et al., 1980). These data suggest that ST is cleared fairly rapidly from the animal and that a fairly narrow window of ST protection exists. This observation has been successfully taken into clinical studies (Howell et al., 1982; Howell et al., 1983; Markman et al., 1985). The most favorable outcomes have resulted in protocols in which cisplatin is administered intraperitoneally and ST is administered IV. Little or no renal toxicity was observed in patients receiving up to 270 mg/m^2 of cisplatin when ST was administered as an IV bolus of 4 gm/m^2 followed by an infusion of ST (12 gm/m^2 over 6 hr). Although less dramatic, a doubling of cisplatin dosage can be administered IV when accompanied by IV ST compared to cisplatin alone (Pfeifle et al., 1985; Hirosawa et al., 1989). No toxicity attributable to ST was observed in any patient.

Aamdal et al. have reported when both cisplatin and thiosulfate were administered IV to tumor-bearing mice, the thiosulfate substantially reduced the antitumor activity of cisplatin resulting in no increase in the therapeutic index of cisplatin (Aamdal et al., 1987). These results produce some doubt as to the advisability of giving these two drugs in combination by the same route of administration. A recent permutation has been the use of the "two-route" approach in which cisplatin is administered intraarterial (IA) and ST is administered IV. With this procedure ST appears to be effective in protecting the kidney without hindering the antitumor activity of cisplatin (Abe et al., 1988).

WR-2721 is an organic thiophosphate which in experimental animal models has been shown to be selectively protective for normal tissues against the toxic effects of radiation and alkylating agents (Yuhas et al., 1980b). Yuhas et al. have further demonstrated that WR-2721 increases the resistance of rat kidneys to the toxicity of cisplatin by a factor of 1.4 to 1.7 (Yuhas et al., 1980c). The mechanism of normal cell protection, while not fully elucidated, appears to be related to the selective sequestration of this drug by normal tissues (Yuhas et al., 1980a). Thus, greater inactivation of cisplatin will occur by the normal tissues thereby sparing these tissues from the cytotoxic activity of cisplatin.

In Phase I studies, Glover et al. clearly demonstrated that escalated doses of cisplatin up to at least 135 mg/m^2 were possible when WR-2721 was administered as an IV infusion over 15 mins (740 mg/m^2), 10 min prior to 30 min infusion of cisplatin (Glover et al., 1984; 1986). In all studies using WR-2721 patients were prehydrated and diuresed. Toxicities associated with WR-2721 were relatively mild and well-tolerated by the patient and included nausea, vomiting, flushing, and sporadic somnolence. Recently, Glover et al. completed a Phase II trial of WR-2721 and cisplatin against advanced metastatic melanoma and observed a slight enhancement of activity of the combination compared to cisplatin alone (Glover et al., 1989). Studies such as these await confirmation by other investigators but they suggest that WR-2721 may both protect the patient and enhance tumor cell kill.

A metabolite of disulfiram (Antabuse), DDTC, was shown to protect rats against cisplatin nephrotoxicity without diminishing the antitumor activity of cisplatin (Borch et al., 1979; 1980). The mechanism of this renal protectant appears to be quite different from the other sulfhydryl protectants in that DDTC can actually remove monoadducted platinum from all biologically relevant binding sites (Dedon and Borch, 1987). The timing of DDTC administration with respect to cisplatin is quite different than for TS or WR-2721 in that DDTC is most effective when given after cisplatin.

Presently, only limited clinical data exist on this chemoprotectant. Qazi et al. reported recently the results of a Phase I study in which 10 patients were hydrated and diuresed prior to receiving DDP (50–120 mg/m^2) which was followed exactly 45 min later with a 90 min infusion of DDTC (75 or 150 mg/m^2) (Qazi et al., 1988). The acute toxic effects observed during DDTC infusion, which included numbness in the infusion arm, severe diaphoresis, discomfort, and a generalized feeling of agitation and flushing, ceased upon completion of the infusion. No nephrotoxicity was observed in any patient and nausea and vomiting were ameliorated in three patients. Similar toxicities were observed by Rothenberg et al. when DDTC was combined with high-dose CBDCA (Rothenberg et al., 1988). However, a significant amount of hematologic and autonomic toxicities were encountered with this combination. A study performed at M.D. Anderson Hospital raises questions about the effectiveness of DDTC as a chemoprotective agent since DDTC did not significantly reduce the renal toxicity of DDP nor did it improve the efficacy of DDP (Paredes et al., 1988). Whereas it is too early to state with certainty the eventual place of DDTC in preventing renal damage the preclinical and early clinical studies do look promising.

Platinum Analogs

A great deal of effort has gone into the development of second and third generation platinum analogs. Of the hundreds of such complexes few have progressed to full scale clinical evaluation. At present only CBDCA and CHIP have received sufficient clinical evaluation to establish the relative renal toxicity compared to the parent DDP. In Phase I and II studies completed to date, both complexes appear to be significantly less nephrotoxic than DDP.

The majority of studies performed thus far have used CBDCA although a few have compared CBDCA and CHIP. CBDCA has been administered as a single bolus IV injection at four-week intervals (Motzer et al., 1987), or 30 to 60 min infusions repeated every four weeks (Cantwell et al., 1986; Koeller et al., 1986; Anderson et al., 1988; Skillen et al., 1988; Tueni et al., 1988). These studies have clearly demonstrated that CBDCA is relatively free of nephrotoxic potential. CHIP has been administered as 30 to 120 min infusions (Pendyala et al., 1985; Cantwell et al., 1986; Anderson et al., 1988; Sessa et al., 1988; Skillen et al., 1988) and was similarly found to be relatively nonnephrotoxic. There is a report that CHIP is possibly slightly more nephrotoxic than CBDCA (Skillen et al., 1988) but to date the preponderance of data indicate that the second-generation platinum complexes are renal sparing.

Because neither complex caused marked acute or chronic changes in kidney function, it would appear that these complexes are viable candidates to be used in place of DDP. Caution must be taken in this regard, however, since occasionally patients experience subclinical tubular damage that may lead to overt nephrotoxicity if therapy is continued. Further studies are required to establish whether these complexes have sufficient anti-tumor activity to warrant inclusion of either one or both of these second generation complexes as first line agents.

Based upon the interest shown in CBDCA at a recent meeting of the American Society for Clinical Oncology (San Francisco, CA, 1989), at which more than 30 abstracts were presented on the toxicity and efficacy of CBDCA, it would appear that these data will be available in the near future for CBDCA. Indeed, if the results of these reports are confirmed there is little doubt that CBDCA will soon be considered a relatively nonnephrotoxic first-line platinum agent.

Nausea and Vomiting

One of the major side effects associated with the use of oncolytics is nausea and vomiting. The most emetogenic of the anticancer drugs include doxorubicin, Dacarbazine, nitrogen mustard, high-dose cyclophosphamide, and cisplatin (Laszlo, 1983). Indeed, cisplatin has been referred to as the most nauseating drug administered to humans. To better understand the mechanism of this toxicity a brief discussion of the physiology of vomiting is included.

Vomiting can be divided into three separate stages: nausea, retching, and emesis (Borison and Wang, 1953). Nausea, defined as the feeling of a need to vomit, is associated with the loss of gastric and pyloric tone, decreased peristalsis and the loss of the duodenal-gastric reflux. Retching, defined as the synchronized, labored movement of the diaphragm and muscles of the stomach and chest, precedes and follows emesis. Finally emesis, defined as the forceful and sustained contraction of diaphragm and abdominal muscles coordinated with opening of the pyloric valve, results in the emptying of stomach contents.

Whereas nausea is under the control of autonomic efferent, retching and emesis are coordinated through the somatic nervous system. Within the central nervous system reside two distinct areas directly involved in the control of emesis. Both the chemotactic trigger zone (CTZ) and the emetic center (EM) are located in the medulla oblongata (Wang and Borison, 1952). The CTZ is found in the area prostrema in the floor of the fourth ventricle and is, therefore accessible to stimuli present in either the blood or the cerebral spinal fluid. For this reason the CTZ is generally considered to be the primary mediator of drug induced emesis (Borison, 1974). Once stimulated, the CTZ activates the emetic center which ultimately induces emesis. Problems associated with invoking the CTZ as the control center for cisplatin induced emesis include the fact that this drug has very poor penetration through the blood–

brain barrier (Smith and Taylor, 1974) and that emesis is most frequently delayed in onset (Rozencweig et al., 1977; Sridhar et al., 1985). Because of these facts, it is possible that a peripheral component in emetic control may regulate cisplatin-induced emesis.

Of concern for this discussion are the cholinergic and dopaminergic receptors as they appear to be involved in modulating both the peripheral and CTZ components of chemical induced nausea and vomiting. Indeed, many of the effective antiemetic agents used to control cisplatin induced emesis have as part of their pharmacologic action the blockade of these receptors. Direct correlation of these actions and the antiemetic activity has yet to be established.

The clinical impact of this toxicity ranges from patient discomfort to loss of patient compliance and in some cases physical injury. Severe nausea and vomiting causes fatigue and anorexia which can result in depression, anxiety, and anticipatory emesis (defined as emetic episodes initiated by the prospect of receiving cisplatin). The effects have an obvious negative impact on the patient's quality of life and can lead to major psychosocial problems (Maguire et al., 1980; Morrow, 1984; Laszlo, 1983). Uncontrolled vomiting results in patients refusing subsequent therapy or at least a significant delay in scheduled courses of therapy (Jacobs et al., 1980; Penta, et al., 1983). Because there is a direct correlation between intensity of therapy and the overall effectiveness of this therapy, any such delay would have a detrimental effect on potentially curative regimen. Finally, medical complications directly related to cisplatin induced emesis such as esophageal tears, fractures, wound dehiscence, and malnutrition can compromise the patient's tolerance to subsequent therapy (Enck, 1977; Whitehead, 1975).

Obviously, proper clinical management of nausea and vomiting is of utmost importance to insure maximum antitumor efficacy of cisplatin. Such management can be divided into direct patient support and pharmacological interventions. Although the latter represents the mainstay of clinical practice the importance of the former must not be underestimated.

Prior to the initiation of therapy, the patient is given proper hydration and electrolyte disturbances are corrected. Alleviation of the anxiety associated with cancer chemotherapy should be attempted by providing good lines of communication between the professional staff (Stoudmire et al., 1984) and the patient as well as the opportunity for a change in environment for patients who develop anticipatory emesis (Laszlo, 1983).

A wide variety of antiemetic agents are available for the pharmacologic control of cisplatin induced emesis. Whereas the management of emesis has met with greatest success using combinations of antiemetics a brief discussion of the individual classes of these drugs is included below.

Inhibitors of Dopaminergic Transmission

Within this class of drugs are three of the most widely used antiemetics which include prochlorperazine, droperidol, and metoclopramide. Both prochlorperazine, a phenothiazine derivative, and droperidol, a butyrophenone, appear to act by inhibiting dopaminergic transmission in the CTZ (Wampler, 1983), whereas metoclopramide, a substituted benzamide, blocks the dopamine receptor in the CTZ and the upper gastrointestinal track (Albibi and McCallum, 1983).

Prochlorperazine has been the subject of the largest number of clinical investigations and although it is more effective than placebo when administered as a single agent few patients respond adequately to the drug (Wampler, 1983). Most studies investigating the efficacy of single agent antiemetics use prochlorperazine as a control (Johansson et al., 1982; Sallan et al., 1980). Recent clinical data suggest that earlier studies using conventional doses of prochlorperazine 10 to 15 mg orally (po) or intramuscular were insufficient to prevent cisplatin induced nausea and vomiting (Carr et al., 1985). By increasing the dose of prochlorperazine to 30 to 40 mg, a marked increase in efficacy was attained if the patient had been pretreated with diphenhydramine to prevent the extrapyramidal effects of high dose prochlorperazine (Carr et al., 1987). Other major complications associated with prochlorperazine include hypotension and drowsiness. This later effect may in actuality be beneficial since it may decrease the anxieties of the patient (Robins et al., 1979). The major role for this drug and for all of the antiemetics appears when in combination with other antiemetics; remarkable control of emesis caused by conventional doses of cisplatin is attained.

Droperidol is structurally and pharmacologically related to prochlorperazine. The data available for droperidol as a single agent are sparse but the efficacy of the drug appears to be somewhat higher than that of prochlorperazine (Jacobs et al., 1980; Ronan and Buchsbaum, 1981). The greatest usefulness of droperidol is in combination with other antiemetics, such as metoclopramide and dexamethasone. When used in such combinations, rather impressive control of nausea and vomiting has been reported (Sridhar and Donnelly, 1988; Kelley et al., 1986; Donowitz et al., 1984). Droperidol must be administered IV thus limiting the use of the drug to the clinical setting. The major side effect of conventional doses of droperidol is sedation but significant hypotension and tachycardia can be encountered with high-dose droperidol (>10 mg, IV loading dose and 4 mg, IV every hour as a maintenance dose) (Kelley et al., 1986). Although extra pyramidal effects have been observed they are less frequent than with prochlorperazine.

Metoclopramide has significant antiemetic activity as a single agent when administered either IV or po (orally). As a single agent administered at a relatively high dose (1–3 mg/kg IV) the emesis will be controlled in approximately 40% of the patients treated with cisplatin (Gralla et al., 1981; 1984; Raila et al., 1985). Because metoclopramide acts both centrally and peripherally (Akarwi, 1983; Harrington et al., 1983) this may explain the superiority of the antidopaminergic drug over prochloperazine and droperidol. As with the other antiemetics the effects of dose modulation and drug combinations are being evaluated to maximize efficacy (Pariknh et al., 1988). The primary toxicities of metoclopramide are mild sedation, diarrhea, and extrapyramidal effects (Albibi and McCallum, 1983). The latter toxicity is dose and age related but is manageable with diphenhydramine administered prophylactically (Kris et al., 1985). An interesting observation reported by Saller et al. (1986) was that transdermal electrical nerve stimulation not only enhanced the antiemetic activity of metoclopramide but also diminished the extrapyramidal effects of the drug.

Domperidone entered clinical trials as a possible replacement for high dose metoclopramide because of claimed advantages of fewer side effects. Much of this hope was based on preclinical studies in which it was shown that domperidone crossed the blood–brain barrier much less effectively than did other antidopaminergics (Ladruon and Leysen, 1979; Heykantis et al., 1981). To date, clinical trials have failed to substantiate the increased safety of this drug nor has any increased efficacy been shown for domperidone (Weaving et al., 1984; Tonato et al., 1985). Therefore, the future of this drug appears doubtful.

Corticosteriods

Both dexamethasone and methylprednisolone have demonstrated antiemetic activity in cisplatin-treated patients (Rich et al., 1980; D'Olimipio et al., 1985). Comparing the efficacy of these drugs to the antidopaminergics is difficult as optimal doses are still being established for the latter. Although the corticosteriods are superior to conventional doses of the antidopaminergics, high-dose metoclopropramide is clearly better than either corticosteroid.

The mechanism of action of these drugs is not understood but appears to be related in some way to their effects on prostaglandins (Rich et al., 1980). Currently, corticosteriods are only used in combination with other antiemetics to control cisplatin-induced emesis. Whereas methylprednisolone must be given parenterally at doses of 125 to 250 mg/kg every four hr to be effective, dexamethasone has been shown to be active whether given IV or po at doses of 10 to 20 mg/kg.

There are several toxicities associated with the use of the corticosteroids but the most prominent are euphoria, fluid retention, anxiety, and insomnia. A concern that may only be of academic interest since it has never been substantiated is the immunosuppressive activity of the cortiocosteroids and the concomitant possibility of increased infection and even tumor promotion (Paine, 1984; Haid, 1981).

Benzodiazepines

Several benzodiazepines have been tested as antiemetics with little success. In 1984, Bishop et al. reported lorazepam, a minor tranquilizer, improved the effectiveness of other antiemetics when combined with these active agents (Bishop et al., 1984). The mechanism of this adjunct activity appears not to be result of antiemetic properties of lorazepam but rather due to its amnestic and anxiolytic properties (Laszlo et al., 1985; Gordon et al., 1989). Thus, the addition of lorazepam (2–4 mg, given po just prior to cisplatin administration) as an antiemetic results in a marked increase in the subjective response of the patient to cisplatin therapy and may have a major role in decreasing anticipatory vomiting experienced by many patients.

Antihistamines

Whereas the antihistamines are effective in controlling nausea and vomiting induced by vestibular activity, these compounds appear to have no activity against cisplatin-induced vomiting. Diphenhydramine, an antihistamine with anticholinergic properties, is used frequently in combination with the antidopaminergics. In these circumstances the primary role for diphenhydramine (50 mg every 4–6 hr, IV) is in the control of the extrapyramidal effects of the antidopaminergics (Sridhar and Donnelly, 1988). However, the extrapyramidal effects in patients <20 years old and agitated depression in older patients remain a dose limiting toxicity of the antidopaminergics even when combined with diphenhydramine (Agonstinucci et al., 1988; Grunberg et al., 1988).

Cannabinoids

The cannabinoids were first used to control emesis induced by low-to-moderate doses of cisplatin as marijuana cigarettes. The active component of marijuana was demonstrated to be tetrahyrocannabinol (THC) (Sallan et al., 1975) and since that time THC has been made available to cancer patients (Kluin-Neleman et al., 1979; Orr et al., 1980). More recently two synthetic cannabinoids, nabilone, or levonantradol, have been shown to have clinical efficacy (Vincent et al., 1983; Citron et al., 1985). The cannabinoids, although quite effective antiemetics, cause several side effects such as dysphoria, ataxia, confusion, orthostatic hypotension, and sedation and has met with poor acceptance in many patient populations (Vincent et al., 1983). The addition of phenothiazine to THC has effectively controlled many of the adverse reactions to THC and has resulted in increased acceptance of the cannabinoids as antiemetic agents (Artim and Dibella, 1983).

Platinum Analogs

Both CBDCA and CHIP are emetogenic. The severity and incidence of this toxicity is dose related but not as great as that encountered with cisplatin. Whether CBDCA is more or less emetogenic than in CHIP remains to be established but with either complex the toxicity appears to be readily manageable for the patient.

Neurotoxicity

Although peripheral neuropathies had been observed in clinical and experimental studies using conventional dosages of cisplatin, the advent of high-dose cisplatin has truly brought this toxicity forward (Ozols and Young, 1985). Several clinical studies have clearly established an important dose–response relationship with cisplatin in head and neck, testicular, and ovarian cancer patients (Dembo, 1987; Forastiere et al., 1987; Bruckner et al., 1981). As discussed above, doses beyond 100 to 120 mg/m^2 were not routinely possible because of dose-limiting nephrotoxicity.

With the advent of hydration and diuresis and hypertonic saline with chloresis, doses of cisplatin as high as 200 mg/m^2 are possible without significant renal toxicity. Unfortunately, these interventions have little or no effect on toxicities not related to the kidney. Consequently, a large number of patients receiving high-dose cisplatin will develop some degree of peripheral neurotoxicity (Ozols and Young, 1985; Panici et al., 1987).

Whereas incidence and severity of neurotoxicity has been significantly increased with the use of high-dose cisplatin, the clinical manifestations are similar to those reported for more conventional dose of the drug. The most frequent complaint is a numbness and tingling in the distal extremities (Kedar et al., 1978; Reinstein et al., 1980). After cessation of drug treatment, the neuropathy often improves (Hadley and Herr, 1979). If the cisplatin therapy is continued, more severe neurologic toxicities are noted, including ataxia, gait disturbances, loss of manual dexterity, and becoming wheelchair bound. These latter toxicities are primarily caused by a marked loss of proprioception. The prognosis of these severe neurologic disorders is not good as little recovery has been observed to date in these patients (Ozols and Young, 1985).

Patients have been evaluated using neurophysiologic methods including electromyography, motor conduction velocities, and sensory conduction velocities (Carenza et al., 1986; Thompson et al., 1984). The most common changes in these patients included a reduction of the interference pattern of the motor unit potentials and abundant fibrillation at rest as measured by electromyogram (EMG) and a marked decrease in sensory neuronal conduction velocities (Carenza et al., 1986; Thompson et al., 1984). Interestingly, the conduction velocities of motor neurons appears to remain relatively intact. Histologic examination of peripheral neuronal tissue revealed axonal degeneration gradually progressing from the periphery to the cell body, with secondary myelin breakdown (Thompson et al., 1984). The description of this toxicity is quite similar to that reported for the "dying-back neuropathies" commonly linked to such metals as arsenic (LeQuesne et al., 1977) and thallium (Cavanagh, 1974).

The mechanism of this toxicity is not known. Tissue distribution studies have demonstrated that little platinum is in central nervous tissue (Smith and Taylor, 1974; Sternson et al., 1984). These data provide a possible explanation for the apparent sparing of the CNS by cisplatin. Recent work by Oakes et al. reported that cisplatin caused a dose dependent reversible inhibition of the Ca^{++} dependent action potential whereas transplatinum and platinic (IV) chloride, both of which lack cytotoxic activity, failed to produce any significant inhibition of this action potential (Oakes et al., 1987).

No effective method of diminishing this dose-limiting toxicity of cisplatinum has been conclusively established thus far. Selected studies have reported that divided doses of cisplatin given on days 1 and 8 produce less neurotoxicity than five daily doses of the same drug when compared on a total drug delivered basis (Gandara et al., 1986). Glover et al. reported that WR2721 appeared to decrease the incidence and severity of cisplatin-induced neurological complications (Glover et al., 1986). Although not currently in clinical trials, experimental data indicate that Org.2766, an $ACTH_{4\text{-}9}$ analog prevented the slowing of sensory nerve conduction rates in rats but had no effect on the antitumor activity of cisplatin (de Konig et al., 1987; Gerritsen van der Hoop et al., 1988). Clinical trials designed to determine the toxicities of Org.2766 have recently begun in the Netherlands (Gerritsen van der Hoop et al.,

1989) and once determined it is planned that clinical trials in combination with cisplatin will be initiated. At present, careful monitoring of the patient for the onset of neurotoxic effects is the only recourse available when cisplatin is administered.

Although peripheral neurotoxicity is observed relatively frequently, and may be a major dose-limiting toxicity, there are few reports of CNS involvement. The symptoms of a sudden electrical shock traveling from the spine to the legs following flexion of the neck, commonly referred to as Lhermitte's sign, have been observed in a few patients receiving cisplatin (Eeles et al., 1986; Walther et al., 1987). As with the peripheral neuropathies, Lhermitte's sign is thought to result from demyelination of the nerve tract.

Visual disturbances, including blurred vision and altered color perception, have been reported in patients after receiving platinum based chemotherapy for germinal cell tumors (Wilding et al., 1985; Kupersmith et al., 1988). These effects may be accompanied by seizures and encephalopathy and appear to be related to the total dose of cisplatin administered (Berman and Mann, 1980; Cohen and Cuneo, 1983; Hitchings and Thompson, 1988). Berman and Mann (1980) observed that concentration of platinum in the CSF and the serum were virtually identical. As stated above the intact blood–brain barrier represents a fairly impenetrable barrier for cisplatin and consequently little platinum is found in the CNS. It is possible that patients developing CNS toxicity have had the blood–brain barrier manipulated either through the disease, the high-dose platinum or by the use of mannitol diuresis.

These CNS toxicities appear to be relatively rare and somewhat reversible following cessation of drug therapy but must be watched for in patients receiving cisplatin therapy. Whether the second generation platinum complexes cause similar toxicities has yet to be established.

Platinum Analogs

Results coming from Phase I and Phase II studies on CBDCA and CHIP have shown both complexes to be less neurotoxic than cisplatin while maintaining comparable antitumor activity (Mbidde et al., 1986; Fuks et al., 1987; Anderson et al., 1988). Whether this apparent decrease in toxic potential will remain as doses of these complexes increase in future clinical trials remains to be seen. In this vein, Ozols et al. have recently reported that high-dose CBDCA in refractory ovarian cancer patients did not cause clinically apparent neurotoxicity (Ozols et al., 1987). Thus, the second generation platinum complexes appear to have significant advantages over the parent cisplatin with respect to the toxicologic complications.

Ototoxicity

Ototoxicity was detected in preclinical toxicity studies involving the Rhesus monkey (Standnicki et al., 1975), and thereafter substantiated in early clinical trials. This toxicity appears to be directly related to damage to the organ of Corti. Wright and Schaefer studied the inner ear changes in postmortem tissue samples taken from five patients (1982). They reported destruction of outer hair cells in all rows of the basal turn of the cochlea but that the severity of damage decreased in the direction of apical turns. Similar cochlear abnormalities have been observed in other clinical and experimental animal studies (Tange, 1987; Kohn et al., 1988; Towfight et al., 1983) and appear quite comparable to those seen with aminoglycoside cochlear damage (Schweitzer et al., 1984).

In humans, the incidence of ototoxicity has ranged from 0 to 90% depending upon a number of factors including: the method used to evaluate hearing loss, the individual dose administered, the total dose administered, the method of drug administration, and predisposing patient characteristics, such as age, prior hearing status, previous therapy. Those studies reporting a low incidence of hearing loss have relied almost exclusively on subjective hearing loss by the patient. In contrast, those studies reporting a high incidence of ototoxicity relied primarily on audiometric testing procedures. The majority of studies have measured only the conventional frequencies (250–8000 Hz) and reported hearing losses to occur most frequently three to four days after cisplatin administration. In these studies the greatest hearing loss is observed in the high frequency range of 4000 to 8000 Hz (Rybak, 1981; Fausti et al., 1984; Helson et al., 1979). More recently, clinicians have included the ultra-high frequency (UHF) range (9000–20,000 Hz) measurements and have found that the initial, and sometimes only, changes in hearing occur in frequencies above the normal test range (van der Hulst et al., 1988; Kopelman et al., 1988).

When low-to-moderate doses of cisplatin (50–100 mg/m^2) were administered, toxicities were most marked in patients receiving bolus injections. Whether administered as an infusion or as a bolus hearing loss appears to be rare when low doses were administered (50 mg/m^2 given every 3–4 weeks) but became clinically important when dose accumulation exceeded 500 mg/m^2 (Chiuten et al., 1981). Recently, Kopelman et al. (1988) reported that high-dose cisplatin administered to patients with advanced disease but normal hearing resulted in 100% of the patients having hearing loss in the UHF range after one to two doses. With repeated doses hearing loss became evident in the high frequency range as well. Several reports have demonstrated that hypertonic saline used in conjunction with high-dose saline was ineffective in diminishing either the incidence or the severity of cisplatin-induced ototoxicity (Bajorin et al., 1987; Pollera et al., 1988; Haines et al., 1987). Finally, while five-day continuous infusion of cisplatin reduced the myelosuppression and hypomagnesemia seen with a similar dose of the drug administered as five daily bolus injections, no effect on the ototoxicity was noted.

To date no pharmacologic intervention has had any success in decreasing this troublesome toxicity. Although the use of diuretics, hydration, and hypertonic saline have had dramatic effects on the nephrotoxicity of cisplatin, patients receiving these renal protectants still develop ototoxicity. Schweitzer and co-workers have demonstrated that fosfomycin, an inhibitor of aminoglycoside ototoxicity, had marked effect in reducing cisplatin induced morphologic and functional changes in the guinea pig inner ear (Schweitzer et al., 1986). This intriguing observation has not been confirmed in clinical studies.

Platinum Analogs

Conflicting data exist for the ototoxic potential of the platinum analogs. In the guinea pig model neither CBDCA nor CHIP produced measurable changes in the inner ear (Schweitzer et al., 1986). In clinical studies, van der Hulst et al. (1988) reported little difference between CBDCA and cisplatin in hearing loss observed in patients treated with clinically equivalent doses of the two drugs. In contrast, Tamura et al. (1988) observed no ototoxicity with CBDCA administered at doses equivalent to those used by van der Hulst et al. However, far less stringent auditory assessment was used in the former study. Finally, Biship et al. (1987) noted only minimal ototoxicity when CBDCA was administered as three daily injections of 100 mg/m^2 in combination with VP-16. The ultimate determination of the ototoxicity of CBDCA awaits large-scale clinical trials but at present it would appear safe to conclude that CBDCA is at least no more ototoxic than the parent cisplatin.

In summary, ototoxicity remains problematic for the patient receiving platinum complexes. The most effective means of diminishing this toxicity appears to be through careful audiometric evaluation (at both high frequency and UHF ranges) of the patient prior to initiation of therapy and at frequent intervals throughout the therapeutic regimen.

Vascular Disorders

The treatment of testicular carcinoma requires rather intensive therapy combining vinblastine, bleomycin, and cisplatin most frequently. A surprisingly high incidence of acute vascular disorders including Raynaud's phenomenon, angina pectoris, transient ischemia of the toes, cerebrovascular accidents, and myocardial infarction in this patient population (Edwards et al., 1979; Kukla et al., 1982; Samuels et al., 1987; Doll et al., 1986). Whether these vascular events result from cisplatin alone or only in combination with other drugs has not been established.

What is known is that nearly 40% of the patients receiving curative platinum vinblastive-bleomycin (PVB) therapy will experience one or more of these toxicities and can result in life-threatening events. A recent study by Stefenelli et al. (1988) was designed to evaluate the frequency of cardiovascular complaints and the time of onset and duration of ischemic events in different vascular beds of 21 patients treated for testicular cancer. No correlation was found between the dose of drugs administered or the duration of therapy but arterial occlusive events, resulting in angina pectoris (38%), Raynaud's phenomenon (33%), and transient ischemia (29%), were frequent and common toxicities.

The mechanism of this toxicity is not known. Several hypotheses have been put forth. High levels of circulating von Willibrand's factor antigen have been associated with occurrence of Raynaud's phenomenon and have been reported in patients who subsequently suffer cerebrovascular accidents following cisplatin-containing chemotherapy (Kahaleh et al., 1981; Licciardello et al., 1984). Hypomagnesemia is a common toxicity of cisplatin, occurring in approximately 75 to 85% of patients treated with this drug (Vogelzang et al., 1985; Schilsky and Anderson, 1979). Because magnesium plays a significant role in the maintenance of vascular smooth muscle tone alterations in magnesium levels could have a marked effect on the vasculature (Altura et al., 1984). Indeed, Turlapaty and Altura reported that magnesium deficiency caused spasms of the coronary vessels in dogs (1980). Another possible cause of vascular complications is dysfunction of the autonomic nervous system, particularly, increased alpha-adrenergic activity. It is likely that more than one of these mechanisms is responsible for vascular complications associated with cisplatin administration. Smoking seems to increase the incidence of vascular complications (Vogelzang et al., 1981). Unfortunately, little is known about effective clinical management of these toxicities.

The platinum complexes are effective in the treatment of several forms of human malignancies. As with all antitumor drugs this efficacy comes at a rather severe cost of host toxicity. The parent complex, cisplatin, causes a number of significant and, at times, life-threatening toxicities. As a result of intensive clinical and preclinical investigations many of these toxicities are now preventable or at least controllable. The introduction of second-generation platinum complexes may further diminish the adverse effects of this important class of anticancer drugs.

REFERENCES

Aamdal S, Fodstad O, and Pihl A Some procedures to reduce cis platinum toxicity reduce antitumor activity. Cancer Treat Rev 1987 14:389–395.

Abe R, Akiyoshi T, Koba F, Tsuji H, and Baba T "Two route chemotherapy" using intra-arterial cisplatin and intravenous thiosulfate, its neutralizing agent, for hepatic malignancies. Eur J Cancer Clin Oncol 1988 24:1671–1674.

Agostinucci WA, Gannon RH, Golub GR, Martin RS, Schauer PK, and Dinonno EB Continuous i.v. infusion versus multiple bolus doses of metoclopramide for the prevention of cisplatin-induced emesis. Clin Pharmacol 1988 7:454–457.

Akwari OE The gastroinestinal tract in chemotherapy induced emesis: A final common pathway. Drugs 1983 25:18–34.

Albibi R and McCallum R Metoclopramide: Pharmacology and clinical application. Ann Intern Med 1983 98:86–95.

Al-Sarraf M, Fletcher W, Oishi N, Pugh R, Hewlett JW, Balducci L, McCracken J, and Padilla F Cisplatin hydration with and without mannitol diuresis in refractory disseminated malignant melanoma. Cancer Treat Rep 1982 66:31–35.

Al-Sarraf M, Metch B, Kish J, Rinehart JJ, Schuller DE, and Coltman CA Jr Platinum analogs in recurrent and advanced head and neck cancer: A Southwest Oncology Group and Wayne State University study. Cancer Treat Rep 1987 71:723–726.

Altura BM, Altura BT, and Gebrewold A Magnesium deficiency and hypertension: Correlation between magnesium deficient diets and microcirculatory changes in situ. Science 1984 223:1315–1317.

Anderson H, Wagstaff J, Crowther D, Swindell R, Lind MJ, McGregor J, Timms MS, Brown D, and Palmer P Comparative toxicity of cisplatin, carboplatin (CBDCA) and iproplatin (CHIP) in combination with cyclophosphamide in patients with advanced epithelial ovarian cancer. Eur J Cancer Clin Oncol 1988 24:1471–1479.

Artim R and DiBella N Tetrahydrocannabinol plus prochlorperazine for refactory nausea and vomiting. Proc ASCO 1983 2:85.

Bajorin D, Bosl GJ, and Fein R Phase I trials of escalating doses of cisplatin in hypertonic saline. J Clin Oncol 1987 5:1589–1593.

Baum ES, Gaynon P, Greenberg L, Krivit W, and Hammond D Phase II trial of cisplatin in refractory childhood cancer: Children's Cancer Study Group report. Cancer Treat Rep 1981 65:815–822.

Berman IJ and Mann MP Seizures and transient cortical blindness associated with cisplatinum (II) diamminedichloride (PDD) therapy in a thirty year old man. Cancer 1980 45:764–766.

Bhuchar VK and Lanzotti VJ High dose cisplatin for lung cancer. Cancer Treat Rep 1982 66:375–376.

Biship JF, Olver I, Wolf M, Matthews J, Long M, Bingham J, Hillcost B, and Cooper I A randomized double-blind cross over study of a new antiemetic in patients receiving cytotoxic agents and prochlorperazine. J Clin Oncol 1984 2:691–695.

Bishop JF, Raghavan D, Stuart-Harris R, Morstyn G, Aroney R, Kefford R, Yuen K, Lee J, Gianoutsos P, and Olver IN Carboplatin (CBDCA, JM-8) and VP-16-213 in previously untreated patients with small cell lung cancer. J Clin Oncol 1987 5:1574–1578.

Borch RF and Pleasant ME Inhibition of cis-platinum nephrotoxicity by diethyldithiocarbamate rescue in a rat model. Proc Natl Acad Sci USA 1979 76:6611–6614.

Borch RF, Katz JC, and Lieder PH Effect of diethyldithiocarbamate rescue on tumor response to cis-platinum in a rat model. Proc Natl Acad Sci USA 1980 77:5442–5444.

Borch RF, Dedon PC, and Montine TJ Experimental approaches to reducing platinum induced kidney toxicity. In: Organ Directed Toxicities of Anticancer Drugs Hacker MP, Lazo JS, and Tritton TR Eds Martinus-Nijhoff Publishers, Boston 1988 pp. 189–202.

Borison H Area prostrema: Chemoreceptor trigger zone for vomiting—is that all? Life Sci 1974 14:1807–1817.

Borison H and Wang S Physiology and pharmacology of vomiting. Pharmacol Rev 1953 5:193–230.

Bozinno JM, Prasad V, and Koriech OM Avoidance of renal toxicity by 24 hour infusion of cisplatin. Cancer Treat Rep 1981 65:351–352.

Bruckner HW, Wallach R, Cohen CJ, Deppe G, Kabakow B, Ratner L, and Holland JF High dose cisplatin for the treatment of refractory ovarian cancer. Gynecol Oncol 1981 12:61–67.

Cafruny EJ, Farah A, and DiStefano HS Effects of mercurial diuretic mersalyl on protein bound sulfhydryl groups in the cytoplasm of rat kidney cells. J Pharmacol Exp Ther 1955 115:390–401.

Cantwell BMJ, Franks CR, and Harris AL A phase II study of the platinum analogues JM8 and JM9 in malignant pleural mesothelioma. Cancer Chemother Pharmacol 1986 18:286–288.

Carenza L, Villani C, Framarino dei Malatesta ML, ProsperiPorta R, Millefiorini M, Antonini G, Bolasco P, Bandiera G, and Marzetti L Peripheral neuropathy and ototoxicity of dichlorodiammine platinum: Instrumental evaluation. Preliminary results. Gynecol Oncol 1986 25:244–249.

Carr BI, Blaney DW, Goldberg DA, Braly P, Metter GE, and Doroshow HJ High doses of prochlorperazine for cisplatin induced emesis. A prospective random dose response study. Cancer 1987 2165–2169.

Carr BJ, Bertrand M, Browning S, Doroshow JH, Presant C, Pulane B, and Hill LR A comparison of the antiemetic efficacy of prochlorperazine and metoclopramide for the treatment of cisplatin induced emesis: A prospective randomized double blind study. J Clin Oncol 1985 3:1127–1132.

Cavanagh JB The effect of thallium salts with particular reference to the nervous system. Q J Med 1974 43:293–297.

Chiuten D, Vogl SE, Kaplan BH, and Greenwald E Is there a cumulative or delayed toxicity from cis-diamminedichloroplatinum II (DDP). Proc Amer Assoc Cancer Res 1981 22:163.

Cinollo G, Dini G, Lanino E, Sindaco F, and Garaventa A Positive direct antiglobin test in a pediatric patient following high dose cisplatin. Cancer Chemother Pharmacol 1988 21:85–86.

Citron M, Herman T, Vreeland F, Krasno S, Fossiek B, Harwood S, Franlin R, and Cohen M Antiemetic efficacy of levonantradol compared to delta-9-tetrahydrocannabinol for chemotherapy induced nausea and vomiting. Cancer Treat Rep 1985 69:109–112.

Clavel M, Monfardini S, Gundersen S, Kaye S, Siegenthaler P, Renard J, van Glabekke M, and Pinedo H Phase II study of iproplatin (CHIP, JM-9) in advanced testicular cancers progressing after prior chemotherapy. Eur J Cancer Clin Oncol 1988 24:1345–1348.

Cohen AI, Harberg J, and Citrin DL Measurement of urinary beta-2-microglobulin in the detection of cisplatin nephrotoxicity. Cancer Treat Rep 1981 65:1083–1085.

Cohen RJ and Cuneo RA Transient left homonymonous hemianopsia and encephalopathy following treatment of testicular carcinoma with cisplatinum, vinblastine and bleomycin. J Clin Oncol 1983 1:392–393.

Daugaard G, Abildgaard U, Holstein-Rathlou N, Bruunshuus I, Bucher D, and Leyssac PP Renal tubular function in patients treated with high dose cisplatin. Clin Pharmacol Ther 1988 44:164–172.

Dedon PC and Borch RF Characterization on the reactions of platinum antitumor agents with biologic and nonbiologic sulfur containing nucleophiles. Biochem Pharmacol 1987 36:1955–1964.

de Konig P, Niejt JP, Jennekens FGI, and Gispen WH Org.2766 protects from cisplatin induced neurotoxicity in rats. Exp Neurol 1987 97:746–750.

Dembo AJ Time-dose factors in chemotherapy: Expanding the concept of dose-intensity. J Clin Oncol 1987 3:694–696.

Dentino M, Luft FC, Yum MN, Williams SD, and Einhorn LH Long term effect of cis- diamminedichloride platinum (CDDP) on renal function and structure in man. Cancer 1978 41:1274–1281.

Diener U, Knoll E, Langer B, Rautenstrauch H, Ratge D, and Wisser H Urinary excretion of N-acetyl-beta-D-glucosaminidase and alanine aminopeptidase in patients receiving amikacin or cisplatinum. Clin Chim Acta 1981 112:149–157.

D'Olimpio J, Camacho F, Chandra P, Lesser M, Maldonado M, Wollner D, and Wiernik P Antiemetic efficacy of high dose dexamethasone versus placebo in patients receiving cisplatin based chemotherapy: A randomized double blind controlled clinical trial. J Clin Oncol 1985 3:1133–1135.

Dobyan DC, Bull JM, Strebel FR, Sunderland BA, and Bulger RE Protective effects of O-(beta-hydroxyethyl)-rutoside on cis-platinum-induced acute renal failure in the rat. Lab Invest 1986 55:557–563.

Doll DC, Ringenberg QS, and Yarbro JW Vascular toxicity associated with antineoplastic agents. J Clin Oncol 1986 4:1405–1417.

Donowtiz GS, O'Quinn AG, and Smith ML Antiemetic efficacy of high dose corticosteroids and droperidol in cisplatin emesis. Gynecol Oncol 1984 18:320–325.

Edwards GS, Lane M, and Smith FE Long term treatment with cis-dichlorodiammineplatinum(II)-vinblastine-bleomycin: Possible association with severe coronary artery disease. Cancer Treat Rep 1979 63:551–552.

Eeles R, Tait DM, and Peckham MJ Lhermitte's sign as a complication of cisplatin containing chemotherapy of testicular cancer. Cancer Treat Rep 1986 70:905–907.

Einhorn L and Furnas B Improved chemotherapy in disseminated testicular cancer. J Clin Hematol Oncol 1976 7:662–671.

Eisenberger M, Hornedo J, Silva H, Donehower R, Spaulding M, and Van Echo D Carboplatin (NCS-241,240): An active platinum analog for the treatment of squamous cell carcinoma of the head and neck. J Clin Oncol 1986 4:1506–1509.

Enck RE Mallory-Weiss lesion following cancer chemotherapy. Lancet 1977 2:927–928.

Erickson LC, Zwelling LA, Ducore JM, Sharkey NA, and Kohn KW Differential cytotoxicity and DNA cross linking in normal and transformed human fibroblasts treated with DDP. Cancer Res 1981 41:2791–2794.

Erye HJ and Ward JH Control of cancer chemotherapy induced nausea and vomiting. Cancer 1984 54:2642–2648.

Fausti SA, Schechter MA, Rappaport BZ, Frey RH, and Mass RE Early detection of cisplatin ototoxicity: Selected case reports. Cancer 1984 53:224–231.

Forastiere AA, Takasugi BJ, Baker SR, Wolf GT, and Kudia-Hatch V High dose cisplatin in advanced head and neck cancer. Cancer Chemother Pharmacol 1987 19:155–158.

Fuks JZ, Wadler S, and Wiernik PH Phase I and II agents in cancer therapy: Two cisplatin analogues and high dose cisplatin in hypertonic saline or with thiosulfate protection. J Clin Pharmacol 1987 27:357–365.

Gandara DR, DeGregorio MW, Wald H, Wilbur B, Kohler W, Lawrence HJ, Deissarth AB, and George CB High-dose cisplatin in hypertonic saline: Reduced toxicity of a modified dose schedule and correlation with plasma pharmacokinetics. A Northern California Oncology Group pilot study in non-small-cell lung cancer. J Clin Oncol 1986 4:1787–1793.

Gandara DR, Mansour R, Wold H, and George C Dose-limiting myelosuppression associated with high dose cisplatin (200 mg/m^2) in hypertonic saline. Cancer Treat Rep 1986 70:820–821.

Gaynon PS, Ettinger LJ, Moel D, Baum ES, Krivit W, and Hammond GD Pediatric phase I trial of carboplatin: A children's cancer study group report. Cancer Treat Rep 1987 71:1039–1042.

Gerritsen van der Hoop R, de Konig P, Boven E, Neijt JP, Jennekens FGI Efficacy of the neuropeptide ORG.2766 in the prevention and treatment of cisplatin induced neurotoxicity in rats. Eur J Cancer Clin Oncol 1988 24:637–642.

Gerritsen van der Hoop R, Vecht C, Elderson A, van den Berg MEL, Haanstra W, Boogerd W, ten Bokkel Huinink W, Heimans J, Vermoken J, Gispen W, and Neijt J ORG.2766, an ACTH(4-9) analog, prevents cisplatin induced neuropathy in ovarian cancer patients. Proc Amer Soc Clin Oncol 1989 8:150.

Getaz EP, Beckley S, and Fitzpatrick J Cisplatin induced amenia. N Engl J Med 1980 303:110–111.

Glover D, Glick JH, Weiler C, Yuhas JM, and Kligerman MM Phase I trials of WR-2712 and cis-platinum. Int J Radiat Oncol Biol Phys 1984 10:1781–1784.

Glover D, Glick JH, Weiler C, Fox K, Turris A, and Kligerman MM Phase I/II trials of WR2721 and cisplatinum. Int J Radiat Oncol Biol Phys 1986 12:1509–1512.

Glover D, Grabelsky S, Fox K, Weiler C, Cannon L, and Glick J Clinical trials of WR-2712 and cis-platinum. Int J Radiat Oncol Biol Phys 1989 16:1201–1204.

Gonzalez-Vitale JC, Hayes DM, Cvitkovic E, and Sternberg SS The renal pathology in clinical trials of cis-platinum (II) diamminedichloride. Cancer 1977 39:1362–1371.

Gordon CJ, Pazdur R, Ziccarelli A, Cummings G, and Al-Sarraf M Metoclopramide versus metoclopramide and lorazepam: Superiority of combined therapy in the control of cisplatin induced emesis. Cancer 1989 63:578–582.

Goren MP, Wright RK, and Horowitz ME Cumulative renal tubular damage associated with cisplatin nephrotoxicity. Cancer Chemother Pharmacol 1986 18:69–73.

Goren MP, Forastiere AA, Wright RW, Horowitz ME, Dodge RK, Kamen BA, Viar MF, and Pratt CB Carboplatin (CBDCA), iproplatin (CHIP) and high dose cisplatin in hypertonic saline evaluated for tubular nephrotoxicity. Cancer Chemother Pharmacol 1987 19:57–60.

Gralla R, Itri L, Pisko S, Squillante A, Kelien D, Braun D, Brodin L, Braun T, and Young C Antiemetic effect of high dose metoclopramide: Randomized trials with placebo and perchlorperazine in patients with chemotherapy-induced vomiting. N Engl J Med 1981 305:905–909.

Gralla R, Tyson L, Bordin L, Clark R, Verlan D, Kris M, Kalman L, and Groshen S Antiemetic therapy: A review of recent studies and a report of a random assignment trial comparing metoclopramide with delta-9-tetrahydrocannabinol. Cancer Treat Rep 1984 68:163–172.

Groth S, Nielsen H, Sorensen JB, Christensen AB, Pedersen AG, and Rorth M Acute and long-term nephro-toxicity of cis-platinum in man. Cancer Chemother Pharmacol 1986 17:191–196.

Grunberg SM, Ehler E, McDermed JE, and Akerley WL Oral metoclopropamide with or without diphenhydramine: Potential for prevention of late nausea and vomiting induced by cisplatin. JNCI 1988 80:864–868.

Guarino AM, Miller DJ, Arnold ST, Pritchard JB, Davis RD, Urbanek MA, Miller TJ, and Litterst CL Platinate toxicity: Past, present and prospects. Cancer Treat Rep 1979 63:1475–1483.

Hadley D, and Herr HW Peripheral neuropathy associated with cis-dichlorodiammineplatinum(II) treatment. Cancer 1979 44:2026–2028.

Haid M Steroid antiemesis may be harmful. N Engl J Med 1981 304:1237.

Haines I, Bosl D, Sprio R, Gerold F, Sessions R, Shah J, Strong E, Vikram B, and Harrison L Very-high-dose cisplatin with bleomycin infusion as initial treatment of advanced head and neck cancer. J Clin Oncol 1987 5:1594–1600.

Hall DJ, Diasio R, and Goplerud DR cis-Platinum in gynecological cancer. III. Toxicity. Am J Obstet Gynecol 1981 141:309–312.

Hannemann J and Baumann K Cisplatin induced lipid peroxidation and decrease of gluconeogenesis in rat kidney cortex: Different effects of antioxidants and radical scavengers. Toxicology 1988 51:119–132.

Harrington RJ, Hamilton CW, and Brogden RN Metoclopramide: An updated review of its pharmacological properties and clinical uses. Drugs 1983 25:451–494.

Hayes DM, Cvitkovic E, Golbey RB, Scheiner E, Helson L, and Krakoff IH High dose cis-diammine dichloride: Ameliolarion of renal toxicity by mannitol diuresis. Cancer 1977 39:1372–1381.

Helson L, Okonkwo E, Anton L, and Cvitkovic Clin Toxicol 1979 13:469–478.

Heykantis J, Knaeps A, Meuldermans W, and Michiels M On the pharmacokinetics of domperidone in animals and man. I. Plasma levels of domperidone in rats and dogs. Age related absorption and passage through the blood brain barrier in rats. Eur J Drug Metab Pharmacokin 1981 6:27–36.

Hirosawa A, Niitani H, Hayashibara K, and Tsuboi E Effects of sodium thiosulfate in combination therapy of cis dichlorodiammineplatinum and vindesine. Cancer Chemother Pharmacol 1989 23:255–258.

Hitchings RN, and Thompson DB Encephalopathy following cisplatin, bleomycin and vinblastine therapy for non-seminomatous germ cell tumour of testis. Aust NZJ Med 1988 18:67–68.

Holleran WM and DeGregorio MW Evolution of high dose cisplatin. Invest New Drugs 1988 6:135–142.

Howell SB and Taetle R Effect of sodium thiosulfate on cis-dichlorodiammineplatinum(II) toxicity and antitumor activity in L1210 leukemia. Cancer Treat Rep 1980 64:611–616.

Howell SB, Pfeifle CL, Wung WE, Olshen RA, Lucas WE, Yon JL, and Green M Intraperitoneal cisplatin with systemic thiosulfate protection. Ann Intern Med 1982 97:845–851.

Howell SB, Pfeifle CE, Wung WE, Olshen RA Intraperitoneal cisplatin with systemic thiosulfate protection. Cancer Res 1983 43:1426–1431.

Jacobs C, Kalman SM, and Tretton M Renal handling of cis dichlorodiammineplatinum (II). Cancer Treat Rep 1980 12:1223–1226.

Jacobs AJ, Deppe G, and Cohen CJ A comparison of the antiemetic effects of droperidol and perchloperazine in chemotherapy with cis-platinum. Gynecol Oncol 1980 10:55–57.

Johannson R, Kikku P, and Groenvoos M A double-blind, controlled trial of nabilone vs prochlroperazine for refactory emesis induced by cancer chemotherapy. Cancer Treat Rev 1982 9:25–33.

Kahaleh MB, Osborn I, and LeRoy EC Increased factor VIII/von Willibrand factor antigen and von Willibrand factor activity in scleroderma and Raynaud's phenomenon. Ann Intern Med 1981 94:482–485.

Kedar A, Cohen ME, and Freeman AI Peripheral neuropathy as a complication of dichlorodiammineplatinum (II) treatment. Cancer Treat Rep 1978 62:819–821.

Kelley SL, Braun TJ, Meyer TJ, Rempel P, and Pearlman NW Trial of droperidol as an antiemetic in cisplatin chemotherapy. Cancer Treat Rep 1986 70:469–472.

Kluin-Neleman JC, Neleman FA, Meuwissen OJ, and Maes RAA Delta-9-tetrahydrocannabinol (THC) as an antiemetic in patients treated with cancer chemotherapy: A double blind cross over study against placebo. Vet Hum Toxicol 1979 21:338–340.

Kociba RJ and Sleight SD Acute toxicologic and pathologic effects of cis-diamminedichloroplatinum (NSC 119875) in the male rat. Cancer Chemother Rep 1971 55:1–8.

Kohn S, Fradis M, Zidan J, Podoshin L, Robinson E, and Nir I Cisplatin ototoxicity in guinea pigs with special reference to toxic effects in the stria vascularis. Laryngoscope 1988 98:865–871.

Koeller JM, Trump DL, Tutsch KD, Earhart RH, Davis TE, and Tormey DC Phase I clinical trial and pharmacokinetics of carboplatin (NSC 241240) by a single monthly 30-minute infusion. Cancer 1986 57:222–225.

Kopelman J, Budnick AS, Kramer MB, Sessions RB, and Wong GY Ototoxicity of high dose cisplatin by bolus administration in patients with advanced cancers and normal hearing. Laryngoscope 1988 98:858–864.

Kovach JS, Moertel CG, Schutt AJ Phase II study of cis-diamminedichloroplatinum in advanced carcinoma of the large bowel. Cancer Chemother Rep 1973 57:357–359.

Krakoff IH Nephrotoxicity of cis-dichloro-diammine platinum (II). Cancer Treat Rep 1979 63:1523–1525.

Kris MG, Gralla RJ, Tyson LB, Clark RA, Kelsen DP, Reilly LK, Groshen S, Bosl GJ, and Kalman LA Improved control of cisplatin induced emesis with high dose metoclopramide and with combinations of metoclopramide, dexamethasone, and diphenyhdramine. Result of consecutive trials in 255 patients. Cancer 1985 55:527–534.

Kuhn JA, Argy WP, Rakowsky TA, Moriarty JK, Schreimer GE, and Schein PS Nephrotoxicity of cis-diamminedichloroplatinum (II) as measured by urinary beta-glucuronidase. Cancer Treat Rep 1980 64:1083–1086.

Kukla LJ, McGuire WP, Lad T, and Saltiel M Acute vascular episodes associated with therapy for carcinomas of the upper aerodigestive tract with bleomycin, vincristine and cisplatin. Cancer Treat Rep 1982 66:369–370.

Kupersmith MJ, Frohman LP, Choi IS, Foo SH, Hiesinger E, Berenstein A, Wise A, Carr RE and Ransohoff J Visual system toxicity following intra-arterial chemotherapy. Neurology 1988 38:284–289.

Ladruon PM and Leysen JE Domperidone, a specific in vitro dopamine antagonist, devoid of in vivo central dopaminergic activity. Biochem Pharmacol 1979 28:2161–2165.

Laszlo J Nausea and vomiting as major complications of cancer chemotherapy. Drugs 1983 25(suppl 1):1–7.

Laszlo J, Clark R, Hanson D, Tyson L, Crumpler L and Gralla R Lorazepam in cancer patients treated with cisplatin: A drug having amnestic, antiemetic and anxiolytic effects. J Clin Oncol 1985 3:864–869.

Legha S, Dimery I, Larson D, Goepfert H, and Bodey G Effect of hypertonic saline on the nephrotoxicity of cisplatin in patients with head and neck cancer. Proc Amer Soc Clin Oncol 1984 3:37.

LeQuesne PM and McLeod JG Peripheral neuropathy following a single exposure to arsenic. J Neurol Sci 1977 32:437–441.

Levi J, Jacobs C, Kalman S, McTigue M, and Weiner MW Mechanism of cis-platinum nephrotoxicity: I. Effects on sulfhydryl groups in rat kidneys. J Pharmacol Exp Ther 1980 213:545–550.

Licciardello J, Moake J, Rudy C, Karp D, and Hong W Increased von Willibrand factor antigen and vascular toxicity following cisplatin based combination chemotherapy. Proc Amer Soc Clin Oncol 1984 3:122C.

Litterst CL Alterations in the toxicity of cis-dichlorodiammineplatinum (II) and in tissue localization of platinum as a function of NaCl concentration in the vehicle of administration. Toxicol Appl Pharmacol 1981 61:99–108.

Maguire G, Tait A, Brooke M, Thomas C, Howat J and Sellwood R Psychiatric morbidity and physical toxicity associated with adjuvant chemotherapy after mastectomy. Br Med J 1980 281:1179–1180.

Maguet JP and Botour JL Platinum amine compounds: Importance of labile and inert ligands for the pharmacologic activities towards L1210 leukemia cells. JNC 1983 70:899–905.

Markman M, Cleary S, and Howell SB Nephrotoxicity of high dose intracavitary cisplatin with intravenous thiosulfate. Eur J Cancer 1985 21:1015–1018.

Mbidde EK, Harland SJ, Calvert AH, and Smith IE Phase II trial of carboplatin (JM8) in treatment of patients with malignant mesothelioma. Cancer Chemother Pharmacol 1986 18:284–285.

Meijer S, Mulder NH, Sleiffer DD, Donker AJM, Sluiter WJ, deJong PE, Schraffordt Koops H, and van der Hem GK Influence of combination chemotherapy with cis-diamminedichloroplatinum on renal function: Long term effects. Oncology 1983a 40:170–173.

Meijer S, Sleijfer DT, Mulder NH, Sluiter WJ, Marrink J, Schraffordt Koops H, Brouwers TM, Oldhoff J, van der Hem GK, and Mandema E Some effects of combination chemotherapy with cis-platinum on renal function in patients with nonseminomatous testicular carcinoma. Cancer 1983b 51:2035–2040.

Milano G, Caldani C, Khater R, Launey J-M, Soummer A-M, Namer M, and Schneider M Time-and dose-dependent inhibition of erythrocyte glutathione peroxidase by cisplatin. Biochem Pharmacol 1988 37:981–982.

Morrow G Clinical characteristics associated with the development of anticipatory nausea and vomiting in cancer patients undergoing chemotherapy treatment. J Clin Oncol 1984 2:1170–1176.

Motzer RJ, Bosi GJ, Tauer K, and Golbey R Phase II trial of carboplatin in patients with advanced germ cell tumors refactory to cisplatin. Cancer Treat Rep 1987 71:197–198.

Oakes SG, Santone KS, and Powis G Effect of some anticancer drugs on the surface membrane electrical properties of differentiated murine neuroblastoma cells. JNCI 1987 79:155–161.

Offerman JJ, Meijer S, Sleijfer DT, Mulder NH, Donker AJ, Koops HS and van der Hem GK Acute effects of cis-diamminedichloroplatinum (CDDP) on renal function. Cancer Chemother Pharmacolo 1984 12:36–38.

Orr, LE, McKernan JF, and Bloome B Antiemetic effect of tetrahyrdocannabinol: Compared with placebo and prochloroerazine in chemotherapy associated nausea and emesis. Arch Intern Med 1980 140:1431–1433.

Ostrow S, Egorin MJ, Hahn D High dose cisplatin therapy using mannitol versus furosemide diuresis: Comparative pharmacokinetics and toxicity. Cancer Treat Rep 1981 65:73–78.

Ozols RF, Corden BJ, Jacob J, Wesley MN, Ostchega Y, and Young RC High dose cisplatin in hypertonic saline. Ann Intern Med 1984 100:19–24.

Ozols RF and Young RC High dose cisplatin therapy in ovarian cancer. Semin Oncol 1985 12(suppl 6):21–30.

Ozols RF, Ostchega Y, Curt G, and Young RC High dose carboplatin in refactory ovarian cancer patients. J Clin Oncol 1987 5:197–201.

Paine T Antiemetic effect of dexamthasone. N Engl J Med 1984 311:1576–1577.

Panici PB, Greggi S, Scambia G, Di Roberto P, Iacobelli S, and Mancuso S High dose (200 mg/m^2) cisplatin induced neurotoxicity in primary advanced ovarian cancer patients. Cancer Treat Rep 1987 71:669–670.

Paredes J, Hong WK, Felder TB, Dimery IW, Choksi AJ, Newman RA, Castellanos AM, Robbins KT, McCarthy K, Atkinson N, Kramer A, Hersh E, and Geopfert H Prospective randomized trial of high dose cisplatin and fluorouracil infusion with or without sodium diethyldithiocarbamate in recurrent and/or metastatic squamous cell carcinoma of the head and neck. J Clin Oncol 1988 6:955–962.

Pariknh PM, Charak BS, Banavali SD, Koppikar SB, Giri N, Nadkarni P, Saikia TK, Gopal R, and Advani SH A prospective randomized double-blind trial comparing metoclopramide alone with metoclopramide plus dexamethasone in preventing emesis induced by high dose cisplatin. Cancer 1988 62:2263–2266.

Pendyala L, Madajewicz S, Lele SB, Arbuck SG, and Creaen PJ Evaluation of the nephrotoxicity of iproplatin (CHIP) in comparison to cisplatin by the measurement of urinary enzymes. Cancer Chemother Pharmacol 1985 15:203–207.

Penta J, Poster D, and Bruno S The pharmacologic treatment of nausea and vomiting caused by cancer chemotherapy: A review. In: Antiemetics and Cancer Chemotherapy. Laszlo J Ed Wilkins and Wilkins, Baltimore 1983 pp. 82–105.

Pfeifle CE, Howell SB, Felthouse RD, Woliver TBS, Andrews PA, Markman M, and Murphy MP High dose cisplatin with sodium thiosulfate protection. J Clin Oncol 1985 3:237–244.

Pollera CF, Marolla P, Nardi M, Ameglio F, Cozzo L, and Bevere F Very high-dose cisplatin-induced ototoxicity: A preliminary report on early and long-term effects. Cancer Chemother Pharmacol 1988 21:61–64.

Qazi R, Chang AY, Borch RF, Montine T, Dedon P, Loughner J, and Bennett JM Phase I clinical and pharmacokinetic study of diethyldithiocarbamate as a chemoprotector from toxic effects of cisplatin. JNCI 1988 80:1486–1488.

Raila F, Tonato M, Basusto C, Canelleti R, Morsia D, Pasalacqua R, DeCortanzo F, Donate D, Colombo N, Baalaton E, DelFavero A, Tognoni G, and Francosi M Antiemetic effect of two different high doses of metoclopramide in cisplatin-treated cancer patients. Cancer Treat Rep 1985 69:1353–1357.

Reed E, Poirier M, Young RC, and Ozols RF High dose cisplatin with hypertonic saline: Toxicity and therapeutic results. In: Organ Directed Toxicities of Anticancer Drugs Hacker MP, Tritton TR, and Lazo JS eds Martinus Nijhoff Publishers, Boston 1988 pp. 203–213.

Reinstein L, Ostrow S, and Weirnik PH Peripheral neuropathy after cis-platinum(II)(DPP) therapy. Arch Phys Med Rehabil 1980 61:280–282.

Rich W, Abdulhaygul G, and Disaia P. Methylprednisone as an antiemetic during cancer chemotherapy. Gynecol Oncol 1980 9:193–198.

Roberts JJ, Knox RJ, Pera MF, Friedlos F, and Lydall DA The role of platinum-DNA interactions in the cellular toxicity and anti-tumor effects of platinum coordination. In: Platinum and Other Coordination Compounds in Cancer Chemotherapy Nicolini M Ed Martinus-Nijhoff Publishing, Boston 1988 pp. 16–31.

Robins HI, Ershler WB, and DeJongh L The antiemetic effect of intravenous diazepam in patients receiving cis-diamminedichloroplatinum (II). Med Pediatr Oncol 1979 7:247–249.

Ronan L and Buchsbaum H Droperidol as an antiemetic in cisplatin chemotherapy. In: The Treatment of Cancer Chemotherapy Induced Nausea and Vomiting Poster DS, Penta JS, and Bruno S Eds Masson, New York 1981 pp. 209–213.

Rosenberg B Anticancer activity of cis-dichlorodiammineplatinum (II) and some relevant chemistry. Cancer Treat Rep 1979 63:1433–1438.

Rosenberg B, Van Camp L, and Krigas T Inhibition of cell division in Eschericia coli by electrolysis products from a platinum electrode. Nature 1965 205:698–699.

Rosenberg B, Van Camp L, Trosko JE, and Mansour VH Platinum compounds: A new class of potent antitumor agents. Nature 1969 222:385–386.

Rossof RH, Slayton RE, and Perlia CP Preliminary clinical experience with cis-diamminedichloroplatinum (II). Cancer 1972 30:1451–1456.

Rothenberg ML, Ostchega Y, Steinberg SM, Young RC, Hummel S, and Ozols RF High dose carboplatin with diethyldithiocarbamate in treatment of women with relapsed ovarian cancer. JNCI 1988 80:1488–1492.

Rozencweig M, Von Hoff DD, Slavik M, and Muggia FM Cis-diamminedichloroplatinum (II): A new anticancer drug. Ann Intern Med 1977 86:803–812.

Rozencweig M, Nicaise C, Beer M, Crespeigne N, Rijmenant MV, Lenaz L, and Kenis Y Phase I study of carboplatin given on a five day intravenous schedule. J Clin Oncol 1983 6:98–105.

Rybak LP Cis-platinum associated hearing loss. J Laryngol Otol 1981 95:745–757.

Safirstein R, Zelent AZ, and Gordon R Cisplatin nephrotoxicity: New insights into the mechanism. In: Organ Directed Toxicities of Anticancer Drugs Hacker MP, Tritton TR, and Lazo JS Eds Martinus-Nijhoff Publishing, Boston 1988 pp. 172–189.

Salem P, Khalyl M, Jabboury K, and Hashimi L Cis diamminedichloroplatinum (II) by 5 day continuous infusion. A new dose schedule with minimal toxicity. Cancer 1984 53:837–840.

Sallan SE, Zinberg NE, and Fei E III Antiemetic effect of delta-9-tetrahydrocannabinol in patients receiving cancer chemotherapy. N Engl J Med 1975 293:795–797.

Sallan SE, Cronin C, Zelen M, and Zinberg NE Antiemetics in patients receiving chemotherapy for cancer: A randomized comparison of delta-9-tetrahydrocannabinol and prochlorperazine. N Engl J Med 1980 302:135–138.

Saller R, Heelenbrecht D, Buhring M, and Hess H Enhancement of the antiemetic action of metoclopramide against cisplatin induced emesis by transdermal electrical nerve stimulation. J Clin Pharmacol 1986 26:115–119.

Samuels BL, Vogelzang NJ, and Kennedy BJ Severe vascular toxicity associated with vinblastine, bleomycin, and cisplatin chemotherapy. Cancer Chemother Pharmacol 1987 19:253–256.

Schaeppi U, Heyman IA, Fleischman RW, Rosenkrantz H, Ilievski V, Phelan R, Cooney D, and Davis R cis-Diamminedichloroplatinum (II)(NSC-119875): Preclinical toxicologic evaluation of an intraveneous injection in dogs, monkeys and mice. Toxicol Appl Pharmacol 1973 25:230–241.

Schilsky RL Renal and metabolic toxicities of cancer chemotherapy. Semin Oncol 1982 9:75–83.

Schweitzer V, Hawkins JE, and Lilly DJ Ototoxic and nephrotoxic effects of combined treatment with cis-diamminedichloroplatinum and kanamycin in the guinea pig. Otolaryngol Head Neck Surg 1984 92:41–49.

Schweitzer VG, Rarey KE, Dolan DF, Abrams G, Litterst CJ, and Sheridan C Ototoxicity of cisplatin vs. platinum analogs CBDCA (JM-8) and CHIP (JM-9). Otolaryngol Head Neck Surg 1986 94:458–470.

Schweitzer VG, Dolan DF, Davidson T, Abrams GE, and Snyder R Amelioration of cisplatin-induced ototoxicity by fosfomycin. Laryngoscope 1986 96:948–958.

Schilsky RL and Anderson T Hypomagnesemia and magnesium wasting in patients receiving cisplatin. Ann Intern Med 1979 90:929–931.

Sessa C, Vermorken J, Renard J, Kaye S, Smith D, ten Bokkel Huinink W, Cavalli F, and Pinedo H Phase II study of iproplatin in advanced ovarian carcinoma. J Clin Oncol 1988 6:98–105.

Skillen, AW, Baumah PK, Cantwell BMJ, Cornell C, Hodson, AW, and Harris AL Urinary protein and enzyme excretion in patients receiving chemotherapy with the cis-platinum analogs carboplatin (CBDCA, JM8) and iproplatin (CHIP, JM9). Cancer Chemother Pharmacol 1988 22:228–234.

Smith PH and Taylor DM Distribution and retention of the antitumor agent 195m Pt cis-dichlorodiamineplatinum(II) in man. J Nucl Med 1974 15:349–351.

Sridhar KS and Donnelly E Combination antiemetics for cisplatin chemotherapy. Cancer 1988 61:1508–1517.

Sridhar KS, Holland JF, Brown JF Doxorubicin plus cisplatin in the treatment of AUPD tumors. Cancer 1985 55:2634–2636.

Stadnicki SW, Gleischman RW, and Schaeppi U Ototoxicity of cisdichlorodiammine platinum (II) (NSC-119875): Hearing loss and other toxic effects in Rhesus monkeys. Cancer Chemother Rev 1975 59:467–480.

Steffenelli T, Kuzmits R, Ulrich W, and Glogar D Acute vascular toxicity after combination chemotherapy with cisplatin vinblastine and bleomycin for testicular cancer. Eur Heart J 1988 9:552–556.

Sternson L, Repta AJ, Shih H, Himmelstein KJ, and Patton TF Distribution of cisplatin vs. total platinum in animals and man. In: Platinum Coordination Complexes in Cancer Chemotherapy Hacker MP, Douple EB, and Krakoff IH Eds Martinus-Nijhoff Publishing, Boston 1984 pp. 126–137.

Stoudmire A, Cotanch P, and Laszlo J Recent advances in the pharmacologic and behavioral management of chemotherapy induced emesis. Arch Int Med 1984 144:1029–1033.

Sugihara K, Nakano S, and Gemba M Effect of cisplatin on in vitro production of lipid peroxides in rat kidney cortex. Jpn J Pharmacol 1987a, 71–76.

Sugihara K, Nakano S, Koda M, Tanaka K, Fukuishi N, and Gemba M Stimulatory effect of cisplatin on production of lipid peroxidation in renal tissues. Jpn J Pharmacol 1987b 43:247–252.

Talley RW, O'Bryan RM, Gutterman JU, Brownlee RW, and McCredie KB Clinical evaluation of the toxic effects of cis-diamminedichloro platinum (NSC-119875) phase I clinical study. Cancer Chemother Rep 1973 57:465–471.

Tamura T, Saijo N, Shinkai T, Eguchi K, Sakurai M, Fujiwara Y, Nakano H, Nakagawa K, and Minato K Phase II study of carboplatin in small cell cancer. Jpn J Clin Oncol 1988 18:27–32.

Tange RA An abnormality in the human cochlear vasculature in a case of cis-platinum ototoxicity. Acta Otolaryngol 1987 436(suppl):133–137.

Thompson SW, Davis LE, Kornfeld M, Hilgers RD, and Standefer JC Cisplatin neurotoxicity: Clinical, electrophysiologic, morphologic and toxicologic studies. Cancer 1984 54:1269–1275.

Tonato M, Roila F, Del Favero A, Tognoni G, Franzosi MG, and Pampallona S A pilot study of high dose domperidone as an antiemetic in patients treated with cisplatin. Eur J Cancer Clin Oncol 1985 21:807–810.

Towflight J, Strauss M, and Lord S Cisplatin ototoxicity: Clinical experience and temporal bone histopathology. Laryngoscope 1983 93:1554–1559.

Tueni E, Sculier J-P, and Klastersky J Phase I study of a carboplatin-etoposide combination in advanced thoracic cancer. Eur J Cancer Clin Oncol 1988 24:963–967.

Turlapaty PD and Altura BM Magnesium deficiency produces spasms of coronary arteries: Relationship to etiology of sudden death in ischemic heart disease. Science 1980 208:198–200.

Van der Hulst RJAM, Drechler WA, and Urbanus NAM High frequency audiometry in prospective clinical research of ototoxicity due to platinum derivatives. Ann Otol Rhinol Laryngol 1988 97:133–137.

Van Echo DA, Egorin MJ, Whitacre MY, Olman EA, and Aisner J Phase I clinical and pharmacological trial of carboplatin daily for 5 days. Cancer Treat Rep 1984 68:1103–1114.

Van Nguyen B, Jaffe N, and Lichtiger B Cisplatin induced anemia. Cancer Treat Rep 1981 65:1121.

Vincent B, McQuiston D, Einhorn L, Nagy C, and Brames M Review of cannabinoids and their antiemetic effectiveness. Drugs 1984 25(suppl 1):52–62.

Vogelzang NJ, Bosl GJ, Johnson K, and Kennedy BJ Raynaud's phenomenon: A common toxicity after combination chemotherapy for testicular cancer. Ann Intern Med 1981 95:288–293.

Vogelzang NJ, Torkelson JL, and Kennedy BJ Hypomagnesemia, renal dysfunction, and Raynaud's phenomenon in patients treated with cisplatin, vinblastine, and bleomycin. Cancer 1985 56:2765–2770.

Vogl SE, Zaravinos T, and Kaplan BH Toxicity of cis-diamminedichloroplatinum (II) given in a two hour outpatient regimen of diuresis and hydration. Cancer 1980 45:11–15.

Von Hoff D, Schilsky R, Reichert CM, Reddick RL, Rozencweig M, Young RC, and Muggia FM Toxic effects of cis-dichlorodiammineplatinum (II) in man. Cancer Treat Rep 1979 63:1527–1531.

Walther PJ, Rossitch E, and Bullard DE The development of Lhermitte's sign during cisplatin chemotherapy. Possible drug induced toxicity causing spinal cord demyelination. Cancer 1987 60:2170–2172.

Wampler G The pharmacology and clinical effectiveness of phenothiazines and related drugs for managing chemotherapy induced emesis. Drugs 1983 25(suppl 1):35–51.

Wang S and Borison H A new concept of organization of the central emetic mechanism: Recent studies on the site of action of apomorphine, copper sulfate, and cardiac glycosides. Gastroenterolgoy 1952 22:1–12.

Ward JM and Fauvie KA The nephrotoxic effects of cis-diammine-dichloroplatinum (II) (NSC-119875) in male F344 rats. Toxicol Appl Pharmacol 1976 38:535–547.

Weaving A, Bezwoda WR, and Derman DP Seizures after antiemetic treatment with dose domperidone: Report of four cases. Br Med J 1984 288:1728.

Whitehead VM Cancer treatment needs better antiemetics. N Engl J Med 1975 293:199–200.

Wilding G, Caruso R, Lawrence TS, Ostchega Y, Ballantine EJ, Young RC, and Ozols RF Retinal toxicity after high dose cisplatin therapy. J Clin Oncol 1985 3:1683–1689.

Wiltshaw E and Kroner T Phase II study of cis-dichlorodiammineplatinum (II) (NSC-119875) in advanced adenocarcinoma of the ovary. Cancer Treat Rep 1976 60:55–60.

Wright CG and Schaeffer SD Inner ear histopathology in patients treated with cis-platinum. Laryngoscope 1982 92:1408–1413.

Yagoda A, Watson RC, Gonzales-Vitale JC, Grabstald H, and Whitmore WF Cis-dichlorodiammineplatinum (II) in advanced bladder cancer. Cancer Treat Rep 1976 60:917–923.

Yuhas JM Active versus passive absorption kinetics as the basis selective protection of normal tissues by WR-2721. Cancer Res 1980a 40:1519–1524.

Yuhas JM, Spellman JM, and Culo F The role of WR-2721 in radiotherapy and/or chemotherapy. In: Radiation Sensitizers Brady L Ed Masson Press, New York 1980b pp. 303–308.

Yuhas JM, Spellman JM, and Jordan SW Treatment of tumors with the combination of WR-2721 and cis-dichlorodiammine platinum or cyclophosphamide. Br J Cancer 1980c 42:574–585.

Zeger G, Smith L, McQuiston D, and Goldfinger D Cisplatinum induced non-immunologic adsorption of immunoglobulin by red blood cells. Transfusion 1988 28:493–495.

CHAPTER 7

Toxicity of Free Radical Forming Anticancer Agents

Garth Powis, D.Phil.

INTRODUCTION

There are currently 40 officially approved anticancer drugs in the U.S.A. excluding steroidal agents (U.S. Pharmacopeia, 1989). Of these drugs, eight have been reported to form free radicals, namely, doxorubicin, daunomycin, mitoxantrone, bleomycin, neocarzinostatin, mitomycin C, actinomycin D, and procarbazine. In this chapter the toxicity of the first five drugs will be covered since there is reasonable evidence to suggest that free radical formation may be linked to at least some of the biological activities of these drugs. The evidence for a free radical mechanism is less convincing for actinomycin D (Flitter and Mason, 1988), mitomycin C (Lown et al., 1978), and procarbazine (Sinha, 1984), and they will not be considered here.

The major toxicities of each of the agents in human subjects is presented although, invariably, some of the more esoteric toxicities often occurring in no more than a few patients will not be covered. An attempt is made to present possible mechanisms for these toxicities as well as the relation of toxicity to antitumor activity. Ways in which toxicities might be prevented or treated are discussed. Animal studies are discussed, where relevant, to understand or prevent human toxicity. Invariably much of the evidence for the mechanism of action of these drugs comes from animal studies which are amenable to experimentation in a way that is not possible with human subjects.

ANTHRACYCLINES

Introduction

Antitumor quinones represent the second largest class of clinically approved anticancer agents in the U.S.A., next only to the chloroethyl alkylating agents. They have been selected from the large number of naturally occurring quinones (Moore et al., 1986; Nohl et al., 1986; Thompson, 1971) and from synthetic quinones (Bruce, 1974). Over 1500 quinones have been tested for antitumor activity since 1955 by the U.S.A. National Cancer Institute's Drug Research and Development Program (Driscoll et al., 1974). The anthracycline glycosides are the largest class of the clinically used antitumor quinones. Some typical anthracycline structures are shown in Fig. 7-1. Daunorubicin (I) was isolated from strains of *Streptomyces* in 1963 (DiMarco et al., 1963; DuBost et al., 1963) followed six years later by doxorubicin (II) (Arcamone et al., 1969). Aclacinomycin A (V) a substantially different type of anthracycline with a three sugar carbohydrate chain was isolated in 1975 (Oki et al., 1975). Several hundred anthracycline analogues have been obtained by partial or total synthesis (Arcamone, 1977; 1984; Henry, 1979; Naff et al., 1982; Nettleton et al., 1977; Oki, 1977) and 17 anthracyclines have been tested clinically (Casazza, 1986). Doxorubicin and daunorubicin are by far the

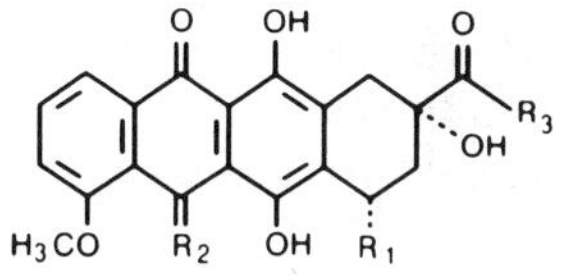

Compound	R_1	R_2	R_3
I Daunorubicin	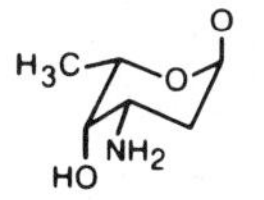	O	CH_3
II Doxorubicin	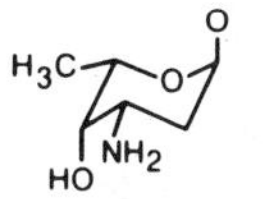	O	CH_2OH
III 4'-Epidoxorubicin	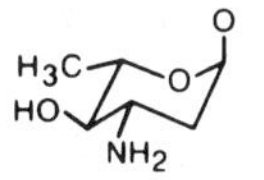	O	CH_2OH
IV MRA-CN	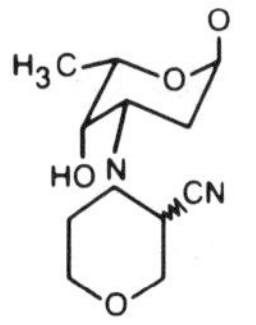	O	CH_2OH

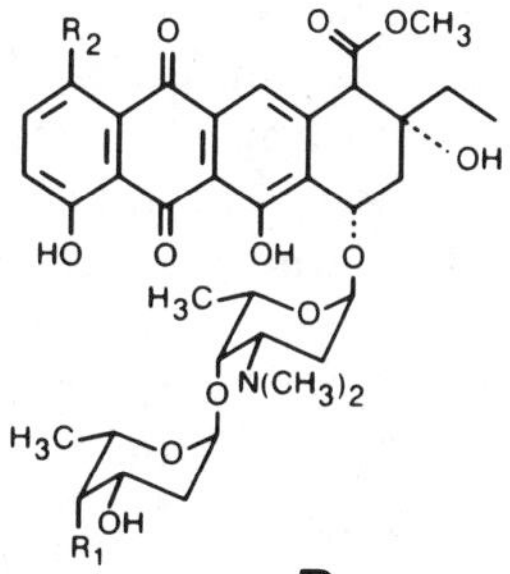

Compound	R_1	R_2
V Aclacinomycin A	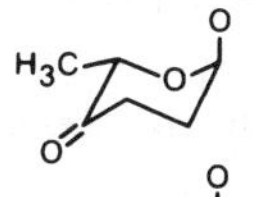	H
VI Marcellomycin	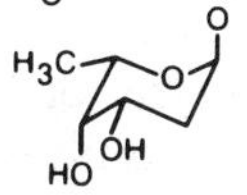	OH

VII Menogaril

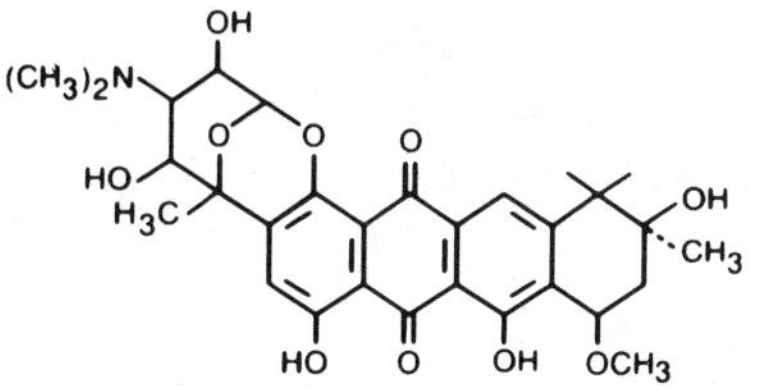

FIGURE 7-1. Structures of some typical antitumor anthracyclines.

most widely used anthracyclines and it is estimated that more than two million cancer patients have received doxorubicin (Arcamone, 1985).

In a little over a decade since their first clinical trials doxorubicin and daunorubicin have gained wide acceptance as major therapeutic agents in the treatment of cancer. They are used extensively as part of combination chemotherapy regimens for the effective treatment of acute non-lymphocytic leukemia, Hodgkin's and non-Hodgkin's lymphomas, breast cancer and sarcomas (Riggs and Sharp, 1987; Young et al., 1981). Doxorubicin has shown activity against human solid tumors including those of breast, lung, ovary, head and neck, endometrium, prostate, and bladder and is the most effective single agent against soft tissue sarcomas in adults. The use of doxorubicin for adjuvant chemotherapy for soft tissue sarcomas and breast and ovarian carcinomas is currently being studied.

The toxic effects of the anthracyclines are dose related. Nausea and vomiting occurs in more than 50% of patients receiving doxorubicin while some degree of alopecia is seen in all patients (Riggs and Sharp, 1987). Somnolence may occur during the first 24 hr after injection and lethargy lasting for several days is often seen in the elderly. Although the anthracyclines are not chemical vessicants their accidental infiltration into the area around an intravenous infusion site can produce severe, painful, progressive ulceration of skin and subcutaneous tissues. Renal toxicity may also occur. Although debilitating these toxicities are not life-threatening. The dose-limiting toxicities of the anthracyclines are myelosuppression, mucositis, and congestive cardiomyopathy.

Mechanism of Antitumor Activity and Toxicity

The mechanism of the antitumor activity of the anthracyclines is not known with certainty. A number of mechanisms have been proposed including intercalation of the anthracycline aglycone moiety between adjacent base pairs in the DNA double helix (Pigram et al., 1972) producing inhibition of DNA, RNA, and protein synthesis (Painter, 1978), protein associated DNA strand breaks due to anthracycline-induced stabilization of the topoisomerase II-DNA complex with the DNA in the open (cleaved) conformation (Pommier et al., 1985; Tewey et al., 1984), and alteration of cell membrane function by anthracyclines (Hickman et al., 1985; Santone et al., 1986; Tritton and Hickman, 1985). Another mechanism for the cytotoxicity of anthracyclines that has received considerable attention is anthracycline free radical mediated alkylation and DNA degradation (Bachur et al., 1978; Berlin and Haseltine, 1981; Powis, 1987). However, none of these mechanisms alone appears adequate to explain all of the cytotoxic properties of the anthracyclines (Bachur et al., 1978; Capranico et al., 1986; Zwelling et al., 1982). It is probably that the mechanism of antitumor activity of the anthracyclines differs from that producing cardiac toxicity since a number of animal and clinical studies, discussed in detail below, have shown that by altering the schedule of administration or by using protective agents it is possible to decrease the cardiotoxicity without reducing the antitumor effects of the anthracyclines. Nausea and vomiting due to anthracyclines can be reduced by decreasing the peak plasma concentration of the drug achieved during bolus administration by going to more frequent bolus administration or to infusions (Hortobagyi et al., 1989; Legha et al., 1982). Myelosuppression, mucositis and alopecia (except where treated locally) appear from clinical studies to be much more difficult to separate from antitumor activity. It is probable that they share a similar mechanism of action to anthracycline antitumor activity. This is, perhaps, not surprising since they all involve inhibition of the growth of rapidly dividing cells.

Myelosuppression and Mucositis

Myelosuppression and mucositis occur seven to 14 days after bolus administration of doxorubicin, with recovery in about seven days (Benjamin et al., 1974). Doxorubicin and daunorubicin myelosuppression is characterized by greater activity against leukocytes, especially neutrophils, than against platelets or erythrocytes. Apthous ulceration, usually of the inner labial and pharyngeal surfaces, may be limited and only mildly to moderately painful but can involve the entire oral cavity and upper aerodigestive mucosa, with bleeding, infection, and the inability to tolerate oral feeding (Benjamin et al., 1974; Riggs and Sharp, 1987). Both the myelosuppression and mucositis caused by the anthracyclines is dose related.

The early clinical trials of doxorubicin showed that certain groups of patients were more likely to experience severe acute toxicities. Severe and sometimes fatal myelosuppression together with severe mucositis were seen in patients who received multiple, sequential injections of doxorubicin and in patients with significantly impaired liver function. Understanding the pharmacokinetics of doxorubicin has allowed clinicians to avert the toxicities of doxorubicin to these high-risk patients. The pharmacokinetics of the anthracyclines is characterized by a rapid and extensive uptake from the plasma followed by slow release back into the plasma (Powis, 1987). Metabolism varies being relatively low for doxorubicin and menogaril and higher for other anthracyclines. Excretion of anthracyclines and anthracycline metabolites occurs predominantly in the bile with only small amounts being found in the urine. The anthracyclines show a very slow terminal phase of elimination and a large apparent volume of distribution indicating extensive tissue uptake (Table 7-1). Benjamin et al. (1974) reported that plasma concentration of doxorubicin in patients with liver dysfunction, measured by bromosulphthalein (BSP) retention, who experienced severe toxicity to doxorubicin were four to five fold higher than in patients with normal liver function, and the elimination of doxorubicin and its metabolites from plasma was delayed. By reducing the dose of doxorubicin given to patients with liver dysfunction plasma concentrations of doxorubicin and metabolites similar to those in patients with normal liver function receiving full doses of doxorubicin could be achieved with a consequent decrease in the severe doxorubicin toxicity (Bachur et al., 1977; Benjamin et al., 1974). Interestingly the therapeutic response to doxorubicin was not increased in patients with delayed doxorubicin elimination suggesting that although toxicity is related to total doxorubicin exposure, measured by the plasma area under the curve (AUC), response is not. Several sets of guidelines have been published for reducing the dose of doxorubicin in patients with liver dysfunction to avoid excessive mucositis and myelosuppression (Benjamin et al., 1974; Brenner et al., 1980; Jacquillot et al., 1977; Reich, 1978). These depend upon the test used to measure liver dysfunction. Serum bilirubin has been reported to be a more reliable index for predicting decreased doxorubicin elimination than BSP retention or serum liver enzyme activity (Benjamin, 1975; Benjamin et al., 1974; Gisselbrecht et al., 1980) (Table 7-2). Doroshow and Chan (1982) reported that indocyanine green clearance give a better indication of delayed doxorubicin elimination than either serum bilirubin or serum liver enzymes. In their study Doroshow and Chan (1982) found some patients with doxorubicin toxicity, despite dose reduction according to established guidelines. Patients with hepatoma may have normal doxorubicin pharmacokinetics

Table 7-1. Pharmacokinetic Parameters of Anthracyclines in Humans*

COMPOUND	TERMINAL HALF-LIFE (hr)	V_d (1/m²)	CL (1/min/m²)
doxorubicin	20–70	310–1088	0.3–0.5
daunorubicin	14–17	1297	0.4–1.8
4′-epidoxorubicin	18–38	516–794	0.4–0.5
4′-demethoxydaunorubicin	25–27	2485	1.2
4′-deoxydoxorubicin	20–90	2994	0.4
4-demethyldaunorubicin	20	139	1.7
menogaril	10–13	197–370	0.2–0.5
aclacinomycin A	2–13	998–2072	2.5–4.0

*Data taken from Powis, 1987. Individual references are omitted.

Table 7-2. Dose Reduction for Doxorubicin in Patients With Liver Dysfunction*

BILIRUBIN mg/dL	AST (SGOT)	REDUCTION IN DOSE† %
< 1.2	< 2 × normal	0
< 1.2	> 2 × normal	25
1.2–3.0	Any	50
> 3.0	Any	75

*Based on Benjamin et al. (1974).
†For a standard dose of 60 mg/m^2.

despite elevated serum bilirubin indicating hepatic dysfunction and dose reduction may result in under treating these patients (Bern et al., 1978; Chan et al., 1980). Although most work has focused on dose reduction of doxorubicin in patients with liver dysfunction the same principles are probably applicable to all the anthracyclines used clinically (Bachur, 1979). Although there is extensive documentation of delayed elimination of many noncancer drugs in patients with hepatic dysfunction (Wilkinson and Branch, 1984) the anthracyclines and a few other cancer drugs (Powis, 1983) are the only examples of dose reduction of therapeutic agents eliminated by the liver commonly used to avoid drug toxicity.

Cardiotoxicity

The toxicity of the anthracyclines that has received, by far, the most extensive study is cardiotoxicity. Doxorubicin shows toxicity to smooth, skeletal, and cardiac muscle but cardiac muscle shows by far the greatest toxicity (Doroshow et al., 1985; Long et al., 1984). Acute cardiovascular effects can develop within minutes but usually within a few hours of doxorubicin administration. Electrocardiographic studies show an incidence of abnormalities in up to 41% of patients receiving doxorubicin (Arena et al., 1972; Herman et al., 1971; LeFrak et al., 1973; Steinberg et al., 1987; Von Hoff et al., 1982; Zbinden and Brandle, 1975; Zweier, 1985). The most common effects were nonspecific ST-T wave changes, sinus tachycardia, premature ventricular and atrial contractions, and low voltage of the QRS complex. These electrocardiographic changes appear to be benign and unrelated to the total dose of doxorubicin administered. They are reversible within a few days to two months and do not appear to be associated with the development of doxorubicin cardiomyopathy. Clinically, the management of patients showing such changes does not usually present a problem, although there is the possibility of sudden death with doxorubicin administration (Wortman et al., 1979).

Congestive cardiomyopathy is the cumulative dose-limiting toxicity of anthracycline therapy and is proportional to the dose of anthracycline administered. With doses of doxorubicin of less than 550 mg/m^2 the incidence of cardiomyopathy has been reported to be no more than 1% (Bonadonna et al., 1975; Cortes et al., 1975; Gottlieb et al., 1973; LeFrak et al., 1975; Praga et al., 1979) whereas for cumulative doses in excess of 550 mg/m^2 (ranges 560–1155 mg/m^2) the incidence is increased to about 30%. There is, however, a continuum of increasing risk of doxorubicin cardiomyopathy as the total dose of drug increases (Fig. 7-2). Even asymptomatic patients who received a total dose of doxorubicin of 480 to 550 mg/m^2 were found upon radionucleide angiography to have a 63% incidence of abnormal scans (Gottdiener et al., 1981). The cardiac damage produced by doxorubicin is not reversible and once clinically overt cardiomyopathy is present the prognosis is grave, with mortality rates as high as 48% (Pratt et al., 1978). Most clinicians adhere to a limit on total doxorubicin dosage of 500 to 550 mg/m^2 for patients with no underlying cardiac diseases and, because of the risk of interactions with thoracic radiation or cyclophosphamide, a total dose of 450 mg/m^2 has been recommended in patients receiving combined methods of therapy. Individual patients may tolerate higher total doxorubicin doses than the recommended maximum but the risk is considerable.

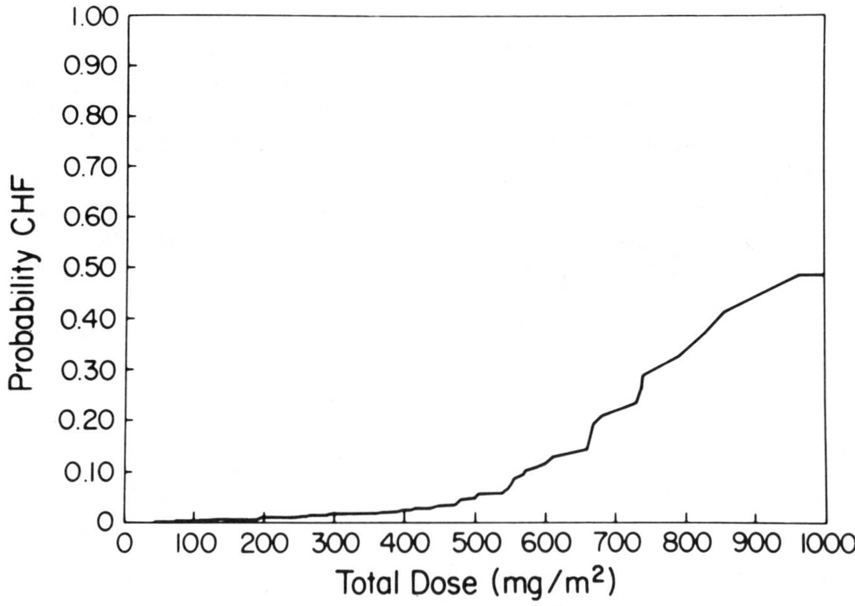

FIGURE 7-2. Continuum of increasing risk of congestive heart failure (CHF) with increasing total dose of doxorubicin. From a study of 3941 patients with 88 cases of CHF by Von Hoff et al. (1979). Reprinted with permission of the American Medical Association and the author.

The clinical presentation of patients with anthracycline induced cardiomyopathy is nonspecific. The first sign may be tachycardia with the patient complaining of shortness of breath or a nonproductive cough, and the usual signs of congestive heart failure include distended neck veins, gallop rhythm, ankle edema, hepatomegaly, cardiomegaly, and pleural effusion (Cortes et al., 1975; Gottlieb et al., 1973; Land et al., 1985; LeFrak et al., 1973; Minow et al., 1975). The onset of symptoms generally occurs about one month after the first dose of doxorubicin but can vary from hours to as long as eight months (Von Hoff et al., 1979). The pathological findings are nonspecific and can be seen with other cardiomyopathies. The lesions include loss of myofibrils, cytoplasmic vacuolization due to swelling of the sarcotubular system, swollen mitochondria, enlarged nuclei with a large distinct nucleolus, increased numbers of lysosomes, and lipid accumulation (Billingham, 1979; Goormaghtigh et al., 1980; LeFrak et al., 1973; Schwartz, 1983; Suzuki et al., 1979). Percutaneous endomyocardial biopsies in patients have demonstrated a direct relationship between the total dose of doxorubicin and pathologic changes in the myocardium (Benjamin et al., 1979; 1981; Billingham et al., 1976; 1978; Bristow et al., 1978). Similar structural changes of doxorubicin cardiomyopathy have been seen in a variety of experimental animals including mice (Lambertenghi-Deliliers et al., 1976; Myers et al., 1977; Rosenhoff et al., 1975), rats (Chalcroft et al., 1973; Singal et al., 1985), pigs (Van Vleet et al., 1979), turkey poults (Bates, 1982), and rabbits (Janke, 1974; Olson et al., 1974). Note that doxorubicin has been found to be more cardiotoxic to spontaneously hypertensive rats than to normal rats (Herman et al., 1985; 1988a).

A variety of methods for the early detection of doxorubicin cardiomyopathy in patients have been studied as an aid to clinicians using the drugs. Serial chest x-ray and serial plasma cardiac enzymes have not proved helpful (Von Hoff et al., 1982). Serial electrocardiogram studies have shown a decreased QRS voltage that coincides with the onset of the congestive heart failure (LeFrak et al., 1973; Minow et al., 1978, 1977; Ali et al., 1979; Friedman et al., 1979). Other tests such as the QRS-Korotkoff sound interval (Greco et al., 1975; Greco, 1978) and echocardiograms (Mason et al., 1978; Ewy et al., 1978; Henderson et al., 1978; Jones et al., 1975; Ramos et al., 1976; Bloom et al., 1978) are not specific or predictive of doxorubicin-induced cardiomyopathy. Monitoring left ventricular function with radionuclide angiography before and during doxorubicin therapy appears to be the most successful noninvasitve method for predicting doxorubicin cardiomyopathy (Fantine and Garnier-Suillerot, 1986; Schwartz et al., 1987). Some loss of left ventricular function occurs in most patients receiving doses of doxorubicin over about 450 mg/m^2 and patients with abnormal baseline function appear to be at greater risk of congestive heart failure after doxorubicin (Anne and Moiroux, 1984). Doxorubicin therapy is discontinued when there is more than a 10% absolute decrease in the left ventricular ejection fraction (LVEF) associated with a decline to an LVEF of $<$ 50% of the baseline value (Schwartz et al., 1987).

Biochemical Changes Produced by the Anthracycline in the Heart

A bewildering array of biochemical changes have been reported for doxorubicin in the heart of experimental animals. They are summarized in Table 7-3. The major problem is to decide which effects might be a cause of, and which effects are secondary to myocardial damage. Many of the effects of anthracyclines in the heart can be explained as secondary to the generation of free radicals which has been suggested by many workers to be the primary cause of anthracycline cardiotoxicity.

Free Radical Formation by Anthracyclines

A characteristic feature of quinones is their ability to undergo reversible oxidation and reduction and when reduced by one electron to form free radicals (see Figure 7-3). Anthracyclines form electron spin resonance (esr) detectable semiquinone free radicals when reduced either chemically (Kleyer and Koch, 1984; Lown and Chen, 1981; Sinha and Chignell, 1979) or enzymatically by a flavoenzyme in the presence of NADPH or NADH (Bachur et al., 1977, 1978; Basra et al., 1985; Berlin and Haseltine, 1981; Gutierrez et al., 1983; Kalyanaraman et al., 1984; Komiyama et al., 1986; Pan et al., 1980; Pollakis et al., 1984; Sato et al., 1977; Schreiber et al., 1987). A wide variety of flavoenzymes catalyze the one-electron reduction of anthracyclines including NADPH-cytochrome P-450 reductase, mitochondrial, NADH dehydrogenase, and nitrate reductase from *Neurospora* (Komiyama et al., 1979; Pan et al., 1981; Pan and Bachur, 1980; Schwartz, 1983; Svingen and Powis, 1981). Under anaerobic conditions the anthracycline semiquinone undergoes deglycosidation to form the anthracycline 7-deoxyaglycone (Oki et al., 1977). The mechanism of anthracycline reductive deglycosidation has been suggested to involve a C-7 carbon centered anthracycline radical (Mason, 1979; Sinha, 1980), or a C-6 carbon centered anthracycline radical (Lown and Chen, 1981). Other workers have suggested a mechanism involving the anthracycline hydroquinone, the two electron reduced form (Anne and Moiroux, 1984; Berg et al., 1982; Fisher et al., 1985; Houee-Levin et al., 1984). In the presence of air doxorubicin semiquinone reacts with oxygen with a bimolecular rate constant of 3×10^8 $M^{-1}s^{-1}$ (Butler et al., 1985; Land et al., 1985). The initial oxygen species formed by this reaction is the superoxide anion radical (Kalyanaraman et al., 1980; 1984; Sinha et al., 1984). Studies using anthraquinonyl glucosaminosides as model compounds have shown that superoxide anion radical formation by rat heart sarcosomes and NADPH increases with the addition of successive hydroxyl groups to the anthraquinone nucleus (Abramson et al., 1986).

Superoxide anion radical formed by redox cycling of anthracycline gives rise by an iron catalyzed reaction to hydroxyl radical that can produce a variety of biological effects including lipid peroxidation (Goodman and Hochstein, 1977; Mimnaugh et al., 1983), degradation of deoxyribose (Gutteridge and Quinlan, 1985; Bates and Winterbourn, 1982), and DNA strand breaks (Rowley and Halliwell, 1983; Sinha et al., 1984; Sugioka et al., 1984). Hemoproteins may be able to replace iron salts in catalyzing anthracycline induced hydroxyl radical formation (Komiyama et al., 1985). Hydroxyl radical, or a species with similar reactivity to

Table 7-3. Biochemical Effects of Doxorubicin on the Heart

EFFECT	RESPONSE	REFERENCES
Free radical formation	Increased oxygen radical formation	Bachur et al., 1977 Costa et al., 1988 Doroshow, 1983 Doroshow et al., 1983 Floyd et al., 1986 Grankvist and Henriksson, 1987 Kalyanaraman et al., 1980 Nohl and Jordan, 1983 Thayer, 1977 Thornalley and Dodd, 1985
	Increased lipid peroxidation	Llesuy et al., 1988 Myers et al., 1977 Ogawa et al., 1987 Singal et al., 1985 Suzuki et al., 1979
	Increased catalase	D'Alessandro et al., 1984 Julicher et al., 1988 Lazzarino et al., 1987
	Increased glutathione	Doroshow and Davies, 1983 Doroshow et al., 1979 Jackson et al., 1984 Julicher et al., 1988 Revis and Marusic, 1978 Tomlinson et al., 1982
	Increased glutathione peroxidase	Doroshow and Davies, 1983 Doroshow et al., 1979 Jackson et al., 1984 Revis and Marusic, 1978 Tomlinson et al., 1982
	Increased DT-diaphorase	Galaris et al., 1985
Membrane effects	Altered adenylatecyclase	Azuma et al., 1981 Robison et al., 1984 Singal and Panagia, 1984
	Increased Ca^{2+} ATPase	Singal and Panagia, 1984
	Decreased guanylate cyclase	Lehotay et al., 1983 Levey et al., 1979
	Altered Na^{+}/K^{+}ATPase	Gosalvez et al., 1979 Kim et al., 1980 Komori et al., 1985 Tomlinson et al., 1985
	Decreased adenine, amino acid deoxyglucose uptake	Reese et al., 1987
	Decreased Ca^{2+}/K^{+} ATPase	Tomilinson et al., 1985
	Sarcolemmal Ca^{2+} release	Tomlinson et al., 1985
	Altered Ca^{2+} fluxes	Azuma et al., 1981 Caroni et al., 1981 Dasida et al., 1979 Singal and Pierce, 1986 Villani et al., 1978
	Increased membrane permeability	LeFrak et al., 1973 Olson et al., 1974 Singal et al., 1985 Suzuki et al., 1979
Mitochondria	Altered Ca^{2+}	Miwa et al., 1986 Revis and Marusic, 1978 Singal and Pierce, 1986

Table 7-3. *(Continued)*

EFFECT	RESPONSE	REFERENCES
Mitochandria *(continued)*	Altered respiratory activity	Aversano and Boor, 1983 Bachman et al., 1987 Cini-Neri and Neri, 1986 Lehninger, 1970 Montali et al., 1985 Mukerhjee et al., 1978 Rinehart et al., 1974
	Decreased high energy phosphate stores	Keller et al., 1986 Nicolay et al., 1987 Pelikan et al., 1986
Lysosomes	Altered lysosomal enzymes	Singal et al., 1985 Gebbis et al., 1985
	Increased size and number	Singal et al., 1985
Myofibrils	Loss	Billingham, 1979 Ferrans, 1978 Janke, 1974 LeFrak et al., 1973 Singal et al., 1986 Suzuki et al., 1979
	Increased F-actin thickness	Lewis et al., 1982
	Increased myosin ATPase	Bergson and Inchiosa, 1985 Lewis et al., 1982

hydroxyl radical, can also be formed by the direct reaction of anthracycline semiquinone radical with hydrogen peroxide (Bates et al., 1982; Bates, 1982; Winterbourn, 1981). High concentrations of oxygen inhibit the process. This occurs because the reaction of doxorubicin semiquinone radical with hydrogen peroxide, $k = 10^4$ to 10^5 $M^{-1}s^{-1}$ (Kalyanaraman et al., 1984), cannot effectively compete with the reaction of oxygen with doxorubicin semiquinone radical to form superoxide anion radical. The reaction appears to require catalytic amounts of iron complexed with the anthracycline, or with ethylene diamine tetraacetic acid (EDTA), or diethylenetriamine pentaacetic acid (DETEPAC) (Gutteridge and Toeg, 1982; Winterbourn et al., 1985). Evidence for the formation of hydroxyl radical when doxorubicin semiquinone radical is mixed with hydrogen peroxide is the esr spin trapping of a hydroxyl radical adduct with 5, 5-dimethylpyroline-N-oxide (DMPO) (Bannister and Thornalley, 1983; Kalyanaraman et al., 1984) and the degradation of methional to ethylene, a reaction known to require hydroxyl radical (Paur et al., 1984). However, other evidence suggests that a species with more limited reactivity than hydroxyl radical may be formed. Breakdown of deoxyribose by doxorubicin semiquinone radical and hydrogen peroxide is inhibited by some, but not all hydroxyl radical scavenging agents (Winterbourn et al., 1984, 1985). The formation of a species that mimics the hydroxyl radical but is more discriminating in its reactivity, a "crypto"-hydroxyl radical, has been described for the reaction of paraquat anion radical, and with hydrogen peroxide under limiting oxygen concentrations (Youngman and Elstner, 1981). A "crypto"-hydroxyl radical may be formed by reaction of doxorubicin semiquinone free radical with hydrogen peroxide (Winterbourn et al., 1985). A summary of the pathways for formation of oxygen radicals by redox cycling of anthracyclines is given in Fig. 7-3.

Free Radical Formation and Anthracycline Cardiotoxicity

The cardiotoxicity of the anthracyclines has frequently been linked to the formation of reactive oxygen species (Adachi et al., 1983; D'Alessandro et al., 1980; Doroshow, 1983a; Doroshow and Davies, 1986; Goodman and Hochstein, 1977; Kalyanaraman et al., 1980;

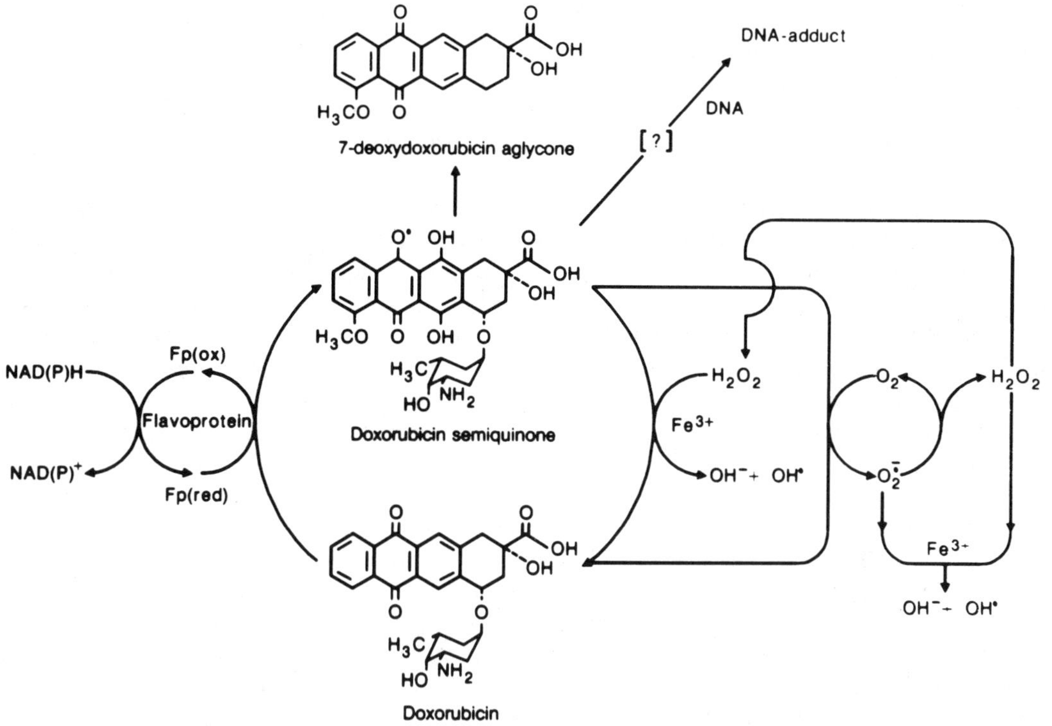

FIGURE 7-3. Formation of oxygen radicals by redox cycling of doxorubicin. From Powis (1989). Reprinted with permission.

Thornalley et al., 1986). Doxorubicin, daunorubicin, and other cardiotoxic anthracyclines stimulate the formation of superoxide anion radical, hydrogen peroxide, and hydroxyl radical by subcellular fractions prepared from heart (Adachi et al., 1983; Doroshow, 1983a, 1983b; Doroshow and Davies, 1986; Gutierrez et al., 1983; Thayer, 1977). The major site of anthracycline-induced oxygen radical formation in the heart is Complex I of the mitochondrial electron transport chain, probably the NADH dehydrogenase (Adachi et al., 1983; Davies et al., 1983; Davies and Doroshow, 1986; Doroshow, 1983a; Thornalley et al., 1986). Doxorubicin, daunorubicin, rubidazone, but not 5-iminodaunorubicin, also directly stimulate oxidation of oxymyoglobin with the formation of reactive oxygen species (Doroshow, 1987).

The major oxygen species formed by redox cycling of anthracyclines in the heart is hydroxyl radical (Pollakis et al., 1984). Using esr flow techniques and respiring heart mitochondria or heart submitochondrial particles incubated with anthracycline, Pollakis et al. (1984) observed short-lived DMPO spin trapped adducts of hydroxyl radical and superoxide anion radical. Superoxide anion was the predominant species formed by intact mitochondria and hydroxyl radical the predominant species formed by sonicated mitochondria. Using esr and spin trapping with DMPO, Thornalley and Dodd (1985) found only hydroxyl radical and no superoxide anion radical formed by rat heart sarcosomes incubated with NADPH and doxorubicin. Hydroxyl radical formation was inhibited by catalase but not by superoxide dismutase, suggesting a direct reduction of hydrogen peroxide to hydroxyl radical. The authors assumed, however, that hydrogen peroxide was being formed by superoxide and that their failure to detect superoxide was due to the much greater efficiency of trapping of hydroxyl radical by DMPO compared to trapping of superoxide anion radical. Nohl and Jordan (1983), also, could find no esr evidence for formation of superoxide anion radical by respiring rat heart mitochondria and doxorubicin using DMPO as a spin trap. In this study, a doxorubicin-derived semiquinone radical signal was seen which was stable even in the presence of oxygen. The signal disappeared on addition of hydrogen peroxide and concomitantly there appeared a DMPO-hydroxyl radical adduct signal. Nohl and Jordan (1983) interpreted their results to indicate that a doxorubicin semiquinone radical was produced during mitochondrial respiration, probably at the lipophilic phase of the mitochondrial inner membrane, in a way which precluded electron transfer to oxygen. This allowed reaction of the anthracycline semiquinone radical with hydrogen peroxide, probably present at relatively high concentrations in the heart because of low levels of catalase (Herzog and Fahimi, 1974) to form hydroxyl radical. Further studies by the same group have suggested that the oxygen-insensitive semiquinone radical is that of 7-deoxydoxorubicin aglycone semiquinone incorporated into the phospholipid of the mitochondrial inner membrane (Nohl et al., 1986). Controlled disruption of the phospholipid membrane exposes the semiquinone radical allowing it to react with oxygen and generate superoxide anion radical.

Electron spin resonance spin trapping has been used to detect doxorubicin dependent hydroxyl radical formation by the isolated perfused rat heart (Rajogopalan et al., 1987). Superoxide dismutase, catalase and ICRF-187, an iron chelator, inhibited hydroxyl radical formation showing the intermediacy of superoxide anion radical and hydrogen peroxide with iron catalysis. Further evidence that links anthracycline-cardiotoxicity to oxygen radical formation is the finding that newer, less cardiotoxic anthracyclines undergo less redox cycling than doxorubicin or daunorubicin. Studies by Lown et al. (1982) have shown a positive correlation between the electrochemical generation of oxygen species from a series of anthracyclines and their cardiotoxicity in the rat. 5-iminodaunorubicin which is less cardiotoxic in animals than either daunorubicin or doxorubicin (Tong et al., 1979; Zbinden et al., 1978) does not undergo enzymatic reduction to form an anthracycline semiquinone radical (Doroshow and Davies, 1986; Pollakis et al., 1984) or produce superoxide or hydroxyl radical (Doroshow and Davies, 1986; Doroshow, 1983b; Peters et al., 1986; Pollakis et al., 1984). 4′-deoxydoxorubicin and 4-demethoxydaunorubicin, which in experimental animals are less cardiotoxic than doxorubicin or daunorubicin, do not generate oxygen free radicals spontaneously in aerated aqueous solution, unlike the parent anthracyclines (Dickinson et al., 1984; 1985). Both compounds are, however, equally active as doxorubicin in stimulating oxygen use when incubated with rat liver microsomes and NADPH (Peters et al., 1986).

Redox cycling of doxorubicin by heart NADH dehydrogenase with formation of hydroxyl radical leads to inhibition of Ca^{2+} uptake by heart sarcoplasmic reticulum (Harris and Doroshow, 1985). N-acetylcysteine and glutathione protect against the inhibition of Ca^{2+} uptake by doxorubicin uptake suggesting that the effect is due to oxidation of critical thiol groups.

Lipid peroxidation is another mechanism by which oxygen radicals can damage critical macromolecules. Studies with rat heart microsomes and NADPH have shown that anthracyclines stimulate lipid peroxidation, but only if the microsomes are prepared from rats fed a diet deficient in α-tocopherol (Mimnaugh et al., 1981, 1982). Mouse heart microsomes, which have low endogenous levels of α-tocopherol, exhibit a marked increase in lipid peroxidation in the presence of anthracyclines (D'Alessandro et al., 1980; Mimnaugh et al., 1983). Even so, some workers have found it necessary to add catalytic Fe(II) to obtain appreciable levels of doxorubicin-stimulated lipid peroxidation in mouse heart microsomes (Daugherty et al., 1982). 5-iminodaunorubicin at low (μM) concentrations inhibits cardiac and hepatic microsomal lipid peroxidation without affecting the rate of NADPH oxidation and inhibits doxorubicin-stimulated NADPH-dependent cardiac microsomal lipid peroxidation (Mimnaugh et al., 1982). The high affinity of 5-iminodaunorubicin for iron could explain its inhibition of lipid peroxidation (Myers et al., 1987). Doxorubicin semiquinone and hydrogen peroxide cause peroxidation of phospholipid liposomes under low oxygen concentrations by a process that is inhibited by iron chelators (Winterbourn et al., 1985). It has been suggested that a "crypto"-hydroxyl radical formed by a doxorubicin-Fe(III) complex in close association with the liposomal phospholipid is responsible for initiating the lipid peroxidation (Winterbourn et al., 1985). A complex of doxorubicin and Fe(III) is a more potent inhibitor of mitochondrial function than doxorubicin alone (Demant, 1983). This has been attributed to inhibition of mitochondrial electron transport by doxorubicin-Fe(III) complex and an increase in lipid peroxidation. Doxorubicin-Fe(III) complex is, however, less toxic to cardiac myocytes in vitro than doxorubicin alone (Lampidis et al., 1987).

Even though anthracyclines stimulate lipid peroxidation by subcellular fractions lipid peroxidation may not be a primary effect of anthracyclines in intact heart tissue. Singal and Pierce (1986) found that increased lipid peroxidation in rat isolated ventricular wall only occurred at a concentration of doxorubicin of 10 μM, which is considerably in excess of therapeutic concentrations, and became maximal at 1 mM doxorubicin. Julicher et al. (1986) found no increase in lipid peroxidation in hearts from α-tocopherol deficient rats treated with doxorubicin despite being able to see doxorubicin-dependent lipid peroxidation in heart mitochondria and microsomal fractions from the same animals. 4′-epidoxorubicin, which is less cardiotoxic than doxorubicin in mice, does not increase lipid peroxidation measured by malondialdehyde formation by mouse heart in vivo (Praet et al., 1986). Praet et al. (1986) have also shown that while both doxorubicin and 4′-epidoxorubicin increase malondialdehyde formation by mouse heart mitochondria in vitro, when administered to intact mice, 4′-epidoxorubicin produces a much smaller increase in malondialdehyde than doxorubicin. Reports of increased in vivo lipid peroxidation following anthracycline administration using malondialdehyde as an indicator of lipid peroxidation (D'Alessandro et al., 1980; Llesuy et al., 1985; Myers et al., 1977; Praet et al., 1986; Stuart et al., 1978; Yamanaka et al., 1979) have to be treated with caution because malondialdehyde formation is not a good measure of in vivo lipid peroxidation (Bus and Gibson, 1979). Studies using breath ethane expiration, which is generally regarded as a more reliable indicator of lipid peroxidation in vivo, have failed to show an increase in lipid peroxidation in rats given lethal doses of doxorubicin (Muliwan et al., 1980). However, several compounds that are believed to exert their toxic effects through generation of active oxygen species and lipid peroxidation, for example nitrofurantoin, paraquat, diquat, and menadione, also did not increase ethane production in vivo in this system (Younes et al., 1985). Thus, the failure to demonstrate a doxorubicin-dependent increase in ethane production in the intact animal cannot be taken as conclusive evidence for a lack of lipid peroxidation by the heart in vivo.

Recent studies in skeletal muscle have shown that anthracyclines are potent stimulators of sarcoplasmic reticulum Ca^{2+} release through a direct interaction with the Ca^{2+} release channel from the triadic junction of muscle (Abramson et al., 1988). This might be caused by direct oxidation of sensitive sulfhydryls on the Ca^{2+} release channel by the anthracycline and could be a mechanism for the cardiotoxicity of the anthracyclines.

Is Cardiotoxicity Due to Anthracycline or Its Metabolites?

The acute cardiotoxicity of the anthracyclines appears to be directly related to the accumulation of the parent drug in the heart (Chen et al., 1987; Sazuka et al., 1987). Uptake of anthracycline probably explains the selective acute toxicity for heart muscle compared to other muscle. In mouse the toxicity of a single dose of doxorubicin was seen in the diaphragm > heart > gastrocnemius, which paralleled the uptake of parent drug into these tissues (Doroshow et al., 1985). Some studies have suggested a link between subacute and chronic anthracycline cardiotoxicity and the formation of C-13 anthracycline alcohols by anthracycline C-13 keto reductase, pH optimum 8.5. The enzyme is present in all tissues except plasma and belongs to a group of widely distributed enzymes classified as $NADP^+$ oxidoreductases (Bachur and Gee, 1971; Felsted et al., 1977). Human and rabbit liver cytosol contain in addition to the pH 8.5 anthracycline keto reductase an anthracycline keto reductase with a pH optimum of 6.0 (Ahmed et al., 1978a; 1978b; 1981). Doxorubicinol (doxorubicin C-13 alcohol) accumulation in the heart following repeated doxorubicin administration to rats appears to coincide with the onset of subacute cardiotoxicity (del Tacca et al., 1985). Doxorubicinol has been reported to be more cardiotoxic to animals in vivo (Olson et al., 1988) and more inhibitory of the sarcoplasmic reticulum Ca^{2+} pump in vitro than doxorubicin (Boucek et al., 1987; Olson et al., 1988). Other studies have, however, found doxorubicin to be less cardiotoxic to rat in vivo than doxorubicin, possibly due to lower cardiac uptake of the more polar doxorubicinol (Danesi et al., 1986; 1987; 1988). At the present time the role of anthracycline C-13 alcohol metabolites in anthracycline cardiotoxicity is unresolved.

Kinins and Acute Anthracycline Cardiotoxicity

Doxorubicin produces a dose dependent histamine release in vitro (Bristow et al., 1983; Decorti et al., 1986; Klugmann et al., 1986). The histamine releases blockers, theophylline and disodium cromoglycate, and the H_1 blocker chlorpheniramine will protect rabbits, mice and dogs against doxorubicin acute cardiotoxicity implicating histamine release in its pathogenesis (Bristow et al., 1983; Gebbia et al., 1987; Klugmann et al., 1986). Histamine release does not, however, appear to be a mechanism for chronic doxorubicin cardiotoxicity (Bristow et al., 1983). Doxorubicin has also been reported to cause an increased vascular sensitivity to vasopressin with activation of the sympathetic and renin-angiotensin systems (Arnolda et al., 1986; Johnston et al., 1986) which could contribute to its acute cardiotoxic effects.

Protection Against Anthracycline Cardiotoxicity Treatments

A wide variety of treatments have been tested for their ability to protect against doxorubicin cardiotoxicity in animals (Table 7-4, pp. 120–121). Several of these treatments have been reported to offer protection against doxorubicin's acute and chronic cardiotoxicity. The treatments fall into three categories, free radical scavengers aimed at preventing free radical damage and lipid peroxidation caused by doxorubicin; drugs, including the Ca^{2+} channel blockers; and biochemical replacement therapy. Only those treatments that have undergone clinical trial will be considered here (Table 7-5, p. 122).

Of the free radical scavengers α-tocopherol appears to offer the best protection against chronic doxorubicin cardiotoxicity in animals. Unfortunately clinical trials of α-tocopherol have not shown it to offer significant protection against doxorubicin cardiotoxicity (Legha et al., 1982; Weitzman et al., 1980; Whittaker and Al-Ismail, 1984). Based on the observation that doxorubicin inhibits ubiquinone (coenzyme Q_{10}) dependent enzymes (Bertazzoli et al., 1976; Iwamoto et al., 1986) and that there is a deficiency of ubiquinone in a variety of myocardial diseases (Folkers and Wolaniuk, 1985) ubiquinone has been studied in animals with some success for its ability to protect against chronic doxorubicin cardiomyopathy (Table 7-4). Clinical studies have reported that ubiquinone decreases the degree of cardiotoxicity in patients with normal cardiac function and allows increased doses of doxorubicin to be given before cardiotoxicity was seen.

The only drugs that have undergone clinical trial for the prevention of doxorubicin's cardiotoxicity are ICRF-187, digoxin, and some Ca^{2+} channel blockers (Table 7-4). ICRF-159 [(±)-1,2-bis-3,5-dioxopeperzainyl-1-yl propane] and its more water soluble (+)-isomer, ICRF-187, were shown to protect against chronic doxorubicin cardiotoxicity in several animal species (Table 7-4). Clinical trials currently under way show promise of significant protection by ICRF-187 against doxorubucin cardiotoxicity in patients (Green et al., 1987; Speyer et al., 1987, 1988). The mechanism of the protective effect may be related to the ability of ICRF-187, a lipid soluble analogue of EDTA, to remove free iron necessary for hydroxyl radical formation and lipid peroxidation by doxorubicin. Although ICRF-187 itself does not bind iron its hydrolysis product has a high affinity for all transition metals including iron (El-Hage et al., 1986). Support for an iron chelating activity of ICRF-187 is found in its ability to decrease alloxan-induced diabetes in animals, which is an iron-dependent free radical process (El-Hage et al., 1986). Studies in a small number of patients have shown that digoxin may protect against changes in left ventricular function caused by doxorubicin (Whittaker and Al-Ismail, 1984). However, no pathologic studies were conducted to confirm this observation. The use of Ca^{2+} channel blockers to prevent doxorubicin cardiotoxicity is based on the hypothesis that doxorubicin causes increased myocardial Ca^{2+} uptake leading to Ca^{2+} overload and cell death (Rabkin et al., 1983). Calcium channel blockers have also been used in combination with doxorubicin in an attempt to improve the therapeutic efficacy of doxorubicin by preventing or overcoming the development of doxorubicin-resistant cells. In vitro, at least, certain Ca^{2+} channel blockers can prevent the increased efflux of doxorubicin from doxorubicin-resistant tumor cells, thus, increasing their drug sensitivity (Ozols et al., 1987). Very high doses of verapamil were found to potentiate doxorubicin cardiotoxicity in rabbits (Rabkin et al., 1983; Stephens et al., 1987). Studies in patients administered doxorubicin together with verapamil in doses sufficient to produce hypotension or heart block showed an unacceptable level of cardiac toxicity with no evidence of increased anthracycline therapeutic efficacy (Ozols et al., 1987). A pilot study by Garbrecht and Müllerleile (1986) using low doses of verapamil in patients receiving doxorubicin showed evidence of protection against cardiotoxicity. Nifedipine was studied clinically in combination with α-tocopherol and found to offer protection against acute cardiac toxic changes caused by doxorubicin (Lenzhofer et al., 1983). Prenylamine, an antianginal drug with calcium antagonistic properties which was shown to protect the rabbit and mouse against chronic doxorubicin cardiotoxicity (Table 7-4) appeared, in a small-scale clinical study, to protect patients in a similar way although no statistical significance could be shown because of the small sample size (Milei et al., 1986). L-carnitine is found in relatively high concentrations in cardiac tissue and plays a critical role in various metabolic functions of the heart including mitochondrial transmembrane transport of long chain fatty acids and regulation of acetyl CoA levels (McFalls et al., 1986). Several animal studies have shown L-carnitine to protect against doxorubicin cardiotoxicity (Table 7-4). Two small-scale studies in which patients receiving doxorubicin were given L-carnitine showed that it could give some protection against doxorubicin cardiotoxicity (DeLeonardis et al., 1985; 1987).

Despite the obvious clinical advantages of reducing doxorubicin cardiotoxicity there have been only a limited number of clinical trials of potential protective compounds. This is not for a lack of promising leads from animal studies. Most of the clinical studies have used relatively few patients and while results showing protection are interesting, they will have to be confirmed by large clinical trials. The most promising agent for protecting against anthracycline cardiotoxicity is ICRF-187, where preliminary results from a large, ongoing clinical trial hold the promise that it may be possible to reduce doxorubicin cardiotoxicity with this agent.

Altered Schedule. An alternative way that has been successfully used to decrease the cardiotoxicity of doxorubicin is to change the schedule of administration. Intermittent bolus administration of doxorubicin every three weeks was originally adopted, in part, because of the long biologic half-life of doxorubicin (Benjamin et al., 1973). Evidence then accumulated that weekly administration of doxorubicin produced less cardiotoxicity, although the incidence of other toxicities was unchanged and therapeutic efficacy was maintained (Anders et al., 1986; Chlebowski et al., 1980; Torti et al., 1983; Valdivieso et al., 1984; Von Hoff et al., 1979; Weiss et al., 1982). It was next reported that giving doxorubicin every three weeks, by 48 hr or 96 hr continuous infusion produced less cardiotoxicity and less nausea and vomiting than bolus administration, whereas myelosuppression was unchanged (Hortobagyi et al., 1989; Legha et al., 1982). Interestingly in these studies the severity of mucositis increased as the duration of the infusion increased. Because of the decreased cardiotoxicity, larger total

Table 7-4. Agents Studied to Protect Against Anthracycline Cardiotoxicity in Animals

AGENT	ACUTE CARDIOTOXICITY			CHRONIC CARDIOTOXICITY		
	SPECIES	EFFECT	REFERENCE	SPECIES	EFFECT	REFERENCE
Radical Scavengers						
α-Tocopherol	Mouse	No effect	Tanigawa et al., 1986	Rabbit/dog	No effect	Breed et al., 1980
	Mouse	Protect	Hermansen and Wassermann, 1986			Van Vleet et al., 1980
			Myers et al., 1976	Rabbit/pig	Protect	Milei et al., 1986
			Mimnaugh et al., 1979			Crescimanno et al., 1988
ascorbate	Mouse/guinea pig	Protect	Fujita et al., 1982			
selenium	Mouse	No effect	Hermansen and Wassermann, 1986	Dog	No effect*	Van Vleet et al., 1980
	Rabbit	Protect	Dimitrov et al., 1987			
glutathione	Mouse	Protect	Yoda et al., 1986			
cysteamine	Mouse	Protect	Olson et al., 1980			
N-acetyl cysteine	Mouse	Protect	Olson et al., 1980	Dog	No effect	Unverferth et al., 1985
			Doroshow et al., 1982			Herman et al., 1985
methylene Blue	Mouse	Protect	Hrushesky et al., 1985			
ubiquinone	Rat, mouse	No effect	Neri et al., 1988	Rabbit	Protect	Domae et al., 1981
			Tàbora et al., 1986			
	Rat, mouse	Protect	Folkers et al., 1978			
			Combs et al., 1977			
Cardiac Drugs						
prenylamine				Rabbit/mouse	Protect	Milei et al., 1985, 1986, 1988
verapamil	Rabbit	Increased toxicity	Stephens et al., 1987			
			Rabkin et al., 1983			
nifedipine	Mouse	Increased toxicity	Nissen et al., 1986			
diltiazem				Rabbit	Increased toxicity	Mochizuki et al., 1987
amrinone				Rat	No effect	Bernardini et al., 1986
trifluoperazine				Rat	No effect	Villani et al., 1988

Miscellaneous Drugs						
ibuprofen	Mouse	No effect	Robison and Giri, 1984			
methylprednisone				Rat	Protect	Dasmahapatra et al., 1984
PEG-400†				Mouse	Protect	Klugmann et al., 1984
solcoseryl				Rat	No effect	Danysz et al., 1986
QMDP-66‡						
bismuth subnitrate	Mice	Protect	Naganuma et al., 1988 ICRF-159§	Mice, Rat	Protect	Fischer et al., 1986
	Rat	Protect	Tian-Hu et al., 1983			Decorti et al., 1983
ICRF-187‖				Rabbit/rat/ dog/pig	Protect	Herman et al., 1988a, 1988b; Herman and Ferrans, 1985; 1983; 1986
Blockers of Histamine Release						
theophylline	Rat	Protect	Klugmann et al., 1986	Rat	Protect	Klugmann et al., 1986
cromoglycate	Rat/rabbit	Protect	Klugmann et al., 1986; Bristow et al., 1983	Rat	Protect	Klugmann et al., 1986
Biochemicals						
L-carnitine	Rat/mouse	Protect	Neri et al., 1988; Neri et al., 1986	Rat, rabbit	Protect	McFalls et al., 1986; Shug, 1987; Green et al., 1984
taurine	Mouse	Protect	Hamaguchi et al., 1988			
inosine				Rat	Protect	Czarnecki and Hinek, 1986
fructose-1,6-bisphosphate	Mouse	Protect	Lazzarino et al., 1987			Scheulen, 1987
isocitrate				Mouse	Protect	Schmitt-Graff and Scheulan, 1986
niacin				Mouse	Protect	Schmitt-Graff and Scheulen, 1986

*With α-tocopherol.
†PEG-400 = polyethylene glycol, mw 400.
‡QMDP-66 = a quinonyl derivative of N-acetylmuramyl dipeptide.
§ICRF-159 = [($\pm$)−1,2-bis-3,5-dioxopeperzainyl-1-yl propane].
‖ICRF-187 = (+) isomer of ICRF-159.

Table 7-5. Clinical Studies of Protection Against Doxorubicin Cardiotoxicity

AGENT	NUMBER OF PATIENTS	EFFECT	REFERENCE
prenylamine	26	Protect*†	Milei et al., 1987
verapamil	8	Increased toxicity‡	Ozols et al., 1987
	35	Protect§,‖,¶	Garbrecht and Müllerlie, 1986
digoxin	18	Protect‖	Whittaker and Al-Ismail, 1984
L-carnitine	9	Protect§*	DeLeonardis et al., 1985
	15		Leonardis et al., 1987
N-acetyl cysteine	20	No effect§ (on acute toxicity)	Unverferth et al., 1983
ubiquinone	22	Protect	Folkers and Wolaniuk, 1985
α-tocopherol	21	No effect	Legha et al., 1982
	19	No effect	Weitzman et al., 1980
	15	No effect‖	Whittaker and Al-Ismail, 1984
α-tocopherol + nifedipine	12	Protect*	Lenzhofer et al., 1983
ICRF-187	82	Protect§,‖	Green et al., 1987 Green, 1987 Speyer et al., 1987, 1988

Based on *ECG, †cardiomyopathy, ‡heart block, §histopathology, ‖left ventricular performance, and ¶echocardiography.

doses of doxorubicin could be given by infusion (600 mg/m^2) than by bolus (465 mg/m^2) administration, which may be responsible for an apparent small increase in therapeutic activity of the infusion schedule of doxorubicin administration. Note however, that the increase in therapeutic activity was small and not statistically significant. It was only seen for those patients who experienced a complete remission where the duration of the remission was prolonged (Hortobagyi et al., 1989). Pharmacokinetic studies showed similar plasma $C \times t$ values for bolus administration of doxorubicin and infusion schedules, but with peak plasma concentrations up to 13-fold higher following bolus administration. The results suggest that high peak plasma concentrations of doxorubicin are a contributing factor in increased cardiotoxicity associated with bolus anthracycline administration. Note that a prediction resulting from theoretical pharmacodynamic models for a cell cycle-nonspecific cytotoxic drug, such as doxorubicin, is that the total cytotoxic effect of a given dose of drug is independent of the schedule of administration (Jusko, 1971).

Studies, so far confined to experimental animals, have shown that combining doxorubicin with a carrier such as poly-L-aspartic acid (Pratesi et al., 1985) or in liposomes (Bellelli et al., 1988; Herman et al., 1983) can decrease cardiotoxicity without altering therapeutic efficacy, probably by producing a slowly releasable form of the anthracyclines.

Less Cardiotoxic Anthracycline Analogues. Attempts to develop less cardiotoxic anthracyclines has provided the main rationale for the extensive isolation and synthetic programs for anthracycline analogs. Anthracyclines that have been reported to have less cardiotoxicity than doxorubicin or daunorubicin in experimental animals include 4′-epidoxorubicin (Fig. 7-1-III, epirubicin), 4′-deoxydoxorubicin (esorubicin), 4-demethoxydaunorubicin (idarubicin), 4-demethyldaunorubicin (carminomycin), aclacinomycin A (Fig. 7-1-V), 4′-0-tetrahydro-pyranyldoxorubicin (THPD), menogaril (Fig. 7-1-VII), 5-iminodaunorubicin, N-trifluoroacetyldoxorubicin-14-valerate (AD-32) and 3′-deamino-3′-13″-cyano-4″-morpholinyldoxorubicin (Acton et al., 1984; Arcamone, 1984; Eliot et al., 1983; Ganzina et al., 1986; Henderson et al., 1978; Müller et al., 1984; Umezawa et al., 1979). Clinical trials have so far confirmed the lower cardiotoxicities of 4′-epidoxorubicin, 4′-deoxydoxorubicin, aclacinomycin A, and THPD (Akman et al., 1985; Cersosimo and Hong, 1986; Dickinson et al., 1984; Eklow et al., 1981; Phillips et al., 1981; Sato et al., 1977). Work to develop less cardiotoxic anthracyclines is based in large part on the belief that the dose limitation caused by cardiotoxicity, limits the therapeutic efficacy of the anthracyclines. However, clinical trials with altered schedules of administration which allowed larger total doses of anthracyclines to be given suggest this may not be the case. Whereas decreased cardiotoxicity may be a desirable property of the newer anthracyclines a more important property may be improved therapeutic efficacy.

Renal Toxicity

Anthracyclines clearly cause renal toxicity in animals but there are very few documented cases of anthracycline renal toxicity in humans (Bernard et al., 1969; Burke et al., 1977; Von Hoff et al., 1978; Weiss and Posner, 1982). This is probably because more severe cardiotoxicity supervenes before renal toxicity becomes a problem. A single or multiple doses of doxorubicin of >100 mg/m^2 to rabbit (Fajardo et al., 1980; Long et al., 1984) causes progressive proteinurea, increased serum creatinine levels, and hyperlipidemia affecting all lipoprotein classes, indicative of renal toxicity (Bizzi et al., 1983; van Hoesel et al., 1986). The first sign of damage is mild proteinurea and histological evidence of epithelial cell damage, followed by distal tubular protein casts (Bertani et al., 1986; Kubosawa et al., 1985; O'Donnell et al., 1985). The glomerular parietal epithelial cells show focal degeneration with blebs and invaginations of the plasma membrane by about one month. The proteinurea becomes worse as endothelial cells detach. Tubular destruction and breakage of the tubular basement membrane causes interstitial damage by six months. Eventually there is diffuse and global glomerular obliteration. The incidence of focal segmental glomerulosclerosis is low at six months but can progress to include most animals by nine months (Bertani et al., 1986). Biochemical changes in the kidney caused by doxorubicin include decreased superoxide dismutase and catalase (Julicher et al., 1988), decreased mitochondrial oxidation of long-chain fatty acids (Bizzi et al., 1983) and increased thromboxane A_2 synthesis (Remuzzi et al., 1985). The histopathological changes in the kidney are related to the dose of doxorubicin (Fajardo et al., 1980) and parallel the time course of myocardial lesions (Fajardo et al., 1980; Van Hoesel et al., 1986). A decreased liver function caused by concomitant administration of nitrosourea increases anthracycline renal toxicity in rats (Raguenez-Viotte et al., 1988). There have been studies to protect against anthracycline renal toxicity in animals. Steroids appear to offer no protection (Bertani et al., 1984), but protection has been seen with aluminum hydroxide (Motomura et al., 1988), a diet of fish oil rich in ω-3 fatty acids (Ito et al., 1988), platelet-activating factor-acether antagonists (David and Speechley, 1987), a thromboxane synthetase inhibitor (Julicher et al., 1988) and ICRF-159 (Tian-Hu et al., 1983). Unfortunately these studies give little indication of the mechanisms of anthracycline renal toxicity. The similar time course and protection by ICRF-159 suggest the mechanism might be similar to that seen in the heart. It appears that the mechanism differs from the renal toxicity seen with the aminonucleoside antibiotics and other causes of glomerular sclerosis (Bertani et al., 1984, 1986; O'Donnell et al., 1985).

Alopecia

A common side effect of anthracycline therapy is shedding of hair (effluvium) and hair thinning or baldness (alopecia). Although not life-threatening the loss of hair can be emotionally devastating for a patient and may lead to a refusal of chemotherapy (Maxwell, 1980; Seipp, 1985; Welch and Lewis, 1980; Wood, 1985). Human scalp hair grows at about 0.3 mm/d and the activity of each hair follicle is independent of adjacent hair follicles (Kligman, 1959). Between 85 and 95% of scalp follicles are in the growing (anagen) phase whereas five to 15% are in the nongrowing or shedding (telogen) phase. Club hair (nongrowing hair with a keratinized club at the base) is retained for about four months before being shed. Cytotoxic drugs are thought to cause alopecia by injuring the mitotically active anagen follicles and, depending on the degree of injury, hair may be shed within a few days due to excessive constriction of the shaft, or hair growth may continue at a slower rate (Flesch, 1963). There may also be excessive shedding of club hairs (telogen effluvium) (Rook, 1965). A correlation has been reported between the toxicity of anticancer drugs to bone marrow and damage to hair follicles (Crounse and Van Scott, 1960). There is currently no standard treatment for anticancer drug-induced alopecia (Dunagin, 1982; Seipp, 1985). Doxorubicin probably causes most problems of hair loss of all the anticancer drugs, and all patients receiving doxorubicin experience some degree of alopecia (Benjamin, 1975). Scalp hypothermia employing ice packs, cooled water, and refrigerated air to produce local vasoconstriction and decreased delivery of doxorubicin to the hair follicles has been used in attempts to prevent doxorubicin-induced alopecia in cancer patients, with varying degrees of success (Anderson et al., 1981; David and Speechley, 1987; Dean et al., 1979, 1983; Guy et al., 1982; Koide et al., 1981; Lawson et al., 1987; Parbhoo and Kelleher, 1985; Symonds et al., 1986; Wheelock et al., 1984). The protection is greater at low doses of doxorubicin (Anderson et al., 1981; David and Speechley, 1987; Lawson et al., 1987) and poor liver function is a significant factor against the success of scalp hypothermia (Anderson et al., 1981; David and Speechley, 1987; Hunt et al., 1982), perhaps because of delayed doxorubicin elimination associated with poor liver function. The technique of scalp hypothermia can only be used in patients who are not at risk of developing subsequent scalp metastases and, thus, excludes patients with leukemia and multiple myeloma (Seipp, 1985). Studies in Angora rabbit, which has a pattern of hair growth similar to that of human hair, have suggested that dietary α-tocopherol may protect against doxorubicin inhibition of new hair growth (Powis and Kooistra, 1987). Legha et al. (1982) reported that α-tocopherol did not protect patients against doxorubicin-induced alopecia, although the patients also received cyclophosphamide which causes alopecia by a mechanism that does not involve free radicals (Dunagin, 1982). A preliminary study by Wood (1985) indicated that large doses of oral α-tocopherol could, perhaps, protect patients against doxorubicin-induced alopecia. Based on this report studies were conducted by Perez et al. (1986) and Martin-Jimenez et al. (1986) on the ability of large doses of oral α-tocopherol to protect patients against doxorubicin-induced alopecia but no protection was found in either study.

Skin Toxicity

Severe toxicity can occur when doxorubicin accidentally leaks into the area around an intravenous (IV) infusion site (Barlock et al., 1979; Labandter and McElwee, 1979; Reilly et al., 1977). The necrosis increases in severity over several weeks and results in slowly healing ulcers. These indolent ulcers are a source of severe pain and even functional impairment for many months. In severe cases, the lesion may extend to deep structures such as underlying tendon and bone, resulting in loss of joint mobility. Estimates of the frequency of doxorubicin extravasation in patients range from 0.5% to over 6% (Svingen et al., 1981). The skin ulceration is a local reaction to the anthracycline and a free radical mechanism in its pathogenesis is suggested by the ability of free radical scavenging agents applied topically to the skin to prevent the skin toxicity. This is seen in animals with the free radical scavenging agents dimethylsulfoxide (Desai and Teres, 1982; Svingen et al., 1981), α-tocopherol (Nobbs and Barr, 1983; Svingen et al., 1981), and butylated hydroxytoluene (Daugherty and Khurana, 1985), or pretreatment of animals with butylated hydroxytoluene (Upton et al., 1986). Dimethylsulfoxide (Lawrence and Goodnight, 1983; Lawrence et al., 1989; Olver and Schwarz, 1983) and a mixture of dimethylsulfoxide and α-tocopherol (Ludwig et al., 1987) have been reported to protect patients against skin ulceration following accidental anthracycline extravasation.

MITOXANTRONE

The search for less cardiotoxic anthracycline-like agents led to the development of *bis*(substituted aminoalkylamino)-anthraquinone antitumor agents (Murdock et al., 1979; Tragenos,

1983; Zee-Cheng and Cheng, 1978). One of these, mitoxantrone (1,4-dihydroxy-5,8-*bis*(2-[(2-hydroxyethyl)amino]ethylamino)-9,10-anthracenedione dihydrochloride) (Fig. 7-4), has undergone extensive clinical evaluation and is now used for the treatment of breast cancer and acute leukemia (Posner et al., 1985; Saletan, 1987; Schenkenberg and Von Hoff, 1986). In mitoxantrone the anthracycline ring is retained but the daunosamine sugar of the anthracyclines has been replaced with an aminoalkylamino group. The *bis*(substituted aminoalkylamino)-anthraquinones have very low redox potentials (Svingen and Powis, 1981) and although they can undergo reduction to a semiquinone free radical (Basra et al., 1984, 1985; Sinha et al., 1983) it is at a much slower rate than anthracyclines (Kharasch and Novak, 1981, 1983c, 1985; Svingen and Powis, 1981). Superoxide anion radical formation is also very low (Basra et al., 1984; Kharasch and Novak, 1983c, 1985; Sinha et al., 1983). Mitoxantrone inhibits oxygen use by cardiac sarcoplasmic reticulum in the presence of NADPH, with no increase in superoxide anion radical formation (Doroshow, 1983a; Doroshow and Davies, 1983). Both in vivo and in vitro the *bis*(substituted aminoalkyl-amino)-anthraquinones cause less lipid peroxidation than anthracyclines (Kharasch and Novak, 1982a, 1983a, 1983b; Mimnaugh et al., 1983; Novak and Kharasch, 1985; Patterson et al., 1983).

Toxicity

The dose-limiting toxicity of mitoxantrone is myelosuppression, usually leukopenia but sometimes thrombocytopenia (Saleton, 1987). Alopecia, stomatitis, and mucositis are also produced but less than with doxorubicin. Mitoxantrone was developed to be less cardiotoxic than the anthracyclines and in preclinical testing in dogs was found to be devoid of cardiotoxic effects (Sparano et al., 1982). However, in mice and guinea pig mitoxantrone produces a spectrum of myocardial toxicity similar to that of doxorubicin (Perkins et al., 1984). In patients, mitoxantrone has been found to be less cardiotoxic than doxorubicin. The incidence of cardiotoxicity with mitoxantrone is 3% in adults and 6% in children (Poirier, 1986). Large scale trials have shown the risk of congestive heart failure to be 0.9% with mitoxantrone compared to 3.0% with doxorubicin (Dukart et al., 1986). The risk of cardiotoxicity with mitoxantrone increases above a cumulative dose of 160 mg/m^2, which is equivalent in terms of myelosuppression to 800 mg/m^2 doxorubicin (Posner et al., 1985). This translates into an improved therapeutic index for mitoxantrone compared to doxorubicin (Saleton, 1987).

BLEOMYCIN

Introduction

The bleomycins are a group of complex glycopeptides produced by *Streptomyces verticillus* that were first discovered in 1959 by Umezawa and his colleagues in Japan (Umezawa et al., 1966; Umezawa, 1979). Although present naturally as a Cu(II) complex, copper-free bleomycin is used clinically to avoid the significant phlebitis caused by the inclusion of copper (Umezawa, 1979). Bleomycin sulfate used clinically is a mixture comprising of 55 to 70% bleomycin A_2, 25 to 32% bleomycin B_2, and small quantities of a number of other bleomycins (Crooke and Bradner, 1976). Several bleomycin analogues have been developed and two

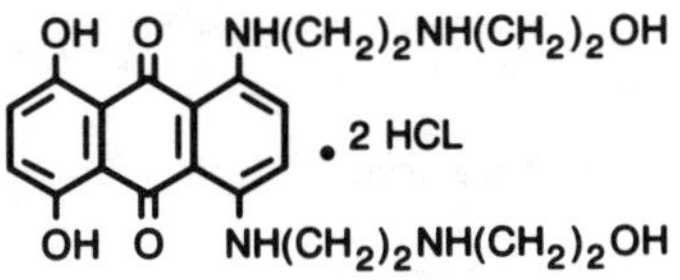

OH O NH$(CH_2)_2$NH$(CH_2)_2$OH

• 2 HCL

OH O NH$(CH_2)_2$NH$(CH_2)_2$OH

FIGURE 7-4. Structure of mitoxantrone.

of them, peplomycin and talisomycin S_{10b}, have undergone clinical trial. The structures of some bleomycins and bleomycin analogues are shown in Fig. 7-5.

Bleomcyin has activity in the treatment of Hodgkin's disease, non-Hodgkin's lymphomas, penile carcinosarcomas, advanced head and neck cancer, cervical cancer, lung cancer, and testicular carcinoma (Baker, 1978; Bonadonna et al., 1975; Einhorn and Donohue, 1977; Folke et al., 1976; Livingston, 1978; Stoter et al., 1979; Wittes et al., 1975). Bleomycin is rarely used alone but is found as part of combination chemotherapy regimens some of which, for germ-cell and testicular carcinomas and lymphomas, are curative. A valuable feature of bleomycin is its lack of significant bone marrow, hepatic, or renal toxicity, thus, allowing it to be combined with other chemotherapeutic agents that possess these toxicities (Bennett and Reich, 1979). The major dose-limiting toxicity of bleomycin is functional and morphological pulmonary injury. Bleomycin also causes significant skin toxicity.

Mechanism of Antitumor Activity

There are two structural features of bleomycin that are important for its biological activity. First, there is a metal binding domain located between the end of the terminal β-aminoalanine and the bithiazole moiety which binds divalent metal ions in the order Fe(II) < Co(II) < Ni(II) < Cu(II) (Sugiura, 1980). X-ray crystallography suggests a square-pyramidal complex with the basal plane comprising the secondary amine nitrogen, the N-4 pyrimidine ring nitrogen, the deprotonated peptide bond nitrogen of the histidine residue, and the imidazole nitrogen. The fifth axial donor is the α-amino nitrogen of the β-aminoalanaine and the sixth axial coordination site can bind molecular oxygen (Antholine et al., 1984; Sugiura, 1980; Umezawa, 1979) (Fig. 7-6). The second important structural feature of bleomycin is a DNA-binding domain comprising the terminal amine and the bithiazole moiety. Bleomycin binds to specific nucleotide sequences such as 5′-GC-3′ and 5′-GT-3′. There may also be preference for other topological features for DNA binding by bleomycin (Mirabelli et al., 1983).

The antitumor activity of bleomycin is thought to depend on the formation of a DNA-

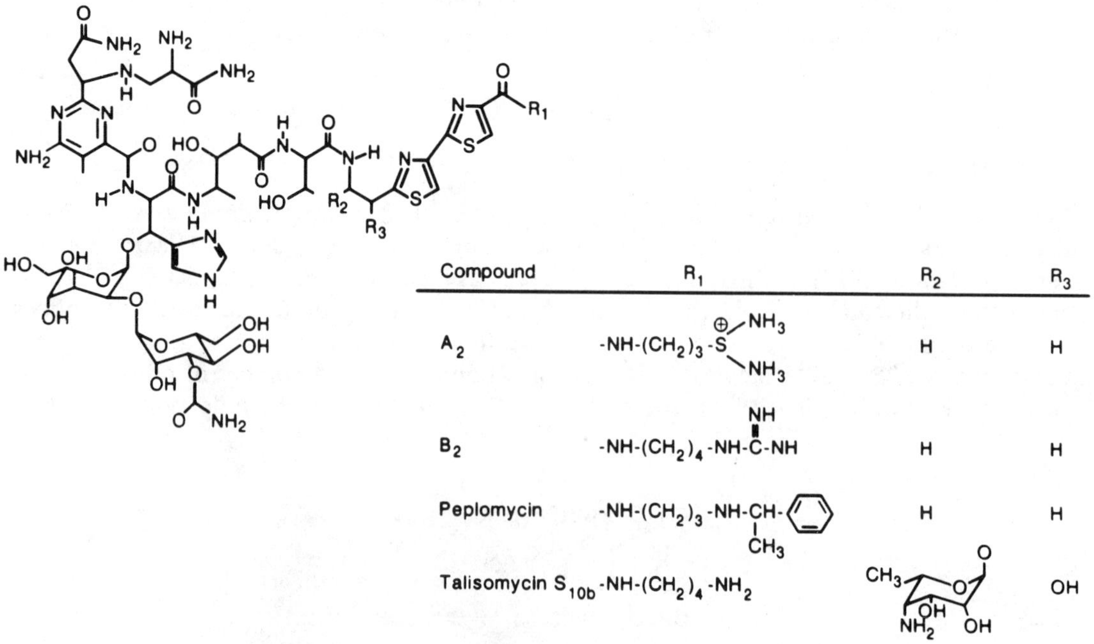

Compound	R_1	R_2	R_3
A_2	$-NH-(CH_2)_3-S^{\oplus}(NH_3)(NH_3)$	H	H
B_2	$-NH-(CH_2)_4-NH-C(=NH)-NH$	H	H
Peplomycin	$-NH-(CH_2)_3-NH-CH(CH_3)-C_6H_5$	H	H
Talisomycin S_{10b}	$-NH-(CH_2)_4-NH_2$	(sugar: CH_3, OH, NH_2, OH)	OH

FIGURE 7-5. Structure of some bleomycins and bleomycin analogues.

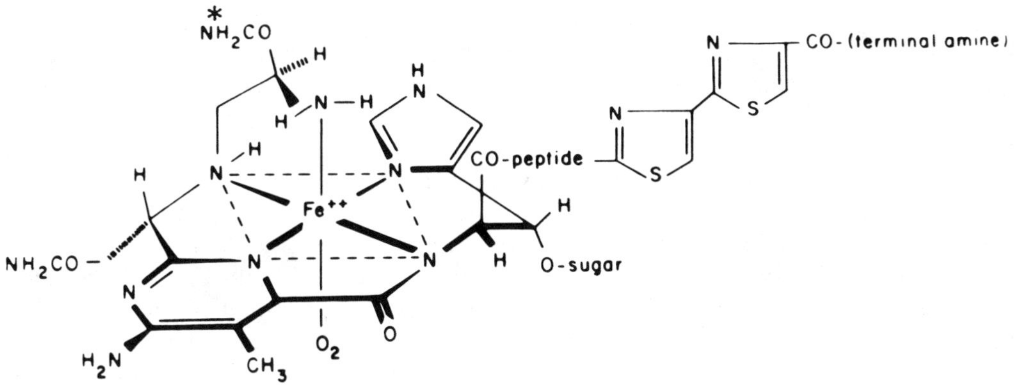

Bleomycin-ferrous-ion complex

FIGURE 7-6. Proposed metal coordination structure of bleomycin. From Lazo et al. (1987). Reprinted with permission.

bleomycin-Fe(II)-O_2 complex (Sausville et al., 1978; Umezawa, 1979). In the presence of appropriate reductants such as sulfhydryl compounds and ascorbate (Burger et al., 1985) there is catalytic formation of hydroxyl and superoxide anion radicals by bleomycin (Lown and Sim, 1977). One mole of bleomycin can turn over 5000 moles of Fe(II) per minute (Caspary et al., 1979). The DNA binding domain of bleomycin presumably allows the metal chelated portion of bleomycin to generate the oxygen radicals in close proximity to DNA, resulting in DNA single and double strand breaks and base release. Bleomycin circulates in the blood (Kanao et al., 1973) and enters the cell as the Cu(II) form (Uehara et al., 1982). Once inside the cell the cupric ion is reduced and the cuprous ion abstracted by sulfhydryl containing macromolecules (Takahashi et al., 1977; Umezawa, 1979). The metal free bleomycin then combines with ferrous (or ferric) ion to produce the biologically active form.

Pulmonary Toxicity

Pulmonary toxicity results in fibrosis as the dose-limiting toxicity of bleomycin. The reported incidence of pneumonitis and fibrosis varies from 10 to 40% of patients (Blum and Carter, 1976; Haas et al., 1976; Sikic, 1985) with progressive fatal pulmonary fibrosis occurring in 1% of patients (Blum and Carter, 1976; Sikic, 1985). The clinical symptoms of bleomycin pneumonitis are seen one to three months after the start of therapy. Typically the symptoms are nonspecific with a nonproductive cough, exertional dyspnea, and fever (DeLena et al., 1972; Van Barneveld et al., 1985). With progressive disease dyspnea at rest, tachypnea, and cyanosis are seen. X-rays show bilateral, bibasilar infiltration, and lower lobe consolidation (Van Barneveld et al., 1985). The risk for serious pulmonary toxicity increases markedly with total cumulative doses of bleomycin over 400 U (Sikic, 1985). Risk factors for the development of pulmonary toxicity with bleomycin are: age (greater than 70 years), preexisting pulmonary or renal disease, thoracic radiation, concomitant chemotherapy, and transient exposure to high oxygen concentrations during anesthesia (Dalgleish et al., 1984; Sikic, 1985; Tryka, 1987; Zabbe et al., 1986). Respiratory function tests have been used to detect early pulmonary toxicity. Carbon monoxide diffusing capacity is probably the most sensitive indicator of subclinical toxicity (Bell et al., 1985; Comis et al., 1979; Srensen et al., 1985) whereas recent studies suggest that quantitative computed tomography may also be useful (Bellamy et al., 1987).

A number of animal models for bleomycin lung toxicity have been developed; in mice (Aso et al., 1976; Harrison and Lazo, 1987; Orr et al., 1986; Sikic et al., 1978), rats (Berend, 1984; Brown et al., 1988; Hay et al., 1987; Wang-Ming and Montgomery, 1980), hamsters (Snider et al., 1978; Tryka, 1987), rabbits (Laurent et al., 1981), and baboons (McCullough et al., 1978). Bleomycin administered either IV, intratracheally, or subcutaneously produces lung fibrosis in animals (Harrison and Lazo, 1987; Lindenschmidt et al., 1986). These models show that the earliest site of bleomycin lung injury is the pulmonary vascular endothelial cells which together with the Type I pneumocytes form the barrier that separates the blood from the air (Catravas, 1987). One week after bleomycin administration diffuse exudative alveolar damage with interstitial edema and sloughing of the alveolar lining and hyaline membrane is apparent (Adamson and Bowden, 1974; Brown et al., 1988; Tryka, 1987). This gives way by two weeks to a proliferative phase of acute toxicity with interstitium thickening by inflammatory cells, hyperplasia of Type II pneumocytes, and alteration in alveolar structure including obliteration, degeneration, collapse, and enlargement. After this acute phase of toxicity the lungs heal with resulting interstitial pulmonary fibrosis. The changes are progressive with repeated doses of bleomycin (Brown et al., 1988).

Studies in animals have confirmed the clinical observation that hyperoxia increases bleomycin lung toxicity (Berend, 1984; Goad et al., 1987; Hay et al., 1987; Tryka et al., 1984) and have demonstrated protection by hypoxia (Berend, 1984). Of potential clinical significance is the observation that the bleomycin damaged lung in mice is a preferential site for metastatic tumor development (Orr et al., 1986). A number of biochemical changes are seen in the lung of bleomycin treated animals including elevated fibroblast polysomal type I procollagen RNA and prolylhydroxylase (Cutroneo et al., 1987), decreased angiotensin-converting enzyme activity and prostaglandin synthesis (Catravas, 1987), decreased serotonin and norepinephrine uptake (Catravas, 1987), increased lipid peroxidation (Giri et al., 1983; Yarbro et al., 1987) and the release by alveolar and interstitial macrophages of immunoregulatory and anabolic monokines (Kelley and Kovacs, 1987).

Mechanism of Bleomycin Lung Toxicity

The basic mechanism of bleomycin damage to the lung is most likely to involve formation of oxygen free radical with subsequent damage to DNA and lipid membranes (Muraoka et al., 1986; Passero and DiSanto, 1988). Several pieces of evidence support a free radical mechanism of lung damage by bleomycin. Patients receiving bleomycin have increased amounts of hydrogen peroxide, a product of free radical formation, in their breath (Yarbro et al., 1987). Free radical protective enzymes in lung, including catalase, glutathione reductase and glutathione peroxidase, are increased by bleomycin administration to animals (Filderman et al., 1988; Giri et al., 1983). There is an increase in thiobarbituric acid reactive material indicative of lipid peroxidation in hamsters given intratracheal bleomycin (Giri et al., 1983). Evidence against the involvement of lipid peroxidation in acute bleomycin lung toxicity is the failure to find an increase in ethane expiration in the breath of rats given a single toxic intraperitoneal (IP) dose of bleomycin (Muliawan et al., 1982). Free radical oxidation of polyunsaturated fatty acids may lead to the formation of chemotactic eicosanoids thus initiating the inflammatory response seen with bleomycin lung toxicity (Passero and DiSanto, 1988).

The reason bleomycin is selectively toxic to the lung and skin appears to be related to a deficiency of an enzyme, bleomycin hydrolase, in these tissues. The biological activity of bleomycin is dependent on the presence of a carboxamide group in the β-aminoalanine moiety (Fig. 7-6). Hydrolysis of the carboxyamide bond to give deamidobleomycin results in a more basic β-amino group of the β-aminoalanine and at physiological pH the carboxylic acid group rather than the now protonated β-amine occupies the fifth coordination site of the bleomycin-Fe(II) complex (Lazo et al., 1987). This results in a decreased efficiency of binding of molecular oxygen and about 1/100th the ability compared to bleomycin of deamidobleomycin to generate free radicals, to cleave DNA and to kill tumor cells (Lazo et al., 1987; Sugiura, 1980; Umezawa, 1979). Deamidobleomycin A_2 does not produce lung toxicity when administered to mice (Lazo and Humphreys, 1983). Lung and skin of animals have low levels of bleomycin hydrolase compared to liver, kidney, spleen, and bone marrow (Ohnuma et al., 1974; Umezawa et al., 1972). A limited study of human tissues has shown lower bleomycin hydroxylase activity in skin compared to the liver, erythrocytes, and spleen (Ohnuma et al., 1974). There also appears to be a genetic basis for sensitivity to bleomycin. Strains of rabbits and mice with increased sensitivity to lung toxicity with bleomycin have very low levels of lung bleomycin hydroxylase (Filderman and Lazo, 1985; Lazo, 1987; Lazo and Humphreys, 1983). Distribution of bleomycin among pulmonary cell types is heterogeneous (Lazo et al., 1984). Bovine lung endothelial cells have low bleomycin hydroxylase activity whereas rabbit lung endothelial cells have significant amounts of the enzyme and type II cells have nearly undetectable activity (Lazo et al., 1987). Lazo and his colleagues (Lazo et al., 1983, 1984; Lazo and Pham, 1984) have proposed a model in which the pulmonary endothelium acts as a physical and metabolic barrier to the entry and bleomycin to the pulmonary interstitium. Damage to the endothelium by factors such as hyperoxia or radiation can injure the pulmonary endothelium allowing increased entry of bleomycin and, thus, increased lung damage.

Protection Against Bleomycin Lung Toxicity

Studies in animals have shown that treatments directed at decreasing oxygen free radical formation by bleomycin can decrease lung toxicity. The treatments studied include hypoxia (Berend, 1984), iron deficiency (Chandler et al., 1987, 1988a), chelation of iron with deferoxamine (Chandler et al., 1988b; Cross et al., 1985; Veninga et al., 1988), or D-penicillamine (Geismar et al., 1986) and free radical scavengers such as dimethylsulfoxide (Pepin and Langner, 1985) and N-acetylcysteine (Ward et al., 1987). Low temperature (4°C) also decreased bleomycin lung toxicity in rat (Berend, 1983). Administration of cis-hydroxyproline partially prevents bleomycin lung fibrosis by decreasing collagen accumulation (Riley et al., 1981) while methylprednisolone decreases total and bleomycin-induced lung collagen synthesis (Phan et al., 1981). Ambroxol, an agent capable of altering the secretory activity of type II pneumocytes, the source of lung surfactant, delayed the appearance of bleomycin lung fibrosis in rats (Luisetti et al., 1987). Clinical studies showed that ambroxol did not protect patients against bleomycin lung toxicity (Luisetti et al., 1987). There have been no other clinical trials of the agents that protect against bleomycin lung toxicity in animals. Currently, patients presenting with bleomycin hypersensitivity pneumonitis are treated with corticosteroids that can cause normalization of symptoms and functional impairment (Holoye et al., 1978). Steroid therapy is only occasionally useful in patients with direct toxic lung damage (Yagoda et al., 1972).

Route and schedule of administration may have an effect on bleomycin lung toxicity. Studies in mice by Sikic et al. (1978) showed that continuous subcutaneous infusion of bleomycin decreased lung toxicity and even increased the antitumor activity of bleomycin. Clinical studies have shown that administering peplomycin by consecutive daily injection (Satake et al., 1985a) or as a continuous subcutaneous infusion (Satake et al., 1985a, 1985b) decreases lung toxicity.

Bleomycin analogues have been studied with the aim of reducing lung toxicity (Takashi et al., 1987). In animals peplomycin (Ekimoto et al., 1984; Hashimoto et al., 1978; Ishii et al., 1985) and liblomycin (Newman et al., 1988) have shown less lung toxicity than bleomycin but talisomycin S_{10b} has shown only marginally decreased lung toxicity compared to bleomycin (Schlein et al., 1981; Schurig et al., 1984). Clinical studies with peplomycin have so far shown no pulmonary toxicity (Villani et al., 1988). New formulations may also help to reduce lung toxicity. Adsorption of peplomycin to carbon particles has been shown to further decrease its lung toxicity when given IP or IV to mice (Hagiwara et al., 1988).

Other Toxicities

Studies in rat have shown that chronic bleomycin administration causes atrophy of sebaceous glands and thickening of the skin which has an increased tensile strength reflecting changes in the total amount and the biochemical properties of the skin collagen (Chandrasekaran et al., 1985, 1987; Mountz et al., 1983). The sensitivity of skin to bleomycin is probably, as in lung, due to the low levels of bleomycin hydrolase compared to other tissues (Ohnuma et al., 1974; Umezawa et al., 1972). Other toxicities of bleomycin are vascular complications, including Raynaud's phenomenon, pulmonary veno-occlusive disease, cerebrovascular accidents, and acute myocardial infarction (Bellmunt et al., 1987). Capillaroscopy has shown signs of capillary damage even in asymptomatic patients and is higher at doses of bleomycin above 100 U. Alopecia occurs in about three quarters of patients (Krakoff, 1986). Mucocutaneous toxicity is also frequently seen (Krakoff, 1986).

NEOCARZINOSTATIN

Introduction

Neocarzinostatin (zinostatin) is a protein antibiotic from *streptomyces carzinostaticus* variant F-41 (Ishida et al., 1965) with antitumor properties in experimental animals (Kikuchi et al., 1974) and, to a limited extent, in humans (Legha et al., 1976; Maeda, 1981). It is a single-chain acidic protein of molecular weight 10,717 with a known amino acid sequence (Kuromitzu et al., 1986; Meienhofer et al., 1972) and a chromophore (Edo et al., 1985) (Fig. 7-7) which fits in a cavity of the protein where it is protected from rapid autoxidation with the generation of superoxide anion radical (Chin and Goldberg, 1986). There is strong circumstantial evidence for a free radical mechanism with damage to DNA being responsible to the antitumor activity of neocarzinostatin. Cells incubated with neocarzinostatin or the neocarzinostatin chromophore show nuclear DNA strand breaks (Hatayama and Goldberg, 1979; Kuo et al., 1984). The addition of thiols greatly stimulates DNA degradation by neocarzinostatin (Beerman and Goldberg, 1974). The chromophore is three to four orders of magnitude more strongly bound to the neocarzinostatin apoprotein than to DNA (Dasgupta et al., 1985) but there is no evidence for the binding of the apoprotein to DNA and the chromophore must first dissociate from the apoprotein before it can bind to the minor groove of DNA (Dasgupta et al., 1985; Jung and Kohnlein, 1981; Povirk and Goldberg, 1980). Reduction of the neocarzinostatin chromophore by thiol generates a free radical species that may be a peroxyl radical or a "crypto" hydroxyl radical (Edo et al., 1980; Sheridan and Gupta, 1981). There is, however, no evidence that free superoxide aniona radical or hydroxyl radical is responsible for DNA damage by neocarzinostatin (reviewed by Chin and Goldberg, 1986). This occurs because the oxygen radical scavengers superoxide dismutase, catalase, and hydroxyl radical scavengers do not prevent the DNA damage by carzinostatin. Despite the inability to identify the critical free radical species it is generally thought that a free radical mechanism is responsible for the antitumor activity of neocarzinostatin (Goldberg, 1987).

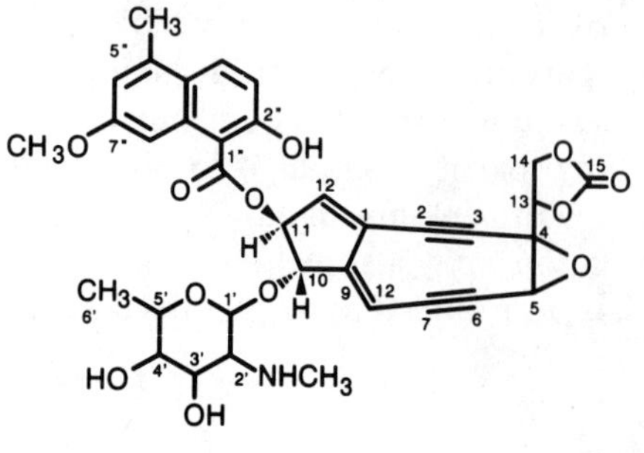

FIGURE 7-7. Structure of the neocarzinostatin chromophore (Edo et al., 1985). Reprinted with permission.

Toxicity

The acute toxicity of neocarzinostatin is nausea and vomiting, fever and chills, rigor hypotension, and mental confusion (Ohnuma et al., 1978; Rivera et al., 1978). These responses are similar to the toxic effects of other proteins used in chemotherapy such as the interferons and tumor necrosis factor (Borden, 1988). The dose limiting toxicity of neocarzinostatin is bone marrow suppression particularly leukopenia and thrombocytopenia (Griffin et al., 1978; Legha et al., 1976; McKelvey et al., 1979; Ohnuma et al., 1978; Rivera et al., 1978). The mechanism of the bone marrow suppression is, presumably, the same as that responsible for antitumor activity, DNA degradation. Thiol containing compounds, gluthathione, sodium thioglycolate, L-cysteine, and N-(2-mercaptopropionyl)-glycine (tiopronin) will block the activity of neocarzinostatin in vivo (Ito et al., 1985). Attempts have been made in animals to increase the therapeutic index of neocarzinostatin by administering the drug IA, IV or directly into the tumor and giving the thiols by another route, in the above cases IV, subcutaneously or IV (Ito et al., 1985; Iwamoto et al., 1986; Ouchi et al., 1988). This has resulted in protection of the bone marrow and decreased toxicity of neocarzinostatin.

Neocarzinostatin causes skin toxicity characterized by pruritis, maculopapular rash, and urticaria in three to 28% of patients (Weiss, 1982). These reactions occur after patients have received at least one course of therapy which would be compatible with the induction of antibodies (Vosika et al., 1983). Attempts to detect formation of antibodies to neocarzinostatin have, however, been unsuccessful (Sakamoto et al., 1978). Pulmonary toxicity has also been reported in patients receiving neocarzinostatin (Calvo et al., 1981; Natale et al., 1980; Seltzer et al., 1978; Weiss and Muggia, 1980). The mechanism for the pulmonary toxicity is not known, but it is tempting to speculate that, as with bleomycin, it is due to free radical damage to the lung. Finally, neocarzinostatin has been shown to cause base substitutions, frame shift mutations, chromosome aberrations and to be mutagenic in a number of test systems (Au et al., 1984; DeGraff, 1984; Povirk and Goldberg, 1987; Tsuda, 1987). Animal studies have shown neocarzinostatin to cause renal carcinoma (Tsuda, 1987) and it has been implicated as a possible cause of multiple secondary tumors in a patient who received neocarcinostatin therapy (Sakamoto et al., 1980).

CONCLUSIONS

Are there any general features to be observed among the toxicities of these free radical forming drugs and can the experience gained from the administration of these drugs to humans be extrapolated to other toxic chemicals? It is clear that although myelosuppression is the acute dose-limiting toxicity of all the drugs except bleomycin, it is reversible, dose related and readily managed in a clinical setting. Clinicians have become extremely well practiced at titrating this form of anticancer drug toxicity. It has also proven very difficult to separate myelosuppression and mucositis from the antitumor effects of the drugs suggesting a common mechanism of action that does not depend on free radical formation. By far the most worrying toxicities are the cumulative, dose-dependent cardiac toxicity exhibited by the anthracyclines and mitoxantrone, and the pulmonary toxicity of bleomycin and neocarzinostatin. These toxicities are most likely related to free radical formation by the drugs in highly vascular, well-oxygenated tissues. The nature of the toxic response suggests there is a threshold cumulative dose below which appreciable human toxicity does not occur.

Human toxic response is variable and clinicians have learned that an understanding of risk factors can do much to lessen the toxic effects of the anticancer drugs. Pharmacokinetic studies have helped to predict which patients may experience cardiac toxicity with the anthracyclines, where the risk of toxicity is correlated with an increased area under the plasma concentration time curve for the drug. Antitumor activity, myelosuppression and mucositis do not show this relationship to pharmacokinetic parameters. Not surprisingly, for drugs that are eliminated by the liver (anthracyclines) or by the kidney (bleomycin) poor hepatic or renal function is associated with an increased risk of toxicity. Age and preexisting disease also predispose to drug toxicity. These simple risk factors could well apply to the human toxicities of a wide number of agents in our environment.

Because of extensive studies conducted in both animals and humans on the toxicity of the radical forming anticancer drugs, we are in a unique position to address the relevance of animal models for predicting human toxicity in a way not possible with most toxic agents. Animals are clearly poor models for predicting alopecia and such subjective toxicities in human as nausea and vomiting. Even when they occur, many even in the health field do not appreciate the devastating psychological impact of these toxicities on the self-image of a patient. Animals have not been useful models for predicting the human cardiac toxicity of mitoxantrone and treatments that protect against anthracycline cardiotoxicity in animals have not proven useful for protecting human subjects. The cardiac toxicity when it occurs in animals seems to be different to that seen in humans. Animal studies have also shown the anthracyclines to be significantly renal toxic but this toxicity is rarely seen in patients. Studies with bleomycin in animals have yielded results more comparable with human toxicity. Work is now emerging showing in mice a genetic basis for bleomycin lung toxicity. Such evidence would be almost impossible to obtain in cancer patients alone.

It cannot be reemphasized too frequently that toxicity need not be an inevitable consequence of cancer chemotherapy. Great advances have been made in reducing toxicity of cancer chemotherapy without compromising therapeutic efficacy. The work on dose modification of anthracyclines to limit cardiac toxicity is an outstanding example. However, continued efforts need to be made to understand the mechanisms underlying anticancer drug toxicity and how it can be reduced.

REFERENCES

Abramson JJ, Buck E, Salama G, Casida JE, and Pessah IN Mechanism of anthraquinone-induced calcium release from skeletal muscle sarcoplasmic reticulum. J Biol Chem 1988 263:18750–18754.

Abramson HN, Banning JW, Nachtman JP, Roginski ET, Sardessai M, Wormser HC, Wu J, Nagia Z, Schroeder RR, and Bernardo MM Synthesis of anthraquinonyl glucosaminosides and studies on the influence of aglycone hydroxyl substitution on superoxide generation DNA binding and antimicrobial properties. J Med Chem 1986 29:1709–1714.

Acton M, Tong GL, Mosher CW, and Wolgemuth RL Intensely potent morpholinyl anthracyclines. J Med Chem 1984 27:638–645.

Adachi T, Nagae T, Ho Y, Hirano K, and Sugiura M Relation between cardiotoxic effect of adriamycin and superoxide anion radical. J Pharmacobiodyn 1983 6:114–123.

Adamson IYR and Bowden DH The pathogenesis of bleomycin induced pulmonary fibrosis in mice. Am J Pathol 1974 77:185–198.

Ahmed NK, Felsted RL, and Bachur NR Heterogeneity of anthracycline antibiotic carbonyl reductases in mammalian livers. Biochem Pharmacol 1978a 27:2713.

Ahmed NK, Felsted RL, and Bachur NR Comparison and characterization of mammalian xenobiotic ketone reductases. J Pharmacol Exper Ther 1978b 209:12–19.

Ahmed NK, Felsted RL, and Bachur NR Daunorubicin reduction mediated by aldehyde and ketone reductases. Xenobiotica 1981 11:131–136.

Akman SA, Dietrich M, Chlebowski R, Limberg P, and Block JB Modulation of cytotoxicity of menadione sodium busulfite versus leukemia L1210 by the acid soluble thiol pool. Cancer Res 1985 45:5257–5262.

Ali MK, Soto A, Maroongroge D, Bekheit-Saad S, Buzdar AU, Blumenschein GR, Hortobagy GN, Tashima CK, Wiseman CL, and Shullenberg CC Electrocardiographic changes after adriamycin chemotherapy. Cancer 1979 43:465–471.

Anders RJ, Shanes JG, and Zeller FP Lower incidence of doxorubicin-induced cardiomyopathy by once-a-week low-dose administration. Am Heart J 1986 111:755–759.

Anderson JE, Hunt JM, and Smith IE Prevention of doxorubicin-induced alopecia by scalp cooling in patients with advanced breast cancer. Br Med J 1981 282:423.

Anne A and Moiroux J One-electron reduction of variously substituted anthraquinones. Reactivity of the radical anions with oxygen in aprotic media. Nouv J Chim 1984 8:259–266.

Antholine WE, Riedy G, Hyde JS, Basosi R, and Petering D ESR parameters for cupric bleomycin in the mobilized state. J Biomol Struct Dynamics 1984 2:469–480.

Arcamone F New antitumor anthracyclines. Lloydia 1977 40:45–66.
Arcamone F Antitumor anthracyclines: Recent developments. Med Res Rev 1984 4:153–158.
Arcamone F Properties of antitumor anthracyclines and new developments in their application; Cain Memorial Award Lecture. Cancer Res 1985 45:5995–5999.
Arcamone F, Franceschi G, Penco S, and Selva A Adriamycin 14-hydroxydaunomycin: A novel antitumor antibiotic. Tetrahedron Lett 1969 13:1007–1016.
Arena E, D'Alessandro N, Dusonchet L, Gebbia L, Gerbasi F, Sanguedolce R, and Rausa L Influence of pharmacokinetic variations on the pharmacologic properties of adriamycin. In: International Symposium on Adriamycin Carter SK, DiMarco A, Ghione M, Krakoff IH, Mathe G Eds Springer-Verlag, Berlin, Heidelberg, New York 1972 pp. 96–116.
Arnolda L, McGrath BP, Cocks M, and Johnston CI Vasoconstrictor role for vasopressin in experimental heart failure in the rabbit. J Clin Invest 1986 78:674–679.
Aso Y, Yoneda K, and Kikkawa Y Morphologic and biochemical study of pulmonary changes induced by bleomycin in mice. Lab Invest 1976 35:558–567.
Au WW, O'Neill JP, Wang W, Luippold HE, and Preston RJ Induction of chromosome aberrations and specific locus mutation but not sister chromatid exchanges in Chinese hamster ovary cells by neocarzinostatin. Teratogenesis Carcinog Mutagen 1984 4:515–522.
Aversano RC and Boor PJ Histochemical alterations of acute and chronic doxorubicin cardiotoxicity. J Mol Cell Cardiol 1983 15:543–555.
Azuma J, Sperelakis N, Hasegawa H, Tanimoto T, Vogel S, Ogura K, Awata N, Sawamura A, Harada H, Ishiyama T, Morita Y, and Yamamura Y Adriamycin cardiotoxicity: Possible pathogenic mechanisms. J Mol Cell Cardiol 1981 13:381–397.
Bachman E, Weber E, and Zbinden G Effects of mitoxantrone and doxorubicin on energy metabolism of the rat heart. Cancer Treat Rep 1987 71:361–366.
Bachur NR Anthracycline antibiotic pharmacology and metabolism. Cancer Treat Rep 1979 63:817–820.
Bachur NR and Gee M Daunorubicin metabolism by rat tissue preparations. J Pharmacol Exp Ther 1971 177:567–572.
Bachur NR, Gee MV, and Gordon SL Enzymatic activation of actinomycin D ACTD to free radical state. Proc Amer Assoc Cancer Res 1978 19:75.
Bachur NR, Gordon SL, and Gee MV Anthracycline antibiotic augmentation of microsomal electron transport and free radical formation. Mol Pharmacol 1977 13:901–910.
Bachur NR, Riggs CE, Green MR, Langaro MR, Van Vurakis JJ, and Levine L Plasma adriamycin and daunorubicin levels by fluorescence and radioimmunoassay. Clin Pharmacol Ther 1977 21:70–77.
Bachur NR, Gordon SL, and Gee MV A general mechanism for microsomal activation of quinone anticancer agents to free radicals. Cancer Res 1978 38:1745–1750.
Baker LA A bleomycin combination for disseminated cervical cancer. In: Bleomycin Current Status and New Developments Carter SK and Umezawa H Eds Academic Press, New York 1978 pp. 173–184.
Bannister JV and Thornalley PJ The production of hydroxyl radicals by adriamycin in red blood cells. FEBS Lett 1983 157:170–172.
Basra J, Brown JR, and Patterson LH Free radical formation in vitro by cytotoxic anthraquinone derivatives; comparison with doxorubicin. Inv New Drugs 1984 2:117.
Basra J, Wolf CR, Brown JR, and Patterson LH Evidence for human liver mediated free-radical formation by doxorubicin and mitoxantrone. Anticancer Drug Design 1985 1:45–52.
Bates DA Evidence for the production of hydroxyl radicals from the adriamycin semiquinone and H_2O_2. FEBS Lett 1982 136:89–94.
Bates DA and Winterbourn CC Deoxyribose breakdown by the adriamycin semiquinone and H_2O_2: Evidence for hydroxyl radical participation. FEBS Lett 1982 145:137–142.
Beerman TA and Goldberg IH DNA strand scission by the antitumor protein neocarzinostatin. Biochem Biophys Res Commun 1974 59:1254–1261.
Bell MR, Meredith DJ, and Gill PG Role of carbon monoxide diffusing capacity in the early detection of major bleomycin-induced pulmonary toxicity. Aust NZJ Med 1985 15:235–240.
Bellamy EA, Nicholas D, and Husband JE Quantitative assessment of lung damage due to bleomycin using computed tomography. Br J Radiol 1987 60:1205–1209.
Bellelli A, Giomini M, Guiliani AM, Giustini M, Lorenzon I, Rusconi V, Sezzi ML, Trotta E, and Belleli L Antitumor effect and cardiotoxicity of a doxorubicin-lecithin association. Anticancer Res 1988 8:177–186.
Bellmunt J, Knobel H, Hidalgo R, Navarro M, Jolis L, Vilardell M, and Sole LA Capillaroscopy: A useful method for detection of bleomycin induced vascular toxicity. ECCO-4 Fourth European Conference on Clinical Oncology and Cancer Nursing 1987 p. 85.

Benjamin RS A practical approach to adriamycin. NSC-123127 toxicology. Cancer Chemother Rep 1975 III 6:191.

Benjamin RS, Wiernik PH, and Bachur NR Adriamycin chemotherapy—efficacy safety and pharmacologic basis of an intermittent single high dosage schedule. Cancer 1974 33:19–27.

Benjamin RS, Ewy MS, Mackay G, Ali MK, Legha SS, and Valdivieso M An endomyocardial biopsy study of anthracycline-induced cardiomyopathy-detection reversibility and potential ameliorations. Proc Amer Soc Clin Oncol 1979 20:372.

Benjamin RS, Legha S, Mackay B, Ewer M, Wallace S, Valdivieso M, Rasmussen S, Blumenschein G, and Freireich E Reduction of adriamycin cardiac toxicity using a prolonged intravenous infusion. Proc Amer Assoc Cancer Res 1981 21:179–198.

Bennett JM and Reich SD Bleomycin. Ann Int Med 1979 90:945–948.

Berend N Low temperature inhibits bleomycin lung toxicity in the rat. Am Rev Respir Dis 1983 128:304–306.

Berend N Protective effect of hypoxia on bleomycin lung toxicity in the rat. Am Rev Respir Dis 1984 130:307–308.

Berg H, Horn G, and Ihn W Electrochemical reduction pathways of anthracycline antibiotics. J Antibiot l982 35:800–805.

Bergson A and Inchiosa MA Jr Cardiac actomyosin ATPase activity after chronic doxorubicin treatment. Res Commun Chem Pathol Pharmacol 1985 48:57–75.

Berlin V and Haseltine WA Reduction of adriamycin to a semiquinone-free radical by NADPH cytochrome P-450 reductase produces DNA cleavage in a reaction mediated by molecular oxygen. J Biol Chem 1981 256:4747–4756.

Bern MM, McDermott W Jr, Cady B, Oberfield RA, Trey C, Clouse ME, Tullis JL, and Parker LM Intraarterial hepatic infusion and intravenous adriamycin for treatment of hepatocellular carcinoma: A clinical and pharmacology report. Cancer 1978 42:399–405.

Bernard J, Paul R, Boiron M, Jacquillat C, and Maral R Rubidomycin: A new agent against cancer. Recent Results Cancer Res 1969 20:101.

Bernardini C, Del Tacca M, Danesi R, and Della-Torre P The influence of amiorinone on cardiac toxicity induced by adriamycin in rats. Arch Int Pharmacodyn Ther 1986 283:243–253.

Bertani T, Cutillo F, Zoja C, Broggini M, and Remuzzi G Tubulo-interstitial lesions mediate renal damage in adriamcyin glomerulopathy. Kidney Int 1986 30:488–496.

Bertani T, Remuzzi G, Rocchi G, Delaini F, Sacchi G, Falchetti M, and Donati MB Steroids and adriamycin nephrosis. Appl Pathol 1984 2:32–38.

Bertani T, Rocchi G, Sacchi G, Mecca G, and Remuzzi G Adriamycin-induced glomerulosclerosis in the rat. Am J Kidney Dis 1986 7:12–19.

Bertazzoli C, Sala L, Ballerini L, Watanabe T, and Folkers K Effect of adriamycin on the activity of the succinate dehydrogenase-coenzyme Q10 reductase of the rabbit myocardium. Res Commun Chem Pathol Pharmacol 1976 15:797–800.

Billingham ME Some recent advances in cardiac pathology. Human Pathol 1979 10:367–386.

Billingham ME, Bristow M, Mason J, and Daniels JR Endomyocardial biopsy findings in adriamycin treated patients. Proc Amer Assoc Cancer Res 1976 17:281.

Billingham ME, Mason JW, Bristow MR, and Daniels JR Anthracycline cardiomyopathy monitored by morphologic changes. Cancer Treat Rep 1978 62:865–872.

Bizzi A, Ceriani L, Gerundino M, Spina A, Tacconi MT, and Veneroni E Adriamycin causes hyperlipemia as a consequence of nephrotoxicity. Toxicol Lett 1983 18:291–300.

Bloom KR, Bini RM, Williams CM, Sonley MJ, and Gribbin MA Echocardiography in adriamycin cardiotoxicity. Cancer 1978 41:1265–1269.

Blum RH, Carter SK, and Agre K A clinical review of bleomycin, a new antineoplastic agent. Cancer 1973 31:903–914.

Bonadonna G and Monfardini A Chemotherapy of non-Hodgkin's lymphomas. Cancer Treat Rev 1974 1:167–181.

Bonadonna G, Beretta G, Tancini G, Brambilla C, Bajetta E, De Palo GM, de Lena M, Fossati Bellceni F, Gasparini M, Valagussa P, and Veronesi U Adriamycin NSC 123127 studies at the Instituto Nasionale Tumori Milan. Cancer Chemother Rep 1975 Part 3 6:231–245.

Bonadonna G, Zucali R, Monfardini S, de Lena M, and Ustenghi C Combination chemotherapy of Hodgkin's disease with adriamycin bleomycin vinblastine and imidazole carboxamide versus MOPP. Cancer 1975 36:252–259.

Borden EC Effects of interferons in neoplastic diseases in man. Pharmacol Ther 1988 37:213–229.

Boucek RJ Jr, Olson RD, Brenner DE, Ogunbunmi EM, Inui M, and Fleischer S The major metabolite of doxorubicin is a potent inhibitor of membrane-associated ion pumps. A correlative study of cardiac muscle with isolated membrane fractions. J Biol Chem 1987 262:15851–15856.

Breed JG, Zimmerman ANE, Dormans JAM, and Pinedo HM Failure of the antioxidant vitamin

E to protect against adriamycin-induced cardiotoxicity in the rabbit. Cancer Res 1980 40:2033–2038.

Brenner D, Chang P, Bachur NR, and Wiernik PH Adriamycin dosing: Relationship to pretreatment liver function, pharmacokinetics and response in leukemia patients. Proc Amer Assoc Cancer Res 1980 21:177.

Bristow MR, Kantrowitz NE, Harrison WD, Minobe WA, Sageman WS, and Billingham ME Mediation of subacute anthracycline cardiotoxicity in rabbits by cardiac histamine release. J Cardiovasc Pharmacol 1983 5:913–919.

Bristow MR, Mason JW, Billingham ME, and Daniels JR Doxorubicin cardiomyopathy evaluation by phonocardiography endomyocardial biopsy and cardiac catheterization. Ann Int Med 1978 88:168–175.

Brown RF, Drawbaugh RB, and Marrs TC An investigation of possible models for the production of progressive pulmonary fibrosis in the rat. The effects of repeated intratracheal instillation of bleomcyin. Toxicology 1988 51:101–110.

Bruce JM Benzoquinones and related compound. In: Rodd's Chemistry of Carbon Compounds Coffey S Ed 2nd ed., Volume III Part 4 1974 pp. 1–306.

Buja LM, Ferrans VJ, Mayer RJ, Roberts WC, and Henderson ES Cardiac ultrastructural changes induced by daunorubicin therapy. Cancer 1973 32:771–778.

Burger RM, Horwitz SB, and Peisach J Stimulation of iron II bleomycin activity by phosphate-containing compounds. Biochemistry 1985 24:3623–3629.

Burke JF, Laucius JF, Brodovsky HS, and Soriano RZ Doxorubicin hydrochloride-associated renal failure. Arch Int Med 1977 137:385–388.

Burlock A, Howser D, and Hubbard S Nursing management of adriamycin extravasation. Am J Nursing 1979 94–95.

Bus JS and Gibson JE Lipid peroxidation and its role in toxicology. In: Reviews in Biochemical Toxicology Hodgson E, Bend JR, and Philpot RM Eds Elsevier/North-Holland, New York 1979 pp. 5–149.

Butler J, Hoey BM, and Swallow AJ Reactions of the semiquinone free radicals of anti-tumour agents with oxygen and iron complexes. FEBS Lett 1985 182:95–98.

Capranico G, Dasdia T, and Zunino F Comparison of doxorubicin-induced DNA damage in doxorubicin-sensitive and resistant P388 murine leukemia cells. Int J Cancer 1986 37:227–231.

Caroni P, Villani F, and Carafoli E The cardiotoxic antibiotic doxorubicin inhibits the Na^+/Ca^{2+} exchange of dog heart sarcolemmal vesicles. FEBS Lett 1981 130:184–186.

Casazza AM Preclinical selection of new anthracyclines. Cancer Treat Rep 1986 70:43–49.

Caspary WS, Niziak C, Lanzo DA, Friedman R, and Bachur NB Bleomycin A_2: A ferrous oxidase. Mol Pharmacol 1979 16:256–260.

Catravas JD Pulmonary toxicity of anticancer drugs. Alterations in endothelial cell function. First International Symposium on Organ-Direct Toxicities of Anticancer Drugs 1987 p. 37.

Cersosimo RJ and Hong WK Epirubicin: A review of the pharmacology clinical activity and adverse effects of an adriamycin analogue. J Clin Oncol 1986 4:425–439.

Chalcroft SCW, Gavin JB, and Herdon PB Fine structure changes in rat myocardium induced by daunorubicin. Pathology 1973 5:99–105.

Chan KK, Chlebowski RT, Tong M, Chen HS, Gross JF, and Bateman JR Clinical pharmacokinetics of adriamycin in hepatoma patients with cirrhosis. Cancer Res 1980 40:1263–1268.

Chandler D, Barton J, Briggs D III, Butler T, Kennedy J, and Fulmer J Effect of iron deficiency on bleomycin-induced fibrosis in hamsters. Fed Proc 1987 46:1149.

Chandler DB, Barton JC, Briggs DD, Butler TW, Kennedy JI, Grizzle WE, and Fulmer JD Effect of iron deficiency on bleomycin-induced lung fibrosis in the hamster. Am Rev Respir Dis 1988a 137:85–89.

Chandler DB, Butler TW, Briggs DD, Grizzle WE, Barton JC, and Fulmer JD Modulation of the development of bleomycin-induced fibrosis by deferoxamine. Toxicol Appl Pharmacol 1988b 92:358–367.

Chandrasekaran L, Ramamurthy U, and Chandrokason G Bleomycin induced alterations in the biophysical properties of rat skin. Fed Proc 1985 44:746.

Chandrasekaran L, Seethalakshmi S, Chandrkasan G, and Dhar SC Alterations in lung and skin compositions of rat in bleomycin-induced fibrosis. Biochem Med Metab Biol 1987 38:205–212.

Chen ZM, Colombo T, Conforti L, Grazia-Donelli M, Fierdorowicz RJ, Marchi S, Paolini A, Riva E, Zuanetti G, and Latini R Effects of three new anthracyclines and doxorubicin on the rat isolated heart. J Pharm Pharmacol 1987 39:947–950.

Chin DH and Goldberg IH Generation of superoxide free radical by neocarzinostatin and its possible role in DNA damage. Biochemistry 1986 25:1009–1015.

Chlebowski RT, Paroly WS, Pugh RP, Hueser J, Jacobs EM, Pajak TF, and Bateman JR Adriamycin given as a weekly schedule without a loading course: Clinical affective with reduced incidence of cardiotoxicity. Cancer Treat Rep 1980 64:47–51.

Cini-Neri G and Neri B Reduction of oxygen uptake in vitro as an index of cardiac toxicity induced by new anthracyclines. Anticancer Res 1986 6:195–197.

Combs AB, Choe JY, Truong DH, and Folkers K Reduction by coenzyme Q10 of the acute toxicity of adriamycin in mice. Res Commun Chem Path Pharm 1977 18:565–572.

Comis RL, Kuppinger MS, Ginsberg SJ, Crooke ST, Gilbert R, Auchincloss JH, and Prestayko AW Role of single-breath carbon monoxide-difusing capacity in monitoring the pulmonary effects of bleomycin in germ cell tumor patients. Cancer Res 1979 39:5076–5080.

Cortes EP, Lutman G, Wanka J, Wang JJ, Pickren J, Wallace J, and Holland JF Adriamycin NSC 123127 cardiotoxicity: A clinicopathologic correlation. Cancer Chemother Rep Part 3 1975 6:215–225.

Crescimanno M, Flandina C, Rausa L, Sanguedolce R, and D'Alessandro N Morphological changes and catalase activity in the hearts of CD_1 mice following acute starvation or single doses of doxorubicin epirubicin or mitoxantrone. Chemioterapia 1988 7:53–59.

Crooke ST A review of carminomycin: A new anthracycline developed in the USSR. J Med 1977 8:295–316.

Crooke ST and Bradner WT Bleomycin: A review. J Med 1976 7:333–427.

Cross CE, Warren D, Gerriets JE, Wilson DW, Halliwell B, and Last JA Deferoxamine injection does not affect bleomycin-induced lung fibrosis in rats. J Lab Clin Med 1985 106:433–438.

Crounse RG and Van Scott EJ Changes in scalp hair roots as a measure of toxicity from cancer chemotherapeutic drugs. J Invest Dermatol 1960 35:83.

Cutroneo KR, Cockayne D, and Sterling KM Jr Biochemical and molecular bases of bleomycin-induced pulmonary fibrosis: Glucocorticoid intervention. First International Symposium on Organ-Directed Toxicities of Anticancer Drugs 1987 p. 41.

Czarnecki A and Hinek A The influence of inosine on adriamycin-induced cardiomyopathy in rats. Eur J Cancer Clin Oncol 1986 22:1357–1363.

D'Alessandro ND, Dusonchet L, Crosta L, Crescimanno M, and Rausa L Does catalase play a role in adriamycin induced cardiotoxicity? Pharmacol Res Commun 1980 12:441–446.

D'Alessandro N, Candiloro V, Crescimanno M, Flandina C, Dusonchet L, Crosta L, and Rausa L Effects of multiple doxorubicin doses on mouse cardiac and hepatic catalase. Pharmacol Res Commun 1984 16:145–151.

Dalgleish AG, Woods RL, and Levi JA Bleomycin pulmonary toxicity its relationship to renal dysfunction. Med Pediatr Oncol 1984 12:313–317.

Danesi R, del Tacca M, Della-Torre P, and Bernardini C General and cardiac toxicity of adriamycinol in rats. Anticancer Res 1986 6:967–972.

Danesi R, del Tacca M, Bernardini C, and Penco S Exogenous doxorubicinol induces cardiotoxic effects in rats. Eur J Cancer Clin Oncol 1987 23:907–913.

Danesi R, Paparelli A, Bernadini N, and del Tacca M Cytoflourescence localization and disposition of doxorubicin and doxorubicinol in rat cardiac tissue. Eur J Cancer Clin Oncol 1988 24:1123–1131.

Danysz A, Czarnecki A, and Hinek A Lack of the protective effect of solcoseryl on adriamycin-induced cardiomyopathy in rats. Acta Pol Pharm 1986 43:504–509.

Dasgupta D and Goldberg IH Mode of reversible binding of neocarzinostatin chromophore to DNA: Evidence of binding via the minor groove. Biochemistry 1985 24:6913–6920.

Dasida T, DiMarco A, Minghetti A, and Necco A Effects of doxorubicin on calcium exchange of cultured heart cells. Pharmacol Res Commun 1979 11:881–889.

Dasmahapatra KS, Vezeridis M, Rao U, Perez-Brett R, and Karakousis CP Prevention of adriamycin ADR-induced cardiotoxicity in rats using methylprednisolone Mp. J Surg Res 1984 36:217–222.

Daugherty JP and Khurana A Amelioration of doxorubicin-induced skin necrosis in mice by butylated hydroxytoluene. Cancer Chemother Pharmacol 1985 14:243–246.

Daugherty JP, Wheat M, Conley S, Cooley E, Vanzant C, Loggins L, and Durant JR Involvement of reactive oxygen species in adriamycin (ADR) cardiotoxicity. Proc Amer Assoc Cancer Res 1982 23:171.

David J and Speechley V Scalp cooling to prevent alopecia. Nurs Times 1987 83:36–37.

Davies KJA and Doroshow JH Redox cycling of anthracyclines by cardiac mitochondria I Anthracycline radical formation by NADH dehydrogenase. J Biol Chem 1986 261:3060–3067.

Davies KJA, Doroshow JH, and Hochstein P Mitochondrial NADH dehydrogenase-catalyzed oxygen radical production by adriamycin and the relative inactivity of 5-iminodaunorubicin. FEBS Lett 1983 153:227–230.

De Leonardis V, Neri B, Bacalli S, and Cinelli P Reduction of cardiac toxicity of anthracyclines by L-carnitine preliminary overview of clinical data. Int J Clin Pharmacol Res 1985 5:137–142.

De Leonardis V, De Scalzi M, Neri B, Bartalucci S, and Cinelli P Echocardiographic assessment of anthracycline cardiotoxicity during different therapeutic regimens. Int J Clin Pharmacol Res 1987 7:307–311.

Dean JC, Griffith KS, and Cetals TC Scalp hypothermia: A comparison of ice packs and the kold kap in the prevention of doxorubicin-induced alopecia. J Clin Oncol 1983 1:33.

Dean JC, Salmon SE, and Griffiths KS Prevention of doxorubicin-induced hair loss with scalp hypothermia. New Engl J Med 1979 301:1427.

Decorti G, Bartoli-Klugmann F, Mallardi F, Klugmann S, Benussi B, Grill V, and Baldini L Effects of ICRF 159 on adriamycin-induced cardiomyopathy in rats. Cancer Lett 1983 19:77–83.

Decorti G, Bartoli-Klugmann F, Candussio L, and Baldini L Characterization of histamine secretion induced by anthracyclines in rat peritoneal mast cells. Biochem Pharmacol 1986 35:1939–1942.

DeGraff WG Mutagenicity of neocarzinostatin in Neurospora crassa. Mutat Res 1984 128:127–135.

del Tacca M, Danesi R, Ducci M, Bernardini C, and Romanini A Might adriamycinol contribute to adriamycin-induced cardiotoxicity? Pharmacol Res Commun 1985 17:1073–1084.

Demant EJF NADH oxidation in submitochondrial particles protects respiratory chain activity against damage by adriamycin-Fe^{3+}. Eur J Biochem 1983 137:113–118.

Desai MH and Teres D Prevention of doxorubicin-induced skin ulcers in the rat and pig with dimethylsulfoxide DMSO. Cancer Treat Rep 1982 66:1371–1374.

Dickinson AC, DeJordy JD and Teres D Absence of generation of oxygen-containing free radicals with 4′-deoxydoxorubicin iron-cardiotoxic anthracycline drug. Proc Amer Assoc Cancer Res 1984 25:296.

Dickinson AC, Boutin MG, Matsunaga N, and Teres D 4′-Deoxydoxorubicin and 4-demethoxydaunorubicin do not generate oxygen free radicals. Proc Amer Assoc Cancer Res 1985 26:225.

DiMarco A, Gaetini M, Dorigotti L, Soldatti M, and Bellini O Studi sperimentali sull'attivita' antineoplastica del neuovo antibiotico daunomicina. Tumori 1963 49:203–217.

Dimitrov NV, Hay MB, Siew S, Hudler DA, Charamell LJ, and Ullrey DE Abrogation of adriamycin-induced cardiotoxicity by selenium in rabbits. Am J Pathol 1987 126:376–383.

Domae N, Sawada H, Matsuyama E, Konishi T, and Uchino H Cardiomyopathy and other chronic toxic effects induced in rabbits by doxorubicin and possible prevention of coenzyme Q10. Cancer Treat Rep 1981 65:79–91.

Doroshow JH Anthracycline antibiotic-stimulated superoxide hydrogen peroxide and hydroxyl radical production by NADH dehydrogenase. Cancer Res 1983a 43:4543–4551.

Doroshow JH Effect of anthracycline antibiotics on oxygen radical formation in rat heart. Cancer Res 1983b 43:460–472.

Doroshow JH Effect of anthracycline antibiotics on reactive oxygen production by cardiac myoglobin. Proc Amer Assoc Cancer Res 1987 28:262.

Doroshow J and Chan K Relationship between doxorubicin clearance and indocyanine green dye pharmacokinetics in patients with hepatic dysfunction. Proc Amer Assoc Clin Oncol 1982 1:11.

Doroshow JH and Davies KJA Comparative cardiac oxygen radical metabolism by anthracycline antibiotics mitoxantrone bisantrene 4′-9-acridinylamino-methesulfon-m-anisidine and neocarzinostatin. Biochem Pharmacol 1983 32:2935–2939.

Doroshow JH and Davies KJA Redox cycling of anthracyclines by cardiac mitochondria. II. Formation of superoxide anion hydrogen peroxide and hydroxyl radical. J Biol Chem 1986 261:3068–3074.

Doroshow JH, Locker GY, Ifrim I, and Myers CE Prevention of doxorubicin cardiac toxicity in the mouse by N-acetylcysteine. J Clin Invest 1982 68:1053–1064.

Doroshow JH, Tallent C, and Schechter JE Ultrastructural features of Adriamycin-induced skeletal and cardiac muscle toxicity. Am J Pathol 1985 118:288–297.

Driscoll JS, Hazard GF, Wood HB, and Goldin A Structure antitumor activity relationships among quinone derivatives. Cancer Chemother Rep 1974 Part 2 4:1–363.

DuBost M, Ganter P, Maral R, Ninet L, Pinnert S, Preu'dhomme J, and Werner GH Un novel antibiotique à propriétés cytostatiques la rubidomycine. CR Acad Sci Paris 1963 257:1813–1815.

Dukart G, Posner L, Henry D, and Weiss A Comparative cardiotoxicity of mitoxantrone vs doxorubicin. Proc Amer Soc Clin Oncol 1986 5:48.

Dunagin WG Clinical toxicity of chemotherapeutic agents dermatologic toxicity. Semin Oncol 1982 9:14.

Edo K, Iseki S, Ishida N, Horie T, Kusano G, and Nozoe S An electron spin resonance study of a spin adduct of the non-protein component NPC of neocarzinostatin. J Antibiot 1980 33:1586–1589.

Edo K, Mizugaki M, Koide Y, Seto H, Furikata K, Otake N, and Ishida N The structure of neocarzinostatin chromophore possessing a novel bicyclo[7,3,0]dodecadiyne system. Tetrahedron Lett 1985 26:331–334.

Egido J, Robles A, Ortiz A, Ramirez F, Gonzalez E, Mampaso F, Sanchez-Crespo M, Braquet P, and Hernando L Role of platelet-activating factor in adriamycin-induced nephropathy in rats. Eur J Pharmacol 1987 138:119–123.

Einhorn LH and Donohue J Cisdiammino dichloro platinum vinblastine and bleomycin combination chemotherapy in disseminated testicular cancer. Ann Inter Med 1977 87:293–298.

Ekimoto H, Takahashi K, Matsuda A, and Umezawa H Changes of anticancer activity and pulmonary toxicity of bleomycins in differences of administration schedules and routes in mice. Gan To Kagaku Ryoho 1984 11:853–857.

Eklow L, Thor H, and Orrenius S Formation and efflux of glutathione disulfide studied in isolated rat hepatocytes. FEBS Lett 1981 127:125–128.

El-Hage A, Herman EH, Yang GC, Crouch RK, and Ferrans VJ Mechanism of the protective activity of ICRF-187 against alloxan-induced diabetes in mice. Res Commun Chem Path Pharm 1986 52:341–360.

Eliot H, Gianni L, and Myers CE Oxidative destruction of DNA by the adriamycin-iron complex. Biochemistry 1983 23:928–936.

Ewy GA, Jones SE, Friedman JJ, Gaines J, and Cruze D Non-invasive cardiac evaluation of patients receiving adriamycin. Cancer Treat Rep 1978 62:915–922.

Fajardo LF, Eltringham JR, Stewart JR, and Kaluber MR Adriamycin nephrotoxicity. Lab Invest 1980 43:242–253.

Fantine EO and Garnier-Suillerot G Interaction of 5-iminodaunorubicin with Fe II and with cardiolipin-containing vesicles. Biochim Biophys Acta 1986 856:130–136.

Fasske E Renal carcinoma due to neocarcinostatin. Dtsch Med Wochensehr 1980 105:1488–1489.

Felsted RJ, Richter DR, and Bachur NR Rat liver aldehyde reductase. Biochem Pharmacol 1977 26:1117–1124.

Ferrans VJ Overview of cardiac pathology in relation to anthracycline cardiotoxicity. Cancer Treat Rep 1978 62:955–961.

Filderman AE and Lazo JS Murine strain variation in bleomycin BLM metabolism in vitro. Am Rev Resp Dis 1985 131:A381.

Filderman AE, Genovese LA, and Lazo JS Alterations in pulmonary protective enzymes following systemic bleomycin treatment in mice. Biochem Pharmacol 1988 37:1111–1116.

Fisher J, Abdella BRJ, and McLane KE Anthracycline antibiotic reduction by spinach ferredoxin $NADP^+$ reductase and ferredoxin. Biochemistry 1985 24:3562–3571.

Fischer VW, Wang GM, and Hobart NH Mitigation of an anthracycline-induced cardiomyopathy by pretreatment with razoxane, a quantitative morphological assessment. Virchows-Arch 1986 51:353–361.

Flesch P Inhibition of keratinizing structures by systemic drugs. Pharmacol Rev 1963 15:653.

Flitter WD and Mason RP The enzymatic reduction of actinomycin D to a free radical species. Arch Biochem Biophys 1988 267:632–639.

Folke E Combined treatment with bleomycin in penile carcinomas. In: Fundamental and Clinical Studies of Bleomycin Carter SK, Ichikawa T and Mathe G Eds Gann Monogr Cancer Res 1976 19:231–233.

Folkers K and Wolaniuk A Research on coenzyme Q10 in clinical medicine and in immunomodulation. Drugs Exptl Clin Res 1985 ll:539–545.

Folkers K, Choe JY, and Combs AB Rescue by coenzyme Q10 from electrocardiographic abnormalities caused by the toxicity of adriamycin in the rat. Proc Natl Acad Sci USA 1978 75:5178–5180.

Friedman JJ, Ewy GA, Jones SE, Cruze D, and Moon FE 1-year followup of cardiac status after adriamycin therapy. Cancer Treat Rep 1979 63:1809–1816.

Fujita K, Shinpo K, Yamada K, Sato T, Niimi H, Shamoto M, Nagatsu T, Takeuchi T, and Umezawa H Reduction of adriamycin toxicity by ascorbate in mice and guinea pigs. Cancer Res 1982 42:309–316.

Ganzina F, Pacciarini MA, and DiPietro N Idarubicin 4-demethoxydaunorubicin. A preliminary overview of preclinical and clinical studies. Inv New Drugs 1986 4:85–105.

Garbrecht M and Müllerlie U Verapamil in the prevention of adriamycin-induced cardiomyopathy. Klin Wochenschr 1986 64:132–134.

Gebbia N, Leto G, Gagliano M, Tumminello FM, and Rausa L Lysosomal alterations in heart and liver of mice treated with doxorubicin. Cancer Chemother Pharmacol 1985 15:26–30.

Gebbia N, Flandina C, Leto G, Tumminello FM, Sanguedolce R, Candiloro V, Gagliano M, and Rausa L The role of histamine in doxorubicin and teniposide-induced cardiotoxicity in dog and mouse. Tumori 1987 73:279–287.

Geismar LS, Hennessey S, Reiser KM, and Last JA D-penicillamine prevents collagen accumulation in lungs of rats given bleomycin. Chest 1986 89:153S–154S.

Giri SN, Chen ZL, Younker WR, and Schiedt MJ Effects of intratracheal administration of bleomycin on GSH-shuttle, enzymes, catalase, lipid peroxidation, and collagen content in the lungs of hamsters. Toxicol Appl Pharmacol 1983 71:132–141.

Gisselbrecht C, Likiec F, Marty M, Mignot L, Belpomme D, Najean Y, and Boiron M Adriamycin pharmacokinetics and abnormal liver function tests. Cancer Chemother Pharmacol 1980 5(Suppl):20.

Goad ME, Tryka AF, and Witschi HP Acute respiratory failure induced by bleomycin and hyperoxia pulmonary edema cell kinetics and morphology. Toxicol Appl Pharmacol 1987 90:10–22.

Goldberg IH Free radical mechanisms in neocarzinostatin-induced DNA damage. Free Rad Biol Med 1987 3:41–54.

Goodman J and Hochstein P Generation of free radicals and lipid peroxidation by redox cycling of adriamycin and daunomycin. Biochem Biophys Res Commun 1977 77:797–803.

Goormaghtigh E, Chatelain P, Caspers J, and Ruysschaert JM Evidence of a specific complex between adriamycin and negatively-charged phospholipids. Biochim Biophys Acta 1980 597:1–14.

Gosalvez M, van Rossum GDV, and Blanco MF Inhibition of sodium-potassium activated adenosine 5′-triphosphatase and ion transport by adriamycin. Cancer 1979 39:257–261.

Gottdiener JS, Mathisen BJ, Borer JS, Bonow RO, Myers CE, Barr LH, Schwartz DE, Bacharach SL, Green MV, and Rosenberg SA Doxorubicin cardiotoxicity: Assessment of late left ventricular dysfunction by radionuclide cineangiography. Ann Intern Med 1981 94:430–435.

Gottlieb JA, LeFrak EA, O'Bryan RM, and Burgess MA Fatal adriamycin cardiomyopathy prevention by dose limitation abstract. Proc Am Assoc Cancer Res 1973 14:88.

Greco FA Subclinical adriamycin cardiotoxicity: Detection by timing the arterial sounds. Cancer Treat Rep 1978 62:901–905.

Greco FA, Merrill RM, Brereton HD, and Rodbard D Noninvasive monitoring of subclinical adriamycin cardiotoxicity by "sphygmo-recording" of the QRS-Korotkoff interval. Clin Res 1975 23:595A.

Green MD, Speyer JL, and Muggia FM Cardiotoxicity of anthracyclines. Eur J Cancer Clin Oncol 1984 20:293–296.

Green MD Rationale and strategy for prevention of anthracycline cardiotoxicity with the bisdioxopiperazine ICRF-187. Path Biol 1987 35:49–53.

Green MD, Speyer JL, Stecy P, Rey M, Kramer E, Sanger J, Feit F, Blum RH, Wernz JC, Ward C, London C, Dubin N, and Muggia FM ICRF-187. ICRF prevents doxorubicin (Dox) cardiotoxicity (Ctox). Results of a randomized clinical trial. Proc Am Soc Clin Oncol 1987 6:A104.

Griffin TW, Comis RL, Lokich JJ, Blum RH, and Canellos GP Phase I and preliminary Phase II study of neocarzinostatin. Cancer Treat Rep 1978 62:2019–2025.

Gutierrez PL, Gee MV, and Bachur NR Kinetics of anthracycline antibiotic free radical formation and reductive glycosidase activity. Arch Biochem Biophys 1983 223:68–75.

Gutteridge JMC and Toeg D Adriamycin-dependent damage to deoxyribose: A reaction involving iron hydroxyl and semiquinone free radicals. FEBS Lett 1982 149:228–232.

Gutteridge JMC and Quinlan GJ Free radical damage to deoxyribose by anthracycline, aureolic acid and aminoquinone antitumor antibiotics. An essential requirement for iron semiquinones and hydrogen peroxide. Biochem Pharmacol 1985 34:4099–4103.

Guy R, Parker H, Shah S, and Geddes D Scalp cooling by thermocirculator. Lancet 1982 1:937.

Hagiwara A, Takahashi T, Ueda T, and Torii T Reduced pulmonary toxicity of peplomycin in a new drug-delivery system. Anticancer Drug Des 1988 2:319–324.

Hallett N Preventing fall-out. Nurs Mirror 1981 152:32–33.

Hamaguchi T, Azuma J, Awata N, Ohta H, Takihara K, Harada H, Kishimoto S, and Sperelakis N Reduction of doxorubicin-induced cardiotoxicity in mice by taurine. Res Commun Chem Pathol Pharmacol 1988 59:21–30.

Harris RN and Doroshow JH Effect of doxorubicin-enhanced hydrogen peroxide and hydroxyl radical formation on calcium sequestration by cardiac sarcoplasmic reticulum. Biochem Biophys Res Commun 1985 130:739.

Harrison JH Jr and Lazo JS High dose continuous infusion of bleomycin in mice: A new model for drug-induced pulmonary fibrosis. J Pharmacol Exp Ther 1987 243:1185–1194.

Hashimoto Y, Yamashita T, Koyu A, Ebihara K, Suzuki H, Kumagai M, Yoshioka O, and Matsuda A Toxicological studies of pepleomycin sulfate. V. Short term intermittent toxicity in dogs. Jpn J Antibiot 1978 31:837–858.

Hatayama T and Goldberg IH DNA damage and repair in relation to cell killing in neocarzinostatin-treated HeLa cells. Biochim Biophys Acta 1979 563:59–71.

Hay JG, Haslam PL, Dewar A, Addis B, Turner-Warwick M, and Laurent GJ Development of acute lung injury after the combination of intravenous bleomycin and exposure to hyperoxia in rats. Thorax 1987 42:374–382.

Henderson IC, Billingham M, Israel M, Krishnan A, and Frei E Comparative cardiotoxicity studies with adriamycin (ADR) and AD32 in rabbits. Proc Amer Assoc Cancer Res 1978 19:158.

Henderson IC, Sloss LJ, Jaffe N, Blum RH, and Frei E III Serial studies of cardiac function in patients receiving adriamycin. Cancer Treat Rep 1978 62:923–929.

Henry DW Structure-activity relationships among daunorubicin and adriamycin analogs. Cancer Treat Rep 1979 63:845–854.

Herman EH and Ferrans VJ Influence of vitamin E and ICRF-187 on chronic doxorubicin cardiotoxicity in miniature swine. Lab Invest 1983 49:69–77.

Herman EH and Ferrans VJ Pretreatment with ICRF-187 provides long-lasting protection against chronic daunorubicin cardiotoxicity in rabbits. Cancer Chemother Pharmacol 1986 16:102–106.

Herman EH, Matre RM, Lee IP, Vick J, and Warardekar VS A comparison of the cardiovascular actions of daunomycin adriamycin and N-acetyl- daunomycin in hamsters and monkeys. Pharmacology 1971 6:230–241.

Herman EH, Rahman A, Ferrans VJ, Vick VA, and Schein PS Prevention of chronic doxorubicin cardiotoxicity in beagles by liposomal encapsulation. Cancer Res 1983 43:5427–5432.

Herman EH, El-Hage AN, Ferrans VJ, and Ardalan B Comparison of the severity of the chronic cardiotoxicity produced by doxorubicin in normotensive and hypertensive rats. Toxicol Appl Pharmacol 1985 78:202–214.

Herman EH, Ferrans VJ, Myers CE, and Van Vleet JF Comparison of the effectiveness of +1−1,2-bis 3,5-dioxo-piperazinyl-1-yl propane ICRF-187 and N-acetylcysteine in preventing chronic doxorubicin cardiotoxicity in beagles. Cancer Res 1985 45:276–281.

Herman EH, El-Hage A, and Ferrans VJ Protective effect of ICRF-187 on doxorubicin-induced cardiac and renal toxicity in spontaneously hypertensive (SHR) and normotensive (WKY) rats. Toxicol Appl Pharmacol 1988a 92:42–53.

Herman EH, Ferrans VJ, Young RSK, and Hamlin RL Effect of pretreatment with ICRF-187 on the total cumulative dose of doxorubicin tolerated by beagle dogs. Cancer Res 1988b 48:6918–6925.

Hermansen K and Wassermann K The effect of vitamin E and selenium on doxorubicin adriamycin induced delayed toxicity in mice. Acta Pharmacol Toxicol Copenh 1986 58:31–37.

Herzog V and Fahimi HD Microbodies peroxisomes containing catalase in myocardium: Morphologic and biochemical evidence. Science 1974 185:271–273.

Hickman J, Chahwala SB, and Thompson MG Interaction of the antibiotic adriamycin with the plasma membrane. Adv Enzym Reg 1985 24:263–274.

Holoye PY, Luna MA, MacKay B, and Bredrossia CWM Bleomycin hypersensitivity pneumonitis. Ann Inter Med 1978 88:47–49.

Hortobagyi GN, Frye D, Buzdar AU, Ewer MS, Fraschini G, Hug V, Ames F, Montague E, Carrasco CH, MacKay B, and Benjamin RS Decreased cardiac toxicity of doxorubicin administered by continuous intravenous infusion in combination chemotherapy for metastatic breast carcinoma. Cancer 1989 63:37–45.

Houée-Levin C, Gardès-Albert M, and Ferradini C Reduction of daunorubicin aqueous solutions by COO-free radicals. Reactions of reduced transients with H_2O_2. FEBS Lett 1984 173:27–30.

Hrushesky WJM, Wood P, Olshefski R, Meshnick S, and Eaton JW Modifying intracellular redox balance: An approach to improving therapeutic index. Lancet 1985 1:565–566.

Hunt JM, Anderson JE, and Smith IE Scalp hypothermia to prevent adriamycin-induced hair loss. Cancer Nurs 1982 5:25–31.

Ishii Y, Ekimoto H, Nishikawa K, Takahashi K, Matsuda A, and Umezawa H Experimental studies on peplomycin: A new derivative of bleomycin. Future Trends Chemother 1985 6:433–438.

Ito A, Koide Y, Haneda I, Toriyama K, Ouchi M, Matsumoto T, and Baba T Screening for the antagonizing agents against lethal toxicity of neocarzinostatin. I. Inhibitory effects of various drugs on the toxicity of neocarzinostatin in vitro and in vivo. Jpn J Antibiot 1985 38:137–144.

Ito Y, Barcelli U, Yamashita W, Weiss M, Glas-Greenwalt P, and Pollak VE Fish oil has beneficial effects on lipids and disease of nephrotic rats. Metabolism 1988 37:352–357.

Iwamoto Y, Kuroiwa T, Aoki K, and Baba T "Two-route chemotherapy" using high-dose intra-arterial neocarzinostatin and systemic tiopronin, its antidote, for rat limb tumor. Cancer Chemother Pharmacol 1986 17:247–250.

Jackson JA, Reeves JP, Muntz K, Kruk D, Prough RA, Willerson JR, and Buja IM Evaluation of free radical effects and catecholamine alterations in adriamycin cardiotoxicity. Am J Pathol 1984 117:140–153.

Jacquillat CL, Weil M, Auclerc M-F, Maral J, Schaison G, Boiron M, and Bernard J Survey of anthracyclines in haematology. Nouve Press Med 1977 7:2061–2066.

Janke RA An anthracycline antibiotic-induced cardiomyopathy in rabbits. Lab Invest 1974 30:292–303.

Johnston CI, Arnolda L, Abrahams J, and McGrath B Role of vasopressin in experimental congestive cardiac failure. J Cardiovasc Pharmacol 1986 8:S96–100.

Jones SE, Ewy GA, and Grove BM Electrocardiographic detection of adriamycin heart disease. Proc Amer Soc Clin Onc 1975 16:228.

Julicher RHM, Sterrenberg L, Bast A, Riksen ROW, Koomen JM, and Noordhoek J The role of acute doxorubicin-induced cardiotoxicity studied in rat isolated heart. J Pharm Pharmacol 1986 38:277–282.

Julicher RHM, Sterrenberg L, Haenen GR, Bast A, and Noordhoek J The effect of chronic adriamycin treatment on heart kidney and liver tissue of male and female rat. Arch Toxicol 1988 61:275–281.

Jung G and Kohnlein W Neocarzinostatin: Controlled release of chromophore and its interaction with DNA. Nucleic Acids Res 1981 5:2959–2967.

Jusko WJ Pharmacodynamics of chemotherapeutic effects. Dose-time-response relationships for phase-nonspecific agents. J Pharm Sci 1971 60:892–895.

Kalyanaraman B, Perez-Reyes E, and Mason RP Spin-trapping and direct electron spin resonance investigations of the redox metabolism of quinone anticancer drugs. Biochim Biophys Acta 1980 630:119–130.

Kalyanaraman B, Sealy RC, and Sinha BK An electron spin resonance study of the reduction of peroxides by anthracycline semiquinones. Biochim Biophys Acta 1984 799:270–275.

Kanao M, Tomita S, Ishida S, Murakami A, and Okada H Chelation of bleomycin with copper in vivo. Chemotherapy 1973 21:1305–1310.

Kanter MM, Hamlin RL, Unverferth DV, Davis HW, and Merola AJ Effect of exercise training on antioxidant enzymes and cardiotoxicity of doxorubicin. J Appl Physiol 1985 59:1298–1303.

Keller AM, Jackson JA, Peshock RM, Rehr RB, Willerson JT, Nunnally RL, and Buja LM Nuclear magnetic resonance study of high-energy phosphate stores in models of adriamycin cardiotoxicity. Magn Reson Med 1986 3:834–843.

Kelley J and Kovacs EJ Immunoregulation of growth factor release in bleomycin induced lung disease. First International Symposium on Organ-Directed Toxicities of Anticancer Drugs 1987 p. 35.

Kharasch ED and Novak RF Anthracenedione activation of NADPH-cytochrome P-450 reductase comparison with anthracyclines. Biochem Pharmacol 1981 30:2881–2884.

Kharasch ED and Novak RF Inhibition of adriamycin-stimulated microsomal lipid peroxidation by mitoxantrone and ametantrone, two new anthracenedione antineoplastic agents. Biochem Biophys Res Commun 1982 108:1346–1352.

Kharasch ED and Novak RF Mitoxantrone and ametantrone metabolic activation and effects on lipid peroxidation. Proc Amer Assoc Cancer Res 1983a 24:257.

Kharasch ED and Novak RF Structural and mechanistic differences in quinone inhibition of microsomal drug metabolism inhibition of NADPH-cytochrome P-450 reductase activity. In: Cytochrome P-450 Biochemistry Biophysics and Environmental Implications Hietanen J Ed Elsevier/North-Holland, Amsterdam 1983b pp. 80–97.

Kharasch ED and Novak RF Bis alkylamino anthracenedione antineoplastic agent metabolic activation diminished activity elative to anthracyclines. Arch Biochem Biophys 1983c 224:682–694.

Kharasch ED and Novak RF Mitoxantrone and ametantrone inhibit hydroperoxide-dependent initiation and propagation reactions in fatty acid peroxidation. J Biol Chem 1985 260:10645–10652.

Kikuchi M, Shoij M, and Ishida N Pre-neocarzinostatin: A specific antagonist of neocarzinostatin. J Antibiot 1974 27:766–774.

Kim DH, Akera T, and Brody TM Inotropic actions of doxorubicin in isolated guinea pig atria, Evidence for lack of involvement of Na+ K+-adenosine triphosphate. J Pharmacol Exp Ther 1980 214:368–374.

Kleyer DL and Koch TH Mechanistic investigation of reduction of daunomycin and 7-deoxydaunomycinone with bi-3,5,5-trimethyl-2-oxomorpholin-3-yl. J Am Chem Soc 1984 106:2380–2387.

Kligman AM The human hair cycle. J Inv Dermatol 1959 33:307.

Klugmann FB, Decorti G, Mallardi F, Klugmann S, and Baldini L Effect of polyethylene glycol 400 on adriamycin toxicity in mice. Eur J Cancer Clin Oncol 1984 20:405–410.

Klugmann FB, Decorti G, Candussio L, Grill V, Mallardi F, and Baldini L Inhibitors of adriamycin-induced histamine release in vitro limit adriamycin cardiotoxicity in vivo. Br J Cancer 1986 54:743–748.

Koide H, Soeda N, and Ohno J Biochemical properties of glomerular basement membrane in daunomycin nephrosis and nephrotoxic serum nephritis. Renal Physiol 1981 4:102–107.

Komiyama T, Oki T, and Inui T A proposed reaction mechanism for the enzymatic reductive cleavage of glycosidic bond in anthracycline antibiotics. Gann 1979 32:1219–1222.

Komiyama T, Sawada MT, Kobayashi K, and Yoshimoto A Enhanced production of ethylene from methional by iron chelates and heme containing proteins in the system consisting of quinone compounds and NADPH-cytochrome P-450 reductase. Biochem Pharmacol 1985 34:977–983.

Komiyama T, Kikuchi T, and Sugiura Y Interaction of anticancer quinone drugs, aclacinomycin A, adriamycin, carbazilquinone, and mitomycin C with NADPH-cytochrome P-450 reductase xanthine oxidase and oxygen. J Pharmacobio-Dyn 1986 9:651–654.

Komori A, Takahashi K, Nakamura I, Shikano T, Ohkubo T, and Nagano M Membrane alterations of myocardial sarcolemma in adriamycin cardiomyopathy. J Mol Cell Cardiol 1985 11:65–67.

Krakoff IH Pharmacology and therapeutic efficacy of bleomycin administered by continuous infusion. In: Clinical Applications of Continuous Infusion Chemotherapy and Concomitant Radiation Therapy Rosenthal CJ and Rotman M Eds Plenum Press, New York 1986 pp. 13–17.

Kubosawa H, Akikusa B, and Kondo Y Daunomycin-induced nephropathy in rats. Acta Pathol Jpn 1985 35:109–123.

Kuo WL, Meyn RE, and Haidle CW Neocarzinostatin-mediated DNA damage and repair in wild-type and repair-deficient Chinese hamster ovary cells. Cancer Res 1984 44:1748–1751.

Kuromizu K, Tsunasawa S, Maeda H, Abe O, and Sakiyama F Reexamination of the primary structure of an antitumor protein neocarzinostatin. Arch Biochem Biophys 1986 246:199–205.

Labandter HP and McElwee T Adriamycin extravasation: Case reports and review. J Lab State Med Soc 1979 131:255–258.

Lambertenghi-Deliliers G, Zanon PL, Pozzoli EF, and Bellini O Myocardial injury by a single dose of adriamycin an electron microscopic study. Tumori 1976 62:517–528.

Lampidis TJ, Garnier-Suillerot A, and Tapiero H Reduced toxicity of non-free radical forming adriamycin in cardiac cells. Proc Amer Assoc Cancer Res 1987 28:270.

Land EJ, Mukherjee T, Swallow AJ, and Bruce JM Possible intermediates in the action of adriamycin—A pulse radiolysis study. Br J Cancer 1985 51:515–523.

Laurent GJ, McAnulty RJ, Corrin B, and Cockerill P Biochemical and histological changes in pulmonary fibrosis induced in rabbits with intratracheal bleomycin. Eur J Clin Invest 1981 11:441–448.

Lawrence HJ and Goodnight SH Dimethylsulfoxide and extravasation of anthracycline agents. Ann Intern Med 1983 98:1025.

Lawrence HJ, Walsh D, Zapotowski KA, Denham A, Goodnight SH, and Gandra DR Topical dimethylsulfoxide may prevent tissue damage from anthracycline extravasation. Cancer Chemother Pharmacol 1989 23:316–318.

Lawson N, Adams L, Symonds RP, and Maxted KJ Epirubicin 50 mg/m^2 alopecia prevented by cold air scalp cooling. Fourth Europ Conf Clin Oncol Cancer Nursing 1987 p. 316.

Lazo JS Pulmonary metabolism of bleomycin and its role in drug induced lung injury. First International Symposium on Organ-Directed Toxicities of Anticancer Drugs 1987 p. 39.

Lazo JS and Humphreys CJ Lack of metabolism as the biochemical basis of bleomycin-induced pulmonary toxicity. Proc Natl Acad Sci USA 1983 80:3064–3068.

Lazo JS and Pham ET Pulmonary fate of [^{3}H] bleomycin A_2 in mice. J Pharmacol Exp Ther 1984 228:13–18.

Lazo JS, Merrill WW, Pham ET, Lynch TJ, McCallister J, and Ingbar DH Bleomycin hydroxylase activity in pulmonary cells. J Pharmacol Exp Ther 1984 231:583–588.

Lazo JS, Sebti SM, and Filderman AE Metabolism of bleomycin and bleomycin-like compounds. In: Metabolism and Action of Anti-Cancer Drugs Powis G and Prough RA Eds Taylor & Francis, London 1987 pp. 194–210.

Lazzarino G, Viola AR, Mulieri L, Rotilio G, and Mavelli I Prevention by fructose-1,6-bisphosphate of cardiac oxidative damage induced in mice by subchronic doxorubicin treatment. Cancer Res 1987 47:6511–6516.

LeFrak EA, Pitha J, Rosenheim S, and Gottlieb J A clinicopathologic analysis of adriamycin cardiotoxicity. Cancer 1973 32:302–314.

LeFrak EA, Pitha J, Rosenheim S, O'Bryan RM, Burgess MA, and Gottlieb JA Adriamycin NSC 123127 cardiomyopathy. Cancer Chemother Rep 1975 Part 3 6:203–208.

Legha SS, von Hoff DD, Rosencweig M, Abraham D, Slavik M, and Muggia M Neocarzinostatin NSC 157365 a new cancerostatic compound. Oncology 1976 33:265–270.

Legha SS, Wang YM, Mackay B, Ewer M, Hortobagy GN, Benjamin RS, and Ali MK Clinical and pharmacologic investigation of the effects of α-tocopherol on adriamycin cardiotoxicity. Ann NY Acad Sci 1982 393:411.

Lehninger AL Mitochondria and calcium ion transport. Biochem J 1970 119:129–138.

Lehotay DC, Levey BA, and Levey GS Inhibition of cardiac guanylate cyclase by doxorubicin and some of its analogs. Biomed Pharmacoth 1983 37:312–316.

Lenzhofer R, Ganzinger U, Rameis H, and Moser K Acute cardiac toxicity in patients after doxorubicin treatment and the effect of combined tocopherol and nifedipine pretreatment. J Cancer Res Clin Oncol 1983 106:143–147.

Levey GS, Levey A, Rutz E, and Lehotay DC Selective inhibition of rat and human cardiac guanylate cyclase in vitro by doxorubicin adriamycin: Possible link to anthracycline cardiotoxicity. J Mol Cell Cardiol 1979 11:591–599.

Lewis W, Kleinerman J, and Puszkin S Interaction of adriamycin in vitro with cardiac myofibrillar proteins. Circ Res 1982 50:547–553.

Lindenschmidt RC, Tryka AF, Godfrey GA, Frome EL, and Witschi H Intratracheal versus intravenous administration of bleomycin in mice: Acute effects. Toxicol Appl Pharmacol 1986 85:69–77.

Livingston RB Bleomycin in the treatment of lung cancer. In: Bleomycin Current Status and New Developments Carter SK, Crooke ST, and Umezawa H Eds Academic Press, New York 1978 pp. 165–171.

Llesuy SF, Milei J, Molina H, Boveris A, and Milei S Comparison of lipid peroxidation and myocardial damage induced by adriamycin and 4′-epiadriamycin in mice. Tumori 1985 71:241–249.

Long HJ, Diamond SS, Raflo CP, and Burningham RA Dose-response relationships of chronic adriamycin toxicity in rabbits. Eur J Cancer Clin Oncol 1984 20:129–135.

Lown JW and Chen HH Electron paramagnetic resonance characterization and conformation of daunorubicin semiquinone intermediate implicated in anthracycline metabolism cardiotoxicity and anticancer action. Can J Chem 1981 59:3212–3218.

Lown JW and Sim SK The mechanism of the bleomycin-induced cleavage of DNA. Biochem Biophys Res Commun 1977 77:1150–1157.

Lown JW, Sim SK, and Chen HH Hydroxyl radical production by free and DNA-bound aminoquinone antibiotics and its role in DNA degradation. Electron spin resonance detection of hydroxyl radicals by spin trapping. Can J Biochem 1978 56:1042–1047.

Lown JW, Chen HH, Plambeck JA, and Acton EM Further studies on the generation of reactive oxygen species from activated anthracyclines and the relationship to cytotoxic action and cardiotoxic effects. Biochem Pharm 1982 31:575–581.

Ludwig CU, Stoll H-R, Obrist R, and Obrecht J-P Prevention of cytotoxic drug induced skin ulcers with dimethylsulfoxide DMSO and α-tocopherol. Eur J Cancer Clin Oncol 1987 23:327–329.

Luisetti M, Pozzi E, Salmona M, and Villani F Ambroxol and bleomycin BLM induced pulmonary toxicity, experimental and clinical aspects. First International Symposium on Organ-Directed Toxicities of Anticancer Drugs, 1987, p. 57.

Maeda H Neocarzinostatin in cancer chemotherapy review. Anticancer Res 1981 1:175–186.

Martin-Jimenez M, Diaz-Rubio E, Gonzalez Larriba JL, and Sangro B Failure of high-dose tocopherol to prevent alopecia induced by doxorubicin. N Engl J Med 1986 315:894.

Mason JW, Bristow MR, Billingham ME, and Daniels JR Invasive and noninvasive methods of assessing adriamycin cardiotoxic effects in man: Superiority of histologic assessment using endomyocardial biopsy. Cancer Treat Rep 1978 62:867–864.

Mason RP Free radical metabolites of foreign compounds and their toxicological significance. In: Reviews in Biochemical Toxicology Hodgson E, Bend JR, and Philpot RM Eds Part 1, Elsevier/North-Holland, Amsterdam 1979 pp. 151–200.

Maxwell MB Scalp tourniquets for chemotherapy-induced alopecia. Am J Nursing 1980 80:900.

McCullough B, Collins JF, Johanson Jr WG, and Grover FL Bleomycin induced diffuse interstitial pulmonary fibrosis in baboons. J Clin Invest 1978 61:79–88.

McFalls EO, Paulson DJ, Gilbert EF, and Shug AL Carnitine protection against adriamycin-induced cardiomyopathy in rats. Life Sci 1986 38:497–505.

McKelvey EM, Burgess MA, McCredie KB, Murphy WK, and Bodey GP Neocarzinostatin: A Phase I clinical trial with five-day intermittent and continuous infusions. Cancer 1979 44:1182–1188.

Meienhofer J, Maeda H, Glaser CB, Czombos J, and Kuromizu M Primary structure of neocarzinostatin: An antitumor protein. Science 1972 178:875–876.

Milei J, Boveris A, Molina H, Llesuy S, Storino R, and Milei SE Prenylamine inhibition of adriamycin-induced myocardiopathy. Acta Cardiol Brux 1985 40:383–396.

Milei J, Boveris A, Llesuy S, Molina HA, Storino R, Ortega D, and Milei SE Amelioration of adriamycin-induced cardiotoxicity in rabbits by prenylamine and vitamins A and E. Am Heart J 1986 111:95–102.

Milei J, Marantz A, Ale J, Vazquez A, and Buceta JE Prevention of adriamycin-induced cardiotoxicity by prenylamine—a pilot double blind study. Cancer Drug Deliv 1987 4:129–136.

Milei J, Vazquez A, Boveris A, Llesuy S, Molina HA, Storino R, and Marantz A The role of prenylamine in the prevention of adriamycin-induced cardiotoxicity. A review of experimental and clinical findings. J Int Med Res 1988 16:19–30.

Mimnaugh EG, Siddik ZH, Drew R, Sikic BI, and Gram T The effects of alpha-tocopherol on the toxicity disposition and metabolism of adriamycin in mice. Toxicol Appl Pharmacol 1979 49:119–126.

Mimnaugh EG, Trush MA, Ginsburg E, and Gram TE Differential effects of anthracycline drugs on rat heart and liver microsomal reduced nicotinamide adenine dinucleotide phosphate-dependent lipid peroxidation. Cancer Res 1982 42:3574–3582.

Mimnaugh EG, Trush MA, and Gram TE Stimulation of adriamycin of rat heart and liver microsomal NADPH-dependent lipid peroxidation. Biochem Pharm 1981 30:2797–2804.

Mimnaugh EG, Gram EG, and Trush MA Stimulation of mouse heart and liver microsomal lipid peroxidation by anthracycline anticancer drugs: Characterization and effects of reactive oxygen scavengers. J Pharmacol Exp Ther 1983 226:806–816.

Mimnaugh EG, Gram EG, and Trush MA Stimulation of mouse heart and liver microsomal lipid peroxidation by anthracycline anticancer drugs characterization and effects of reactive oxygen scavengers. J Pharmacol Exp Ther 1983 226:806–816.

Minow RA, Benjamin RS, and Gottlieb JA Adriamycin NSC 123127 cardiomyopathy—An overview with determination of risk factors. Cancer Chemother Rep 1975 Part 3 6:195–201.

Minow RA, Benjamin RS, Lee ET, and Gottlieb JA Adriamycin cardiomyopathy—risk factors. Cancer 1977 39:1397–1402.

Minow RA, Benjamin RS, Lee ET. and Gottlieb JA QRS voltage change with adriamycin administration. Cancer Treat Rep 1978 62:931–934.

Mirabelli CK, Huang CH, and Crooke ST Role of deoxyribonucleic acid topology in altering the site/sequence specificity of cleavage of deoxyribonucleic acid by bleomycin and talisomycin. Biochemistry 1983 22:300–306.

Miwa N, Kanaide H, Meno H, and Nakamura M Adriamycin and altered membrane functions in rat hearts. Br J Exp Pathol 1986 67:747–755.

Mochizuki T, Okazaki T, Ishikura H, Izumi Y, Tashima M, Sawada H, Uchino H, Konishi T, Ikeguchi S, and Takasu K Effect of diltiazem on the cardiotoxicity induced by adriamycin in rabbits. Nippon Gan Chiryo Gakkai Shi 1987 20:539–549.

Montali U, Del Tacca M, Bernardini C, Segnini D, and Solaini G Cardiotoxic effects of adriamycin and mitochondrial oxidation in rat cardiac tissue. Drugs Exp Clin Res 1985 11:219–222.

Moore HW, Czerniak R, and Hamdan A Natural quinones as quinone methide precursors—ideas in rational drug design. Drugs Expl Clin Res 1986 12:475–494.

Motomura K, Okuda S, Sanai T, Hirakata H, Shimamatsu K, Onoyama K, and Fujishima M Aluminium hydroxide prevents progression in experimental focal glomerular sclerosis. Nephrol Dial Transplant 1988 3:263–268.

Mountz JD, Downs-Minor MB, Turner R, Thomas MB, Richards F, and Pisko E Bleomycin-induced cutaneous toxicity in the rat, analysis of histopathology and ultrastructure compared with progressive systemic sclerosis scleroderma. Br J Dermatol 1983 108:679–685.

Mukerhjee A, Wong TM, Templeton G, Buja LM, and Willerson JT Influence of volume dilution, lactate, phosphate and calcium on mitochondria function. Am J Physiol 1978 237:H224–H238.

Muliawan H, Scheulen ME, and Kappus H Acute adriamycin treatment of rats does not increase ethane expiration. Res Commun Chem Path Pharm 1980 30:509–519.

Muliawan H, Burkhardt A, Scheulen ME, and Kappus H Minor role of lipid peroxidation in acute bleomycin toxicity in rats. J Cancer Res Clin Oncol 1982 103:135–143.

Müller A, Cadenas E, Graf P, and Sies H A novel biologically active seleno-organic compounds-1 Glutathione peroxidase-like activity in vitro and antioxidant capacity of PZ51 Ebselen. Biochem Pharmacol 1984 33:3235–3239.

Muraoka Y, Takita T, and Umezawa H Bleomycin and peplomycin. Cancer Chemother 1986 8:65–72.

Murdock KC, Child RG, Fabio PF, Angier RB, Wallace RE, Durr FE, and Citarella RV Antitumor agents. 1. 1,4-bis[aminoalkyl amino]-9,10-anthraquinones. J Med Chem 1979 22:1024–1030.

Myers CE, McGuire WP, Liss RH, Ifrim I, Grotzinger K, and Young RC Adriamycin, the role of lipid peroxidation in cardiac toxicity and tumor response. Science 1977 19:165–167.

Myers CE, McGuire WP, and Young R Adriamycin amelioration of toxicity by alpha-tocopherol. Cancer Treat Rep 1976 60:961–962.

Myers CE, Muindi JRF, Zweir J, and Sinha BK 5-Iminodaunomycin. An anthracycline with unique properties. J Biol Chem 1987 262:11571–11577.

Naff MB, Plowman J, and Naryanan VL Anthracyclines in the National Cancer Institute Program. In: Anthracycline Antibiotics, El Khadem HS Ed Academic Press, New York 1982 pp. 1–57.

Naganuma A, Satoh M, and Imura N Specific reduction of toxic side effects of adriamycin by induction of metallothionein in mice. Jpn J Cancer Res 1988 79:406–411.

Neri B, Cini-Neri G, Bartalucci S, and Bandinelli M Protective effect of L-carnitine on cardiac metabolic damage induced by doxorubicin in vitro. Anticancer Res 1986 6:659–662.

Neri B, Neri GC, and Bandinelli M Differences between carnitine derivatives and coenzyme Q10 in preventing in vitro doxorubicin-related cardiac damages. Oncology 1988 45:242–246.

Nettleton DE, Bradner WT, Bush JA, Coon AB, Moseley JE, Myllmaki RW, O'Herron FA, Schreiber RH, and Vulcano AL New antitumor antibiotics musettamycin and marcellomycin from bohemic acid complex. J Antibiot 1977 30:525–529.

Newman RA, Siddik ZH, Ayele W, Ho DH, and Krakoff IH Assessment of pulmonary and hematologic toxicities of liblomycin (LIB). A novel bleomycin (BLM) analog. Proc Amer Assoc Cancer Res 1988 29:A1287.

Nicolay K, Aue WP, Seelig J, van Echteld CJ, Ruigrok TJ, and de Kruijff B Effects of the anti-cancer drug adriamycin on the energy metabolism of rat heart as measured by in vivo 31P-NMR and implications for adriamycin-induced cardiotoxicity. Biochim Biphys Acta 1987 929:5–13.

Nissen E, Fichtner I, Weiss H, Arndt D, Oettel P, and Tanneberger S Effects of nifedipine on cell resistance and cardiac toxicity—in vitro and in vivo experiments. Arch Geschwulstforsch 1986 56:169–177.

Nobbs P and Barr RD Soft-tissue injury caused by antineoplastic drugs is inhibited by topical dimethyl sulphoxide and alpha tocopherol. Br J Cancer 1983 48:873–876.

Nohl H and Jordan W OH-generation by adriamycin semiquinone and H_2O_2 and explanation for the cardiotoxicity of anthracycline antibiotics. Biochem Biophys Res Commun 1983 114:197–205.

Nohl H, Jordan W, and Youngman RJ Quinones in biology. Functions in electron transfer and oxygen activation. Adv Free Rad Biol Med 1986 2:211–279.

Novak RF and Kharasch ED Mitoxantrone: Propensity for free radical formation and lipid peroxidation—implications for cardiotoxicity. Invest New Drugs 1985 3:95–99.

O'Donnell MP, Michels L, Kasiske B, Raij L, and Keane WF Adriamycin-induced chronic proteinuria, a structural and functional study. J Lab Clin Med 1985 106:62–67.

Ohnuma T, Nogeire C, Cuttner J, and Holland JF Phase I study with neocarzinostatin tolerance to two hour infusion and continuous infusion. Cancer 1978 42:1670–1679.

Ohnuma T, Holland JF, Masuda H, Waligunda JA, and Goldberg GA Microbiological assay of bleomycin. Inactivation tissue distribution and clearance. Cancer 1974 33:1230–1238.

Oki T, Matsuzawa Y, Yoshimoto A, Numata K, Kitamura I, Hori S, Takamatsu A, Umezawa H, Ishizuka M, Naganawa H, Suda H, Hamada M, and Takeuchi T New antitumor antibiotics aclacinomycin A and B. J Antibiot 1975 28:830–834.

Oki T New anthracycline antibiotics. Jap J Antibiot 1977 30(Suppl):S70–S84.

Olson HM, Young DM, Prieur DJ, LeRoy AF, and Reagan RL Electrolyte and morphologic alterations of myocardium in adriamycin-treated rabbits. Am J Pathol 1974 77:439–454.

Olson RD, McDonald JS, Van Boxtel CJ, Boerth RC, Harbison RD, Slonim AE, Freeman RW, and Oates JA Regulatory role of glutathione and soluble sulfhydryl groups in the toxicity of adriamycin. J Pharmacol Exp Ther 1980 215:450–454.

Olson RD, Mushlin PS, Brenner DE, Fleischer S, Cusack BJ, Chang BK, and Boucek RJ Jr Doxorubicin cardiotoxicity may be caused by its metabolite doxorubicinol. Proc Natl Acad Sci USA 1988 85:3585–3589.

Olver IN and Schwarz MA Use of dimethyl sulfoxide in limiting tissue damage caused by extravasation of doxorubicin. Cancer Treat Rep 1983 67:407–408.

Orr FW, Adamson IY, and Young L Quantification of metastatic tumor growth in bleomycin-injured lungs. Clin Exp Metastasis 1986 4:105–116.

Ouchi M, Toriyama K, Matsumoto T, and Baba T Screening for antagonistic agents to the lethal toxicity of neocarzinostatin. II. Effects of various drugs in inhibiting the toxicity of neocarzinostatin in vivo. Jpn J Antibiot 1988 41:105–115.

Ozols RF, Cunnion RE, Klecker RW Jr, Hamilton TC, Ostchega Y, Parrillo JE, and Young RC Verapamil and adriamycin in the treatment of drug-resistant ovarian cancer patients. J Clin Oncol 1987 5:641–647.

Painter RB Inhibition of DNA replicon initiation by 4-nitroquinoline 1-oxide, adriamycin, and ethyleneimine. Cancer Res 1978 38:4445–4449.

Pan S-S and Bachur NR Xanthine oxidase catalyzed reduced cleavage of anthracycline antibiotics and free radical formation. Mol Pharmacol 1980 17:95–99.

Pan S-S, Pedersen L, and Bachur NR Comparative flavoprotein catalysis of anthracycline antibiotic. Reductive cleavage and oxygen consumption. Mol Pharmacol 1981 19:184–186.

Parbhoo SP and Kelleher SM An improved technique for scalp hypothermia to prevent adriamycin/mitozantrone induced alopecia in patients with advanced breast cancer. 3rd Europ Conf Clin Oncol and Cancer Nursing 1985 p. 232.

Passero MA and DiSanto L Peroxidation of arachidonic acid by bleomycin: A possible mechanism of bleomycin pulmonary toxicity. Proc Amer Assoc Cancer Res 1988 29:A9994.

Patterson LH, Gandecha BM, and Brown JR 1,4-Bis [[2-[2-hydroxyethyl] ethylamino]-9,10-anthracenedione an anthraquinone antitumor agent with daunorubicin. Biochem Biophys Res Commun 1983 110:399–405.

Paur E, Youngman RJ, Lengfelder E, and Elstner EF Mechanisms of adriamycin-dependent oxygen activation catalyzed by NADPH-cytochrome c-ferredoxin-oxidoreductase. Z Naturforsch 1984 39c:261–267.

Pelikan PC, Weisfeldt ML, Jacobus WE, Miceli MV, Bulkley BH, and Gerstenblith G Acute doxorubicin cardiotoxicity; functional metabolic and morphologic alterations in the isolated perfused rat heart. J Cardiovasc Pharmacol 1986 8:1058–1066.

Pepin JM and Langner RO Effects of dimethylsulfoxide DMSO on bleomycin-induced pulmonary fibrosis. Biochem Pharmacol 1985 34:2386–2389.

Perez JE, Macchiavelli M, Leone BA, Romero A, Rabinovich MG, Goldar D, and Vallejo C High-dose alpha-tocopherol as a preventive of doxorubicin-induced alopecia. Cancer Treat Rep 1986 70:1213.

Perkins WE, Schroeder RL, Carrano RA, and Imondi AR Myocardial effects of mitoxantrone and doxorubicin in the mouse and guinea pig. Cancer Treat Rep 1984 68:841–847.

Peters JH, Ross GG, Kashiwase D, Lown JW, Yen SF, and Plambeck JA Redox activities of antitumor anthracyclines determined by microsomal oxygen consumption and assays for superoxide anion and hydroxyl radical generation. Biochem Pharmacol 1986 35:1309–1323.

Phan SH, Thrall RS, and Williams C Bleomycin induced pulmonary fibrosis. Am Rev Respir Dis 1981 124:428–434.

Phillips DR and Carlyle GA The effect of physiological levels of divalent metal ions on the interaction of duanomycin with DNA. Evidence of a ternary daunomycin-Cu^{2+}-DNA complex. Biochem Pharmacol 1981 30:2021–2024.

Pigram WJ, Fuller W, and Hamilton LD Stereochemistry of intercalation. Interaction of daunomycin with DNA. Nature 1972 235:17–19.

Poirier TI Mitoxantrone. Drug Intell Clin Pharmacol 1986 20:97–105.

Pollakis G, Goormaghtigh E, Delmelle M, Lion Y, and Ruysschaert JM Adriamycin and derivatives interaction with the mitochondrial membrane, O_2 consumption and free radicals formation. Res Commun Chem Path Pharm 1984 44:445–459.

Pommier Y, Schwartz RE, Zwelling LA, and Kohn KW Effects of DNA intercalating agents on topoisomerase. II. induced DNA strand cleavage in isolated mammalian cell nuclei. Biochemistry 1985 24:6406-6410.

Posner LE, Dukart G, Goldberg J, Bernstein T, and Cartwright K Mitoxantrone: An overview of safety and toxicity. Invest New Drugs 1985 3:123–132.

Povirk LF and Goldberg IH Binding of the nonprotein chromophore of neocarzinostatin to deoxyribonucleic acid. Biochemistry 1980 19:4773–4780.

Povirk LF and Goldberg IH A role of oxidative DNA sugar damage in mutagenesis by neocarzinostatin and bleomycin. Biochimie 1987 69:815–823.

Powis G Effects of disease states on pharmacokinetics of anticancer drugs. In: Pharmacokinetics of Anticancer Agents in Humans Ames MM, Powis G, and Kovach JS Eds Elsevier Sciences, Amsterdam 1983 pp. 363–397.

Powis G Metabolism and reactions of quinoid anticancer agents. Pharmacol Ther 1987 35:57–162.

Powis G Metabolism of anthracyclines. In: Metabolism and Action of Anti-Cancer Drugs Powis G and Prough RA Eds Taylor and Francis, London 1987 pp. 211–260.

Powis G and Kooistra KL Doxorubicin-induced hair loss in the Angora rabbit: A study of treatments to protect against the hair loss. Cancer Chemother Pharmacol 1987 20:291–296.

Praet M, Laghmiche M, Pollakis G, Goormaghtigh E, and Ruysschaert JM In vivo and in vitro modification of the mitochondrial membrane induced by 4′-epiadriamycin. Biochem Pharmacol 1986 35:2923–2928.

Praga C, Beretta G, Vigo PL, Lenaz GR, Pollini C, Bonadonna G, Canetta R, Castellani R, Villa E, Gallagher CG, von Meichner H, Hayat M, Ribaud P, De Wasch G, Mattson W, Heinz K, Waldner R, Kolaric K, Buehner R, Ten Bokkel-Huyninck W, Pererodchikova NI, Manziuk LA, Senn HJ, and Mayr AC Adriamycin cardiotoxicity; A survey of 1273 patients. Cancer Treat Rep 1979 63:827–834.

Pratesi G, Savi G, Pezzoni G, Ellini O, Penco S, Tinelli S, and Zunino F Poly-L-aspartic acid as a carrier for doxorubicin a comparative in vivo study of free and polymer-bound drug. Br J Cancer 1985 52:841–848.

Pratt CB, Ransom JL, and Evans WE Age-related adriamycin cardiotoxicity in children. Cancer Treat Rep 1978 62:1381–1385.

Rabkin SW, Otten M, and Polimeni PI Increased mortality with cardiotoxic doses of adriamycin after verapamil pretreatment despite prevention of myocardial calcium accumulation. Can J Physiol Pharmacol 1983 61:1050–1056.

Raguenez-Viotte G, Lahoue M, Ducastelle T, Morin JP, and Fillastre JP CCNU-adriamycin association induces earlier and more severe nephropathy in rats. Arch Toxicol 1988 61:282–291.

Rajagopalan S, Politi PM, Sinha BK, and Myers CE Adriamycin-induced free radical formation in the perfused rat heart: Implications for cardiotoxicity. Cancer Res 1987 48:4766–4769.

Ramos A, Meyer RA, Korfhagen, Wong KY, and Kaplan S Echocardiographic evaluation of adriamycin cardiotoxicity in children. Cancer Treat Rep 1976 60:1282–1284.

Reich SD Clinical correlations of adriamycin pharmacology. Pharmacol Ther 1978 Part C 2:239–249.

Reilly JJ, Neifeld JP, and Rosenberg SD Clinical course of management of accidental adriamycin extravasation. Cancer 1977 40:2053–2057.

Remuzzi G, Imberti L, Rossini M, Morelli C, Carminati C, Cattaneo GM, and Bertani T Increased glomerular thromboxane synthesis as a possible cause of proteinuria in experimental nephrosis. J Clin Invest 1985 75:94–101.

Revis N and Marusic N Glutathione peroxidase activity and selenium concentration in the hearts of doxorubicin-treated rabbits. J Mol Cell Cardiol 1978 10:945–951.

Revis N and Marusic N Effects of doxorubicin and its aglycone metabolite on calcium sequestration by rabbit heart liver and kidney mitochondria. Life Sci 1979 25:1055–1064.

Riggs CE and Sharp SA Adriamycin: Review of clinical pharmacology and toxicity of an effective anticancer drug. Iowa Med 1987 77:242–251.

Riley DJ, Kerr JR, Berg RA, Ianni BD, Pietra GG, Edelman NH, and Prockop DJ Prevention of bleomycin induced pulmonary fibrosis in the hamster by cis-4-hydroxy-6 proline. Am Rev Respir Dis 1981 123:388–393.

Rivera G, Howarth C, Aur RJ, and Pratt CB Phase I study of neocarzinostatin in children with cancer. Cancer Treat Rep 1978 62:2105–2107.

Robison TW and Giri SN Effect of ibuprofen on doxorubicin toxicity in mice. Pharmacol Res Commun 1984 16:409–418.

Rook A Abnormal hair growth in man. In: Comparative Physiology and Pathology of the Skin Rook AJ and Walton GS Eds FA Davis Co, Philadelphia, PA 1965 p. 231.

Rosenhoff SH, Olson HM, Young DM, Bostick F, and Young RC Adriamycin-induced cardiac damage in the mouse: A small animal model of cardiotoxicity. J Cancer Inst 1975 55:191–194.

Rowley DA and Halliwell B DNA damage by superoxide-generating systems in relation to the mechanism of action of the anti-tumor antibiotic adriamycin. Biochim Biophys Acta 1983 761:86–93.

Sakamoto S, Maeda H, and Matsumoto T Experimental and clinical studies on the formation of antibodies to neocarcinostatin a new protein antibiotic. Cancer Treat Rep 1978 62:2063–2070.

Sakamoto S, Ueno F, Hamada Y, Kiyosaki H, Nomura H, Ogata J, and Ikegami K A case of primary triple cancers originating from the bladder thyroid and prostate. Gann 1980 26:589–593.

Saletan S Mitoxantrone an active new antitumor agent with an improved therapeutic index. Cancer Treat Rev 1987 14:297–303.

Santone KS, Oakes SG, Taylor SR, and Powis G Anthracycline-induced inhibition of a calcium action potential in differentiated neuroblastoma cells. Cancer Res 1986 46:2659–2664.

Satake I, Tari K, Suzuki F, and Yoshida S Decrease pulmonary toxicity in continuous subcutaneous infusion and consecutive daily injection of peplomycin in testicular tumor patients. Nippon Gan Chiryo Gakkai Shi 1985a 20:2291–2297.

Satake I, Tari K, Honma T, Noguchi Y, and Yoshida K Decreased pulmonary toxicity of peplomycin in elderly patients employing continuous subcutaneous infusion. Nippon Gan Chiryo Gakkai Shi 1985b 20:1349–1356.

Sato S, Iwaizumi M, Handa K, and Tamura Y Electron spin resonance study on the mode of generation of free radicals of daunomycin adriamycin and carboquone in NADPH-microsome system. Gann 1977 68:603–608.

Sausville EA, Stein RW, Peisach J, and Horwitz SB Properties and products of the degradation of DNA by bleomycin and iron II. Biochemistry 1978 17:2746–2754.

Sazuka Y, Yoshikawa K, Tanizawa H, and Takino Y Effect of doxorubicin on lipid peroxide levels in tissues of mice. Jpn J Cancer Res 1987 78:1281–1286.

Schenkenberg TD and Von Hoff DD Mitoxantrone: A new anticancer drug with significant activity. Ann Intern Med 1986 1:67–81.

Schlein A, Schurig JE, and Baca C Pulmonary toxicity studies of bleomycin and talisomycin. Cancer Treat Rep 1981 65:291–297.

Schmitt-Graff A and Scheulen ME Prevention of adriamycin cardiotoxicity by niacin isocitrate or N-acetyl-cysteine in mice. A morphological study. Pathol Res Pract 1986 181:168–174.

Schreiber J, Mottley C, Sinha BK, Kalyanaraman B, and Mason RP One-electron reduction of daunomycin daunomycinone and 7-deoxydaunomycinone by the xanthine/xanthine oxidase system. Detection of semiquinone free radicals by electron spin resonance. J Am Chem Soc 1987 109:348–351.

Schurig JE, Rose WC, Hirth RS, Schlein A, Huftalen JB, Florczyk AP, and Bradner WT Tallysomycin S10b, experimental antitumor activity and toxicity. Cancer Chemother Pharmacol 1984 13:164–170.

Schwartz HS Enhanced antitumor activity of adriamycin in combination with allopurinol. Cancer Lett 1983 20:69–74.

Schwartz RG, McKenzie WB, Alexander J, Sayer P, D'Souza A, Manatunga A, Schwartz PE, Berger HJ, Setano J, Surkin L, Wackers FJ, and Zaret BL Congestive heart failure and left ventricular dysfunction complicating doxorubicin therapy. Am J Med 1987 82:1110–1118.

Seipp CA Adverse effects of treatment—hair loss. In: Cancer Principle and Practice of Oncology DeVita VT, Hellman S, and Rosenberg SA Eds 2nd ed., Lippincott, Philadelphia 1985 p. 2007.

Sheridan RP and Gupta RK Electron spin resonance detection of free radicals in the mercaptan-activation and UV-inactivation of neocarzinostatin. Biochem Biophys Res Commun 1981 99:213–220.

Shimamoto N, Tanabe M, Shino A, Hirata M, Kawaji H, Azuma I, Fukuda T, Kobayashi S, and Yamamura Y Preventive effect of a quinonyl derivative of N-acetylmuramyl dipeptide QMDP-66 against adriamycin-induced ECG abnormalities in rats. Int J Immunopharmacol 1983 5:245–251.

Shug AL Protection from adriamycin-induced cardiomyopathy in rats. Z Kardiol 1987 76:46–52.

Sikic BI In: Bleomycin Chemotherapy Sikic BI, Rozencweig M, and Carter SK Eds Academic Press, New York 1985 pp. 247–254.

Sikic BI, Collins JM, Mimnaugh EG, and Gram TE Improved therapeutic index of bleomycin when administered by continuous infusion in mice. Cancer Treat Rep 1978 62:2011–2017.

Singal PK and Pierce GN Adriamycin stimulates low-affinity Ca^{2+} binding and lipid peroxidation but depresses myocardial function. Am J Physiol 1986 250:H419–425.

Singal PK, Segstro RJ, Singh RP, and Kutryk MJ Changes in lysosomal morphology and enzyme activities during the development of adriamycin-induced cardiomyopathy. Can J Cardiol 1985 1:139–147.

Sinha BK Binding specificity of chemically and enzymatically activated anthracycline anticancer agents to nucleic acids. Chem Biol Int 1980 30:67–77.

Sinha BK Metabolic activation of procarbazine. Evidence for carbon centered free radical intermediates. Biochem Pharmacol 1984 33:2777–2781.

Sinha BK and Chignell CF Binding mode of chemically activated semiquinone free radicals from quinone anticancer agents to DNA. Chem Biol Interact 1979 28:301–308.

Sinha BK, Motten AG, and Hanck KW The electrochemical reduction of 1,4-bis 2[2-hydroxyethyl-amino]ethylamino-anthracenedione and daunomycin biochemical significance in superoxide formation. Chem Biol Interact 1983 43:371–377.

Sinha BK, Trush MA, Kennedy KA, and Mimnaugh EG Enzymatic activation and binding of adriamycin to nuclear DNA. Cancer Res 1984 44:2892–2896.

Snider GL, Celli BR, Goldstein RH, O'Brien JJ, and Lucey EC Chronic interstitial pulmonary fibrosis produced in hamsters by endotracheal bleomycin. Am Rev Respir Dis 1978 117:289–297.

Sparano BM, Gordon G, Hall C, Iatropoulos MJ, and Noble JF Safety assessment of new anticancer compound mitoxantrone in beagle dogs. Comparison with doxorubicin. II. Histologic and ultrastructural pathology. Cancer Treat Rep 1982 66:1145–1148.

Speyer J, Green M, Ward C, Wernz J, Blum R, Muggia F, Meyers M, Rey M, Sanger J, Kramer E et al Rationale and preliminary results of a randomized clinical trial of ICRF 187 as a protective agent against cumulative dose-related anthracycline cardiac toxicity. First International Symposium on Organ-Directed Toxicities of Anticancer Drugs, June 4–6, Burlington, VT, The Vermont Regional Cancer Center 1987 p. 13.

Speyer J, Green M, Ward C, Kramer E, Rey M, Sanger J, Ferrans V, Jacquotte A, Dubin N, Wernz J, Blum R, Meyers M, Stecy P, Feit F, Taubes S, and Muggia F Endomyocardial biopsies EB provided additional evidence for ICRF-187 protection against adriamycin Adria-induced cardiac toxicity Cytox. Proc Amer Soc Clin Oncol 1988 7:A244.

Srensen PG, Rosing N, and Rrth M Carbon monoxide diffusing capacity: A reliable indicator of bleomycin-induced pulmonary toxicity. Eur J Respir Dis 1985 66:333–340.

Steinberg JS, Cohen AJ, Wasserman AG, Cohen P, and Ross AM Acute arrhythmogenicity of doxorubicin administration. Cancer 1987 60:1213–1218.

Stephens LC, Wang YM, Schultheiss TE, and Jardine JH Enhanced cardiotoxicity in rabbits treated with verapamil and adriamycin. Oncology 1987 44:302–306.

Stoter G, Sleijfer DT, Vendrik CPJ, Schraffordt Koops H, Struyvenberg A, Van Oosterom AT, Brouwers TM, and Pinedo HM Combination chemotherapy with cisdiammine dichloro platinum vinblastine and bleomycin in advanced testicular non-seminoma. Lancet 1979 1:941–945.

Stuart MJ, de Alarcon PA, and Barvinchak MK Inhibition of adriamycin-induced human platelet lipid peroxidation by vitamin E. Am J Hematol 1978 5:297–303.

Sugioka K, Nakano H, Tsuchiya J, Nakano M, Sugioka Y, Tero-Kubota S, and Ikegami V Clear evidence for the participation of OH in gamma DNA breakage induced by the enzymatic reduction of adriamycin in the presence of iron-ADP. Importance of local OH concentration for DNA strand cleavage. Biochem Int 1984 9:237–242.

Sugiura Y Bleomycin-iron complexes. Electron spin resonance study ligand effect and implication for action mechanism. J Am Chem Soc 1980 102:5208–5215.

Suzuki T, Kanda H, Kawai Y, Tominaga K, and Murata K Cardiotoxicity of anthracycline antineoplastic drugs—clinicopathological and experimental studies. Jpn Circ J 1979 43:1000–1008.

Svingen BA and Powis G Pulse radiolysis studies on antitumor quinones radical lifetimes reactive with oxygen and one-electron reduction potentials. Arch Biochem Biophys 1981 209:119–126.

Svingen BA, Powis G, Appel PL, and Scott M Protection against adriamycin induced skin necrosis in the rat by dimethylsulfoxide and α-tocopherol. Cancer Res 1981 41:3395–3399.

Symonds RP, McCormick CV, and Maxted KJ Adriamycin alopecia prevented by cold air scalp cooling. Am J Clin Oncol 1986 9:454.

Tàbora O, Lewandowski E, and Combs AB Influence of in vitro ubiquinone antagonists on doxorubicin toxicity in vivo. J Toxicol Environ Hlth 1986 18:231–240.

Takahashi K, Yoskioka O, Matsuda A, and Umezawa H Intracellular reduction of the cupric ion of bleomycin copper complex and transfer of the cuprous ion to a cellular protein. J Antibotics Tokyo Ser A 1977 30:861–869.

Tanigawa N, Katoh H, Kan N, Mizuno Y, Tanimura H, Satomura K, and Hikasa Y Effect of vitamin E on toxicity and antitumor activity of adriamycin in mice. Jpn J Cancer Res 1986 77:1249–1255.

Tewey KM, Rowe TC, Yang L, Halligan BD, and Liu LF Adriamycin-induced DNA damage mediated by mammalian DNA topoisomerase II. Science 1984 226:466–468.

Thayer WS Adriamycin stimulated superoxide formation in submitochondrial particles. Chem Biol Int 1977 19:265–278.

Thompson RH In: Naturally Occurring Quinones. Academic Press, London 1971 pp. 1–669.

Thornalley PJ and Dodd NJF Free radical formation from normal and adriamycin-treated rat cardiac sarcomas. Biochem Pharmacol 1985 34:669–674.

Thornalley PJ, Bannister WH, and Bannister JV Reduction of oxygen by NADH/NADH dehydrogenase in the presence of adriamycin. Free Rad Res Commun 1986 2:163–171.

Tian-Hu S, Brandle E, and Zbinden G Inhibition of cardiotoxic nephrotoxic and neurotoxic effects of doxorubicin by ICRF-159. Pharmacology 1983 26:210–220.

Tomlinson CW, Godin DV, and Rabkin SW Implications of cellular changes in a canine model with mild impairment of left ventricular function. Biochem Pharmacol 1985 34:4033–4041.

Tong GL, Henry DW, and Acton EM 5-Iminodaunorubicin reduced cardiotoxic properties in an antitumor anthracycline. J Med Chem 1979 22:36–39.

Torti FM, Bristow MR, Howes AE, Aston D, Stockdale FE, Carter SK, Kohler M, Brown BW JR, and Billingham ME Reduced cardiotoxicity of doxorubicin delivered on a weekly schedule. Assessment by endomyocardial biopsy. Ann Intern Med 1983 99:745–749.

Trangenos F Dihydroxanthraquinone and related bis-substituted aminoanthraquinones: A novel class of antitumor agents. Pharmacol Ther 1983 22:199–214.

Tritton TR and Hickman JA Cell surface membranes as chemotherapeutic target. Cancer Treat Rev 1985 24:81–131.

Tryka AF Bleomycin induced lung injury. First International Symposium on Organ-Directed Toxicities of Anticancer Drugs 1987 p. 33.

Tryka AF, Godleski JJ, and Brain JD Differences in effects of immediate and delayed hyperoxia exposure on bleomycin-induced pulmonary injury. Cancer Treat Rep 1984 68:759–764.

Tsuda S Chromosome aberrations induced by neocarzinostatin in cultured human lymphocytes. Nippan Ketsueki Gakkai Zasshi Acta Haematologica Jap 1987 50:65–78.

Uehara Y, Hori M, and Umezawa H Specificity of transport of bleomycin and cobalt-bleomycin in L5178Y cells. Biochem Biophys Res Commun 1982 104:416–421.

Umezawa H In: Bleomycin Chemical Biochemical and Biological Aspects Hecht SM Ed Springer-Verlag, New York 1979 pp. 24–36.

Umezawa H, Maeda K, Takeuchi T, and Okami Y New antibiotics bleomycin A and B. J Antibiotics Tokyo Ser A 1966 19:200–209.

Umezawa H, Takeuchi T, Hori S, Sawa T, and Ishizuka M Studies on the mechanism of antitumor effect of bleomycin on squamous cell carcinoma. J Antibot Tokyo Ser A 1972 25:409–420.

Umezawa H, Takahashi Y, Kinoshita K, Naganawa H, Masuda T, Ishizuka M, Tatsuta K, and Takeuchi T Tetrahydropyranyl derivatives of daunomycin and adriamycin. J Antibiot 1979 32:1082–1085.

Unverferth DV, Jagadeesh JM, Unverferth BJ, Magorien RD, Meier CV, and Balcerzak SP Attempt to prevent doxorubicin-induced acute human myocardial morphologic damage with acetylcysteine. JNCI 1983 71:917–920.

Unverferth DV, Leier CV, Balcerzak SP, and Hamlin RL Usefulness of a free radical scavenger in preventing doxorubicin-induced heart failure in dogs. Am J Cardiol 1985 56:157–161.

Upton PG, Yamaguchi KT, Myers S, Kidwell TP, and Anderson RJ Effects of antioxidants and hyperbaric oxygen in ameliorating experimental doxorubicin skin toxicity in the rat. Cancer Treat Rep 1986 70:503–507.

US Pharmacopeia Approved Drugs and Legal Requirements. 9th Edition 1989.

Valdivieso M, Burgess MA, and Ewer MS Increased therapeutic index of weekly doxorubicin in the therapy of non-small cell lung cancer: A prospective randomized trial. J Clin Oncol 1984 2:207–214.

Van Barneveld PW, Mulder NH, Van der Mark TW, and Sleijfer DT Bleomycin and pulmonary toxicity. Neth J Med 1985 28:516–523.

Van Hoesel QG, Steerenberg PA, Dormans JA, de Jong WH, de Wildt DJ, and Vos JG Time-course study on doxorubicin-induced nephropathy and cardiomyopathy in male and female LOU/M/Wsl rats lack of evidence for a causal relationship. JNCI 1986 76:299–307.

Van Vleet JF, Greenwood LA, and Ferrans VJ Pathologic features of adriamycin toxicities in young pigs nonskeletal lesions. Am J Vet Res 1979 40:1537–1552.

Van Vleet JF, Ferrans VJ, and Weirich WE Cardiac disease induced by chronic adriamycin administration in dogs and an evaluation of vitamin E and selenium as cardioprotectants. An J Pathol 1980 99:13–42.

Veninga TS, Vriesendorp R, Blom-Muilwijk MC, Sleyfer DT, and Konings AW Absence of an additional fibrotic response caused by oxygen in the lungs of rats after the intratracheal administration of bleomycin. Br J Anaesth 1988 61:413–418.

Villani F, Piccinini F, Merrelli P, and Favalli L Influence of adriamycin on calcium exchangeability in cardiac muscle and its modification by ouabain. Biochem Pharmacol 1978 27:985–987.

Villani F, Monti E, Piccinini F, Favalli L, Rozza Dionigi A, Laza E, and Poggi P Trifluoroperazine does not affect doxorubicin cardiotoxicity in the rat. Anticancer Res 1988 8:659–663.

Villani F, Pizzini L, and Rossi A Evaluation of pulmonary toxicity induced by pepleomycin. Tumori 1988 74:429–432.

Von Hoff DD, Rozencweig M, and Piccat M The cardiotoxicity of anticancer agents. Semin Oncol 1982 9:23–33.

Von Hoff DD, Rozencweig M, and Slavik M Daunomycin: An antibiotic effective in acute leukemia. Adv Pharmacol Chemother 1978 15:1–50.

Von Hoff DD, Layard MW, Basa P, Davis HL Jr, Von Hoff AL, Rozencweig M, and Muggia FM Risk factors for doxorubicin-induced congestive heart failure. Ann Intern Med 1979 91:710–717.

Vosika GJ, Cooper MR, and Comis R Severe toxicity and death associated with neocarzinostatin administration, 1983.

Wang-Ming T and Montgomery MR Biochemical and morphological assessments of bleomycin pulmonary toxicity in rats. Toxicol Appl Pharmacol 1980 53:64–74.

Ward HE, Nicholson A, and Berend N Failure of systemic N-acetyl cysteine to protect the rat lung against bleomycin toxicity. Pathology 1987 19:358–360.

Weiss RB Hypersensitivity reactions to cancer chemotherapy. Semin Oncol 1982 9:5–13.

Weiss RB and Posner DS The renal toxicity of cancer chemotherapeutic agents. Cancer Treat Rev 1982 9:37–56.

Weitzman SA, Lorell B, Carey RW, Kaufman S, and Stossel TP Prospective study of tocopherol prophylaxis for anthracycline cardiac toxicity. Curr Ther Res 1980 28:682–686.

Welch D and Lewis K Alopecia and chemotherapy. Am J Nursing 1980 80:903.

Wheelock JB, Myers MB, Krebs HB, and Goplerud DR Ineffectiveness of scalp hypothermia in the prevention of alopecia in patients treated with doxorubicin and cisplatin combinations. Cancer Treat Rep 1984 68:1387.

Whittaker JA and Al-Ismail SA Effect of digoxin and vitamin E in preventing cardiac damage caused by doxorubicin in acute myeloid leukemia. Brit Med J 1984 288:283–284.

Wilkinson GR and Branch RA Effects of hepatic disease on clinical pharmacokinetics. In: Pharmacokinetic Basis for Drug Treatment Benet LZ, Massoud N, and Gambertoglio JG Eds Raven Press, New York 1984 pp. 44–62.

Winterbourn CC Evidence for the production of hydroxyl radicals from the adriamycin semiquinone and H_2O_2. FEBS Lett 1981 136:89–94.

Winterbourn CC and Sutton HC Hydroxyl radical production from hydrogen peroxide and enzymatically generated paraquat radicals, catalytic requirements and oxygen dependence. Archiv Biochem Biophys 1984 235:116–126.

Winterbourn CC, Gutteridge JMC, and Halliwell B Doxorubicin-dependent lipid peroxidation at low partial pressures of O_2. J Free Rad Biol Med 1985 1:43–49.

Wittes RE, Brescia F, Young CW, Magill GB, Golbey RB, and Krakoff IH Combination chemotherapy with cisdiammino-dichloroplatinum II and bleomycin in tumours of the head and neck. Oncology 1975 32:202–207.

Wood LA Possible prevention of adriamycin-induced alopecia by tocopherol. New Engl J Med 1985 312:1060.

Wortman JR, Lucas VS Jr, Schuster E, Thiele P, and Logue GL Sudden death during doxorubicin administration. Cancer 1979 44:1588–1591.

Yagoda A, Mukherji B, Young C, Etcubanas E, Lamonte C, Smith JR, Tan CTC, and Krakoff I Bleomycin, an antitumor antibiotic: Clinical experience in 274 patients. Ann Intern Med 1972 77:861–870.

Yamanaka N, Kato T, Nishida K, Fujikawa T, Fukushima M, and Ota K Elevation of serum lipid peroxide level associated with doxorubicin toxicity and its amelioration by [dl]-α-tocopheryl acetate or coenzyme Q10 in mouse doxorubicin, toxicity, lipid peroxide, tocopherol, coenzyme Q10. Cancer Chemother Pharmacol 1979 3:223–227.

Yarbro JW, Conley NS, Patterson WP, and Zeidler RB Hydrogen peroxide in breath condensates of patients receiving bleomycin. Proc Amer Soc Clin Oncol 1987 6:A82.

Yoda Y, Nakazawa M, Abe T, and Kawakami Z Prevention of doxorubicin myocardial toxicity in mice by reduced glutathione. Cancer Res 1986 46:2551–2556.

Younes M, Cornelius S, and Siegers CP Fe^{2+} -supported in vivo lipid peroxidation induced by compounds undergoing redox cycling. Chem Biol Int 1985 54:97–103.

Young RC, Ozols RF, and Myers CF Medical Progress. The anthracycline antineoplastic drugs. N Engl J Med 1981 305:139–153.

Youngman RJ and Elstner EF Oxygen species in paraquat toxicity: The crypto-OH radical FEBS Lett 1981 129:265–268.

Zabbe C, Bellet-Barthas M, Clavier J, Dewitte JD, Andre N, Legrand A, Deredec D, and Nguyen-Huu N Preoperative treatment of bronchial epidermoid cancers: Study of the pulmonary toxicity of bleomcyin. Colloq Inserm 1986 137:519–527.

Zbinden G, Bachmann E, and Holnegger C Model systems for cardiotoxic effects of anthracyclines. Antibiot Chemother 1978 23:255–270.

Zbinden G and Brandle E Toxicologic screening of daunorubicin NSC-82151, aadriamycin NSC-123127 and their derivatives in rats. Cancer Chemother Rep 1975 59:707–715.

Zee-Cheng RKY and Cheng CC Antineoplastic agents. Structure-activity relationship study of bis substituted aminoalkylamino anthraquinones. J Med Chem 1978 21:291–294.

Zweier JL Iron-mediated formation of an oxidized adriamcyin free radical. Biochim Biophys Acta 1985 839:209–213.

Zwelling LA, Kerrigan D, and Michael S Cytotoxicity and DNA strand breaks by 5-iminodaunorubicin in mouse leukemia L1210 cells. Comparison with adriamycin and 4′-9-acridinylamino methanesulfono-m-anisidine. Cancer Res 1982 42:2687–2691.

CHAPTER 8

Toxicity of Vinca Alkaloids

Miles P. Hacker, Ph.D.

INTRODUCTION

The periwinkle plant has been part of medicinal folklore for many years throughout the world. Noble et al. (1958) first observed the neutropenic and marrow-suppressive effects of periwinkle plant in rats while testing the extracts for antidiabetic activity. This observation initiated the purification of a family of compounds commonly referred to as the vinca alkaloids. Two of these natural products, vincristine and vinblastine, are important clinical agents and two semisynthetic derivatives, vindesine and navelbine, are currently undergoing experimental clinical evaluation.

Each of these asymmetric dimeric compounds is quite similar chemically with only minor modifications present on the vindoline ring. Although only minor chemical changes differentiate the four vinca alkaloids, only minor differences are required to cause dramatic changes in the toxicity and efficacy of vinca alkaloids. For example, removal of an acetyl group or addition of an acetyl group at the appropriate site of the dimer can result in complete loss of biologic activity.

All four vinca alkaloids seem to work through the same mechanism and block mitosis with metaphase arrest. While the complete biochemistry of this activity isn't understood it is apparent that there is binding of the vinca alkaloid to the protein tubulin, a major piece of cellular microtubules (Deconti and Creasy, 1975; Dustin, 1978). Whether this interaction results in increasing the instability of the microtubules (Mitchison and Kirschner, 1984) or increasing the loss of subunits as the minus pole (Margolis and Wilson, 1981) is not clear. What is known from microscopic analysis of vinca treated cells is that microtubules dissolve and highly regular crystals form containing 1 mole of vinblastine per mole of tubulin. Why this effect on microtubular formation and function ultimately leads to the death of a cell is not known.

Despite their similarity chemically, there is little cross-resistance between the individual vinca alkaloids. An exception to this clinical generalization is in the experimental situation referred to as multidrug resistance. In this circumstance the tumor cell becomes resistant to a variety of apparently nonrelated antitumor agents. In this circumstance cross-resistance between the vinca alkaloids has been clearly established.

VINCRISTINE

Vincristine, an alkaloid extracted from the periwinkle plant (for structure see Fig. 8-1), has proven efficacy against a variety of human tumors including acute lymphocytic leukemia, lymphomas (lymphocytic, mixed cellular, histiocytic, non-differentiated, nodular, and diffuse types), Hodgkin's disease, rhabdomyosarcoma, neuroblastoma, and Wilm's tumor (Luce et al., 1971; DeVita et al., 1972; Johnson et al., 1973; Rosenthal, 1981; Bloomfield et al., 1985).

Vincristine is administered intraveneously (IV) most frequently on a weekly basis. Clinical

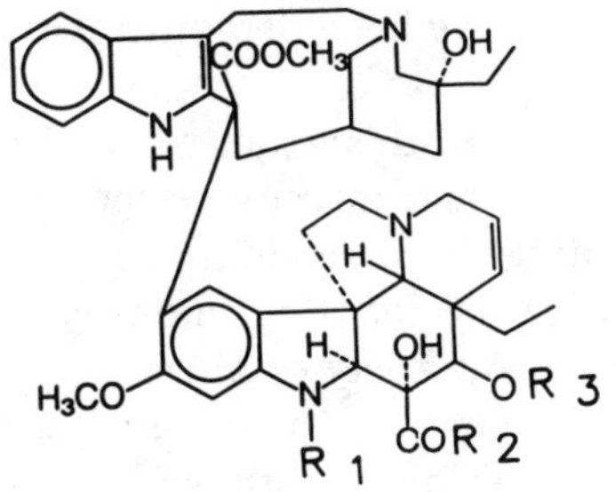

	R_1	R_2	R_3
Vincristine	$-CHO$	$-OCH_3$	$-COCH_3$
Vinblastine	$-CH_3$	$-OCH_3$	$-COCH_3$
Vindesine	$-CH_3$	$-NH_2$	$-H$

FIGURE 8-1. Chemical structures of vincristine, vinblastine and vindesine.

studies involving daily administration in excess of seven days have shown an increased toxicity without enhanced antitumor activity. Interestingly, children seem to tolerate higher doses of vincristine than do adults perhaps due to the increased sensitivity of adults to the neurotoxicity of the drug.

At the usual clinical dose, the peak plasma concentration of vincristine is approximately 0.4 μM, with significant amounts of the drug being bound to plasma proteins (Bender and Chabner, 1982). Vincristine is cleared from the body in a multiphasic pattern with a terminal half-life of approximately 2.5 hr (Bender et al., 1977). The drug is metabolized in the liver to inactive products which may help explain the apparent increase in toxicity observed in patients with obstructive jaundice.

A number of toxicities have been reported in experimental animals and patients treated with vincristine. Of these, the most frequently cited dose-limiting toxicity for this drug is a mixed sensorimotor polyneuropathy (Casey et al., 1973; Rosenthal and Kaufman, 1974; Weiss et al., 1974). The clinical features of this disease include early loss of tendon reflexes at the ankles and distal parasthesias followed by a sensory loss for touch, pain, and vibration (Casey et al., 1973; McLeod and Penny, 1969; Sandler et al., 1969). If the disease becomes sufficiently severe distal extremity weakness can occur (Bradley et al., 1970; Holland et al., 1973). Recovery from most of the neurologic impairment begins shortly after cessation of drug administration, if done soon enough.

The pathogenesis of vincristine-induced neuropathy is poorly understood but it seems likely that microtubular changes play a role since vinca alkaloids have been shown to bind to dimeric tubulin and interfere with microtubular assembly (Dustin, 1984; Himes et al., 1976; Journey and Goldstein, 1965; Malawista et al., 1968; Paulson and McClure, 1974). Histopathologic examination of neuronal tissue has revealed axonal degeneration to be the predominant lesion (Gottschalk et al., 1968; McLeod and Penny, 1968; Sandler et al., 1969). This may explain the vincristine-induced alteration of the axoplasmic transport process (Allen et al., 1985; Brady, 1984; Smith et al., 1975) since axonal degeneration has been shown to accompany axoplasmic transport abnormalities (Green et al., 1977; Ochs et al., 1975). Sahenk et al. (1987) have reported that neurons treated with vincristine have lost portions of axonal microtubules and display a malorientation of microtubules and neurofilaments. These observations could explain the abnormalities in fast axonal transport. The results from several studies indicate that this toxicity is similar to that of other toxic neuropathies where a dying back process has clearly been demonstrated (Guiheneuc et al., 1980; Casey et al., 1973; Sumner, 1978).

Although the clinical importance of this toxicity is well recognized, an appropriate animal model to screen new vinca analogs and investigate the mechanism of toxicity has not been clearly identified. Indeed, as will be discussed in the section on vindesine the standard in vivo preclinical screens, which include the rat, dog, monkey, and chicken, failed to predict the neurotoxic potential of vindesine. A variety of alternatives have been investigated. Recently, Nordino et al. (1988) reported that vincristine administered weekly to rabbits produced functional and microscopic changes similar to those observed in humans and suggest that the rabbit could serve as a predictive model. Others have reported that the cat may show vincristine induced nerve alterations (Goldstein et al., 1981; Cho et al., 1983).

A problem with these studies is that only the known neurotoxic agent vincristine was tested. Thus, the applicability of such models to differentiate between toxic and nontoxic vinca congeners has yet to be established. Brann and Hacker (1983) described an in vivo model in which rats were administered microgram quantities of the drug directly into the substantia nigra and toxicity was assessed by directed contralateral rotations made by the rat. This model was able to differentiate between neurotoxic and nonneurotoxic vinca derivatives (Brann and Hacker, unpublished data).

The applicability of in vitro screens was reviewed recently by Atterwall and Walum (1989). Such screens appear to be acceptable and essential for mechanistic studies but uncertainty exists concerning their use as a means to evaluate drugs for neurotoxic potential. The authors summarized by stating that it is essential for in vitro information to be closely integrated with in vivo data to gain a meaningful neurotoxicity profile.

The clinical sequelae to vincristine related neurotoxicity are quite varied. The earliest motor deficit in this disease process is bilateral wrist-drop or foot-drop and the development of this toxicity has been used as an indicator of maximum vincristine administration. Upon cessation of therapy this deficit usually reverses quite readily. To minimize the incidence of severe weakness or paralysis, the drug is given in a maximum dose of 2 mg and is withdrawn at the first sign of weakness (Kaplan and Wiernik, 1982).

In spite of these precautions vincristine-induced neurotoxicity can result in rather severe manifestations. Variabilities in sensitivity to this toxicity are rather marked. The mechanism of variability is unknown but there appear to be certain factors that may predispose patients to the neurotoxic effects of vincristine. Thant et al. (1982) suggested that preexisting diabetic neuropathy may enhance patient sensitivity to vincristine. Similarly, Griffiths et al. (1985) observed that a patient with Charcot-Marie-Tooth syndrome, a familial disorder in which muscle weakness and wasting of peroneal and intrinsic foot muscles are common, developed severe generalized weakness following a single treatment with vincristine. It has been suggested that patients with Guillan-Barré syndrome may have increased sensitivity to vincristine treatment (Norman et al., 1987). Irradiation of peripheral nerves may accentuate the severity and persistence of vincristine neurotoxicity (Cassady et al., 1980).

Because of the marked variability in the response to vincristine careful clinical management is necessary for patients receiving vincristine. How to best monitor patients for the onset of neurotoxicity has been the focus of clinical investigations. Currently, the degree of patient monitoring appears to be related to the aggressiveness of therapy. Patients receiving less aggressive therapy can be monitored by questions pertaining to feeling in the fingertips or toes, whereas patients receiving more aggressive therapy should be monitored with electrophysiological assays such as nerve conduction velocity or Achilles tendon reflex (Guiheneuc et al., 1980).

The actual manifestations of vincristine induced neurotoxicity other than the wrist-drop and foot-drop described above can be quite varied. Ryan and Emami (1983) reported that five children developed bilateral peroneal nerve palsies with equinocavus deformities. If the foot and ankle were left in the equinocavus position, surgery was required to correct the deformity. If the peroneal palsy is braced as soon as the deformity is diagnosed, then physical therapy without surgery should correct this deficit. Also in children, vincristine, even when given in conventional doses, has been associated with rare instances of seizures (Johnson et al., 1973). The problem with ascribing this toxicity to vincristine has been the lack of pathological confirmation (Rosenthal and Kaufman, 1974). Recently, Hurwitz et al. (1988) reported that an eight-year-old child developed seizures following vincristine for the treatment of acute lymphocytic leukemia (ALL). A brain biopsy revealed neurotubular dissociation which is characteristic of vincristine damage in experimental animals (Bradley, 1970; Cho et al., 1983). When the drug was withheld the symptoms resolved suggesting strongly that these were toxicities directly related to vincristine administration.

Ocular toxicity is not uncommon in vincristine-treated patients (Griffin and Garnick, 1981). Bilateral optic atrophy and blindness have been observed, primarily in patients receiving combination chemotherapy or vincristine in addition to cranial radiation (Norton and Stockman, 1979; Sanderson et al., 1976; Margileth et al., 1977; Byrd et al., 1981). Recovery from this toxicity varied, with some suffering irreversible blindness (Margileth et al., 1977) and others recovering following cessation of drug administration (Norton and Stockman, 1979; Sanderson et al., 1976; Shurin et al., 1982). The relative low frequency of serious central nervous system (CNS) toxicity has been attributed to poor penetration of the blood–brain barrier by vincristine (Jackson et al., 1984). However, such complications as vincristine overdose, impaired drug metabolism, or disruption of the blood–brain barrier can result in increased risk of CNS damage. A less debilitating form of ocular toxicity is a possible correlation between vincristine and night blindness (Ripps et al., 1984). The noninvasive test procedures used suggest a striking similarity between this drug induced toxicity and that seen in subjects with recessively inherited stationary night blindness.

Vincristine neurotoxicity has resulted in urologic complications such as urinary retention (Gottlieb and Cuttner, 1971; Bradley et al., 1970; Hancock and Naysmith, 1975), dysuria (Tan and Aduna, 1961), and impotence (Holland et al., 1973). Wheeler et al. (1983) reported on a patient with urinary retention and documented neuropathic detrusor areflexia after a single dose of vincristine. Incontinence of the bowel and bladder, with electromyogram evidence of denervation of the anal sphincter, has also been observed in a patient treated with vincristine (Raphelson et al., 1983). In each case, recovery followed cessation of drug administration.

The syndrome of inappropriate secretion of antidiuretic hormone is a rare but a well-recognized side effect of vincristine (Young and Ponsner, 1980; Tomiwa et al., 1983). The disease is characterized by hyponatremia with increased urinary salt excretion probably resulting from an effect of vincristine on the hypothalamic nuclei (Rosenthal and Kaufman, 1974). Again, recovery can be expected if vincristine administration is stopped when this toxicity is noted.

Another toxicity, possibly related to hypothalamic stimulation (Kaufman et al., 1976), seen in children within 24 hr after vincristine administration is a febrile response. The episodes are accompanied by fatique and loss of appetite and have a duration of six to 96 hr (Ishii et al., 1988). The fever appears to be amenable to prophylactic administration of an antipyretic (Ishii et al., 1988).

The gastrointestinal tract is often affected by vincristine induced neurotoxicity resulting most frequently in colicky abdominal pain and constipation (Holland et al., 1973; Sandler et al., 1969). The constipation may be severe and can result in fecal impaction (Rosenberg and Caridi, 1983) but is usually readily reversible upon cessation of drug administration. Whereas no specific drug therapy has been approved for this toxicity, metoclopramide administration caused rapid resolution of vincristine induced ileus in three patients (Garewal and Dalton, 1985).

A less-recognized neurotoxicity of vincristine is laryngeal nerve paralysis (Bohannon et al., 1963; Whittaker and Griffith, 1977). The most frequent complaint is hoarseness but this can proceed to paresis and ultimately death in which laryngeal paralysis impairs respiration (Whittaker and Griffith, 1977). The problem with this complication is that when a patient with systemic disease complains of hoarseness it is tempting to suspect the disease as the causative agent. If the hoarseness can be ascribed to the vincristine it is reversible when the drug use is withdrawn (Delaney, 1982).

Given that neurotoxicity is the principal limiting side effect of vincristine, what is available to minimize or prevent these toxicities? Presently, little can be done to intervene other than limiting the dose of vincristine (2 mg per treatment is the standard maximum dose administered), administering the drug on a weekly basis (more frequent treatment seems to enhance the toxicity more than increase the efficacy) and monitoring the patient for developing toxicity.

A systematic exploration of potential modifiers of neurotoxicity has resulted in the identification of glutamic acid as a possible protectant (Jackson et al., 1984). This amino acid was selected because of its reported protection against vinblastine induced myelosuppression without an apparent inhibition of oncolytic activity (Armstrong et al., 1962). In a study involving 42 patients receiving weekly injections of vincristine (1 mg/m^2) alone and 42 patients receiving vincristine plus glutamic acid (500 mg, orally [po], three times daily), there was an indication that glutamic acid decreased vincristine induced neurotoxicity without having adverse side effects (Jackson et al., 1988). The mechanism of this potentially protective activity of glutamic acid is not known but it has been hypothesized that glutamate may either stabilize microtubular structures (Hamel and Lin, 1981) or prevent vincristine uptake by competing at the vincristine transport site (Bleyer et al., 1975; Creasy et al., 1971).

Given that vincristine is a neurotoxic agent, it is not surprising that when the drug is administered intrathecally catastrophic results occur. Indeed, a number of reports have been published in which the drug was inadvertently administered intrathecally and in each case a fatality ensued (Schochet et al., 1968; Slyter et al., 1980; Gaidys et al., 1983; Williams et al., 1983). Attempts at treatment of this iatrogenic complication have included CNS washout, high-dose folinic acid, and symptomatic support but they were of no value.

Vincristine is not generally regarded as a myelotoxic agent. Early studies with the drug reported only infrequent episodes of neutropenia (Holland et al., 1973; Stein et al., 1974). Many times the appearance of granulocytopenia has been ascribed to disease progression when patients are receiving vincristine plus prednisone, another myelosparing drug. Stein and Roth have reported, however, that treatment of chronic myelogenous leukemia in blastic transformation with vincristine/prednisone has resulted in granulocytopenia that may well have resulted from therapy and not disease progression (Stein and Roth, 1976). Thus, although vincristine does not have marked myelotoxic potential its effect on the marrow cannot be disregarded.

One interesting effect of vincristine on the marrow is an apparent increase in the number of circulating platelets (Carbone et al., 1963; Robertson et al., 1973). This observation has been exploited clinically in the treatment of idiopathic thrombocytopenia purpura (Reiquam and Proper, 1966; Sultan et al., 1971; Marmont and Damaios, 1971). While still used clinically, vincristine treatment of IDP is limited.

A number of other toxicities have been reported for vincristine and include a mild and readily reversible alopecia in approximately 20% of the patients. If the drug is inadvertently extravasated serious complications can be encountered. The extent of damage is related to the amount extravasated and can range from mild inflammation and pain to frank tissue necrosis. It has been reported that infiltration of the exposed area with hydrocortisone helps ameliorate the damage (Choy, 1979; Bellone, 1981).

Myocardial infarctions appear to occur in association with the administration of vinca alkaloids (Mandel et al., 1975; Somers et al., 1976; Yancey and Talpaz, 1982; Subar and Muggia, 1986). The mechanism of the cardiac toxicity is not known but does not appear to be related to vinca induced platelet aggregation (Mandel et al., 1975; Yancey and Talpaz, 1982).

Subar and Muggia (1986) have suggested a multifactorial explanation involving coronary spasm and increased sensitivity of the myocardium to hypoxia.

VINBLASTINE

Vinblastine is another antimitotic plant alkaloid closely related to vincristine that has been used clinically for almost 30 years (Frei et al., 1961). Although there are similarities in the structure of the two vinca alkaloids (Fig. 8-1), there is an apparent difference in the spectrum of tumor responses and toxicities associated with vincristine and vinblastine. Whereas the former is used primarily against leukemias and has peripheral neuropathy as the primary dose-limiting toxicity, the latter is used to treat a variety of solid tumors and is limited in most patients by a leukopenia.

In most clinical studies the primary toxicity encountered with vinblastine is a fall in circulating leukocytes (Hertz et al., 1960; Johnson et al., 1963; Warwick et al., 1961). Differential cell counts usually reveal a lymphocyte predominance with generally less than 10% neutrophils (Samuels and Howe, 1970). The nadir of leukocyte count occurs approximately seven to 10 days after treatment and recovers within 21 days posttreatment. Concomitant with the leukopenia is an increased risk of infection which can, for the most part, be managed with appropriate use of antibiotics.

Attempts to minimize vinblastine leukocyte toxicity have been directed primarily at schedule modification. The rationale for this approach comes from experimental data suggesting that vinblastine cytotoxicity is very dependent on the duration of drug exposure (Ludwig et al., 1984), possibly caused by the rapid efflux of the drug from the cells when the drug is removed from the culture medium (Ferguson et al., 1984; Gout et al., 1984). Most clinical protocols administer vinblastine as a single IV injection or daily injections on days 1, 2 or 1, 2, and 3 with a concomitant adjustment in daily dose. With the advent of reliable drug administration pumps, prolonged infusions have been possible (Yap et al., 1980; Ratain and Vogelzang, 1986). Whether this approach will result in a true gain in therapeutic index has yet to be determined but the ultimate dose-limiting toxicity still appears to be myelosuppression (Ratain and Vogelzang, 1986).

Although neutropenia is the most common type of leukocyte toxicity associated with vinblastine therapy, altered platelet counts have also been reported to be correlated to vinblastine administration (Rees et al., 1982; Pedrazzini et al., 1983; Abrahamsen et al., 1986). This toxicity is transient in nature with a nadir occurring within three days of treatment and full recovery by day 14–15. Platelet survival studies indicate an increased destruction of platelets as the mechanism of toxicity (Abrahamsen et al., 1986). Except in critically ill patients with a predilection to bleeding problems, this thrombocytopenia appears to be of little toxicological consequence.

Following retrospective analysis of the pathogenesis of chemotherapy induced anemia in children receiving consolidation therapy for acute leukemia, it appeared as though vinblastine and not other antineoplastic agents caused the characteristic changes in erythrocyte morphology (Barr et al., 1980). In an attempt to ascribe a mechanism to this vinblastine effect, Neville et al. (1982) studied the effect of vinblastine on the morphology and stability of erythrocytes. Only at supratherapeutic concentrations of the drug could reproducible changes in morphology be detected but vinblastine was clearly shown to be stomatocytogenic in this in vitro test.

Although vinblastine has been shown to cause thrombocytopenia in some individuals, it has also been clearly demonstrated that vinblastine can induce a thrombocytosis (Robertson and McCarthy, 1969; Hwang et al., 1969). This response is quite similar to that discussed above for vincristine and is probably related to the same mechanism. Indeed, vinblastine has been administered to patients with idiopathic thrombocytopenia purpura, either as a free drug (Sultan et al., 1971; Marmont et al., 1971) or as vinblastine loaded platelets (Ahn et al.,

1978) with some rather impressive results. The mechanism of this treatment is still not understood but may be related to the autoimmune nature of this disease (Shulman et al., 1965). As with vincristine, the clinical use of vinblastine in the treatment of idiopathic thrombocytopenia purpura is quite limited.

Although not as common as with vincristine, neurotoxicity is seen in patients treated with vinblastine. Occasionally, parasthesias in the hands and feet are noted and if sufficient drug is administered even foot-drop, wrist-drop, or motor difficulty involving voluntary muscles have been reported. Please note the section above for a complete description of the toxic sequelae that can be encountered with vinblastine. The primary difference between the two drugs is that the incidence and severity of neurotoxicity is far less for vinblastine.

Associated with the neurotoxicity of vinblastine are other, less frequent toxicities of neurologic origin. Brook and Schreiber (1971) first described vocal cord paralysis in two patients. When the drug was withdrawn, both patients recovered vocal cord functions within four to six weeks. A number of reports have come out describing the occurrence of Raynaud's phenomenon in patients receiving vinblastine in combination with bleomycin (Mantel 1982; Harvey et al., 1981; Grau et al., 1983; Scheulen and Schmidt, 1982; Teutsch et al., 1977; Vogelzang et al., 1981). This toxicity is not considered to be a hypersensitive response to the combination of vinblastine and bleomycin, it does not appear to be dose related, and is certainly sporadic in occurrence. The mechanism of this toxicity is not understood but may be related to peripheral neurotoxicity of vinblastine or, more likely, an interaction between the two drugs. Rothberg (1978) reported partial symptomatic relief by administering guanethidine.

Pain has been associated with vinblastine injection occurring during the first or second day following treatment (Stark and Fletcher, 1966; Lucas and Huang, 1977). A proposed mechanism of this toxicity has been related to the structural similarities between vinblastine and ergot alkaloids capable of causing vasoconstriction. However, when patients are placed on vincristine because of unbearable pain due to vinblastine, no such pain is noted (Lucas and Huang, 1977). Given that the incidence of this toxicity can range as high as 40% and the severity of pain associated with this toxicity is such that an analgesic such as morphine must be administered or perhaps vincristine should replace vinblastine.

The syndrome of inappropriate antidiuretic hormone secretion has been reported infrequently for children and adults receiving vincristine. With standard doses of vinblastine, the occurrence of this syndrome seems even more infrequent as few reports exist in the clinical literature (Ginsberg et al., 1977). However, if an overdose of vinblastine is administered (Winter and Arbus, 1977) or a more aggressive high-dose vinblastine protocol is administered (Ravikumar and Grage, 1983) this syndrome is more likely to occur. The mechanism of this toxicity may be related to vinblastine induced derangements in neuronal input from volume receptors in the periphery resulting in a "resetting" of the osmoreceptor activity (Robertson et al., 1973).

The differential diagnosis of acute interstitial pneumonitis and pulmonary fibrosis in the patient treated with oncolytics includes a growing list of drugs. Whereas not as yet causally related there have been reports of possible pulmonary toxicity secondary to vinblastine administration. Israel and Olson (1978) first reported pulmonary edema in a patient within two hr after being treated with vinblastine. Exclusion of a number of potential nondrug related causes of edema indicated an etiologic role of vinblastine. More recently Konitis et al. (1982) described pulmonary changes observed in two patients treated with vinblastine and mitomycin-C. Both patients developed diffuse interstitial infiltrates within one hr following drug administration. The infiltrates cleared but recurred in subsequent treatments and ultimately produced chronic lung changes. It would appear that patients receiving vinblastine in combination with known pneumotoxic drugs or thoracic irradiation should be observed carefully for potential pulmonary damage.

Drug-induced photodermatitis may be divided into phototoxic and photoallergic reactions.

Breza et al. (1975) described a photosensitization of the skin in a patient receiving vinblastine. Photoreactions to intradermal injections of vinblastine were produced in five normal controls with suberythema doses of ultraviolet (UV) light. Although the data obtained suggest a phototoxic response to vinblastine, a photoallergic response could not be ruled out due to the pruritic, vesicular nature of the eruption.

Epithelial keratopathy is a recognized complication of chemical injury to the eyes with vinblastine solution. A temporary reduction in vision to hand movements with minute grey opacities identified by ophthalmic examination (Mosci et al., 1967). No permanent damage other than a possible astigmatism was detected in this individual. McLendon and Bron (1978) reported similar acute changes in an individual who splashed vinblastine solution into his eye. Although corneal changes resolved, the patient has persistent complaints of dry eye. Whether this persistent toxicity was a result of vinblastine was not clearly established.

When extravasated vinblastine can cause localized tissue damage similar to that discussed above for vincristine. Therapy for this inadvertent subcutaneous injection of vinblastine is identical for vincristine but as with vincristine treatment is not completely successful. Alopecia will occur in approximately 20 to 30% of the patients treated with vinblastine but recovery is complete following cessation of drug.

VINDESINE

Vindesine (desacetyl vinblastine amide sulfate, see Fig. 8-1 for structure) was derived from vinblastine sulfate at the Lilly research laboratories (Cullinan et al., 1974; Barnett et al., 1978). The differences in chemical structures between the parent compound and vindesine are, as can be seen, relatively minor. Not surprisingly vindesine binds to microtubules resulting in mitotic arrest of chinese hamster ovary cells (Sweeney et al., 1978). Preclinical toxicology studies revealed intestinal, spermatogenic, and bone marrow toxicities (Todd et al., 1976). The compound was entered into clinical trials with a great deal of enthusiasm as no neurotoxicity was detected in animal models for vinca alkaloid induced neurotoxicity (Todd et al., 1979) whereas marked antitumor activity was observed in a wide range of experimental tumors (Dyke et al., 1979).

The first clinical trials of vindesine began in the mid-1970s and shortly thereafter it became obvious many of the toxicities associated with other vinca alkaloids also occurred in patients treated with vindesine. Currie et al. (Currie, 1978) reported myelosuppression, alopecia, parasthesia, aesthesia, myalgia, and hyporeflexia in patients treated with a single IV dose every seven to 14 days or daily doses × five to 10 days. In addition, patients administered vindesine on a daily basis experienced a significant amount of stomatitis, pyrexia, constipation, and paralytic ileus compared to patients receiving weekly injections. Dyke and Nelson (1977) reported similar toxicities but also noted that extravasation of the drug caused produced marked cellulitis.

Based on measurable tumor response in Phase I studies vindesine advanced to efficacy studies. In the main, vindesine has been administered as a single weekly IV injection and has resulted in toxicities generally associated with the vinca alkaloids with myelosuppression and peripheral neuropathy being the most frequent dose-limiting toxicities (Jewkes et al., 1983; Alavi et al., 1984; Bezwoda et al., 1984; Vogl et al., 1984; Rhomberg et al., 1986). Postmus et al. (1987) compared the effect of twice weekly administration to weekly treatments and found no therapeutic advantage for the more intensive regimen. This latter toxicity was both unexpected and disappointing as no preclinical screen detected a neurotoxic potential for vindesine.

Vindesine proved to be rather effective as a single agent in selected tumor combination studies. To date no marked therapeutic advantage for long-term survival has been reported for vindesine when combined with other drugs or radiation (Gralla et al., 1980; DiConstanza et al., 1986; Einhorn et al., 1986). Interstitial lung disease has been reported for vindesine combined with radiation (Bott et al., 1986) or mitomycin-C and cisplatin (Einhorn et al., 1986). Neither the clinical significance nor the mechanism of this interaction has been addressed to date.

The ultimate clinical status of vindesine in the U.S.A. is unknown. Whereas available by prescription in Canada, vindesine remains classified as an experimental agent in the U.S.A. The data accumulated to date suggest that while vindesine has better activity against selected tumors such as non-small cell lung cancer than either vinblastine or vincristine when used as a single agent, no significant advantage has been noted in combination protocols. The profile of host toxicity appears to be similar to that for other vinca alkaloids which includes a peripheral neurotoxicity not predicted by preclinical screens. This dichotomy between clinical experience and preclinical screening points to the need for further development of a predictive neurotoxicity assay.

NAVELBINE

Navelbine (5′-nor-anhydrovinblastine, vinorelbine) is a new semisynthetic compound derived from the vinca alkaloid series that has demonstrated activity against a variety of experimental tumor systems (Maral et al., 1984). The mechanism of action of this drug appears to be similar to that of other vinca derivatives, except that navelbine may not affect the different tau proteins equally. Thus, navelbine may have selectivity for specific microtubular proteins (Fellous et al., 1989) which could explain two potentially important properties of the drug, that is, a reduced neurotoxicity and a different antineoplastic spectrum (Armand and Marty, 1989).

To date limited clinical data are available but those studies completed thus far indicate that myelosuppression is the primary dose limiting toxicity. When administered on a weekly basis the dose-limiting toxicity was leukopenia, primarily of the granulocytic series (Mathe and Reizenstein, 1985; Besenval et al., 1989). Neurotoxicity was observed in a few patients but the severity was mild and the incidence much less than one would expect for any of the other vinca alkaloids. Constipation was frequent in these patients but paralytic ileus was rare. Phase II studies with this interesting drug have been reported (Depierre et al., 1989; Canobbio et al., 1989; George et al., 1989) but it is too early to state whether the oncolytic activity of navelbine will warrant large-scale combination chemotherapy studies. Whether the apparently diminished neurotoxicity and increased spectrum of activity continues with further testing remains to be established.

In summary, the vinca alkaloids represent an important class of antitumor drugs having impressive activity against a variety of human tumors. All of the vinca derivatives studies thus far appear to have their antimitotic activity as result of the interaction with microtubular proteins. There is a commonality among the range of toxicities that can occur following administration of the drugs to humans but the incidence and severities of these toxicities vary between the drugs. Fortunately most of the toxicities encountered during clinical use of the vinca alkaloids appear to be reversible if the drug is stopped once toxicity has been identified. Thus, careful clinical monitoring of patients is essential for favorable patient outcome. For vincristine the primary dose-limiting toxicity is a peripheral neuropathy, for vinblastine the primary dose-limiting toxicity is myelosuppression, and for vindesine both neuropathy and myelosuppression are problematic. The status of vindesine and the most recent vinca alkaloid to enter clinical trials, navelbine, has yet to be established.

REFERENCES

Abrahamsen AF, Klepp O, Fossa SD, and Sonstevold A Transient vinblastine-induced thrombocytopenia during chemotherapy with vinblastine, cisplatinum and bleomycin. Scand J Haematol 1986 37:44–49.

Ahn Y, Byrnes JJ, Harrington WJ, Cayer ML, Smith DS, Brunskill DE, and Pall LM The treatment of idiopathic thrombocytopenia purpura with vinblastine-loaded platelets. N Engl J Med 1978 298:1101–1107.

Alavi JB, Weiler CB, and Bruno LA Phase II evaluation of vindesine in the treatment of malignant glioma. Cancer Treat Rep 1984 68:807–808.

Allen RD, Weiss DG, Hayden JH, Brown DT, Fujiwake H, and Simpson M Gliding movements of and bidirectional organelle transport along single native microtubules from squid axoplasm: Evidence for an active role of microtubules in cytoplasmic transport. J Cell Biol 1985 100:1736–1752.

Armand JP and Marty M Navelbine: A new step in cancer chemotherapy? Semin Oncol 1989 16:41–45.

Armstrong JG, Dyke RW, Foruts PJ, and Gahimer JE Hodgkin's disease, carcinoma of the breast and other tumors treated with vinblastine sulfate. Cancer Chemother Rep 1962 18:49–71.

Atterwall CK and Walum E Neurotoxicology in vitro: Model systems and practical applications. Toxicol in Vitro 1989 3:159–161.

Barnett CJ, Cullinan GJ, Gerzon K, Hoying RC, Jones WE, Newlon WM, Poore GA, Robison RL, Sweeney MJ, and Todd GC Structure activity relationships of dimeric catharanthus alkaloids. 1. Desacetylvinblastine amide (Vindesine) Sulfate J Med Chem 1978 21:88–96.

Barr RD, Davidson AR, Jung LKL, and Pai KRM Erythrocytotoxicity induced by cancer chemotherapeutic agents. In vitro studies of osmotic fragility and methemoglobin generation. Scand J Haematol 1980 25:363–368.

Bellone JD Treatment of vincristine extravasation JAMA 1981 245–343.

Bender RA and Chabner BA Tubulin binding agents. In: Pharmacologic Principles of Cancer Treatment. Chabner BA Ed. W.B. Saunders Co., Philadelphia 1982 pp. 256–268.

Bender RA, Castle MC, Margileth DA, and Oliverio VT The pharmacokinetics of ($_3$H)-vincristine in man. Clin Pharmacol Ther 1977 22:430–438.

Besenval M, Delgado M, Demarez JP, and Krikorian A Safety and tolerance of navelbine in Phase I-II clinical studies. Semin Oncol 1989 16:37–40.

Bezwoda WR, Derman DP, Weaving A, and Nissenbaum M Treatment of esophageal cancer with vindesine: An open trial. Cancer Treat Rep 1984 68:783–785.

Bleyer A, Frisby SA, and Oliverio VT Uptake and binding of vincristine by leukemia cells. Biochem Pharmacol 1975 24:633–639.

Bloomfield CD, Hurd DD, and Peterson BA Leukemias. In: Medical Oncology. Calabresi P, Schein PS, and Rosenberg SA Eds Macmillan Publishing Co., New York 1985 pp. 523–575.

Bohannon RA, Miller DG, and Diamond HD Vincristine in the treatment of lymphomas and leukemias. Cancer Res 1963 23:613–621.

Bott SJ, Stewart FM, and Prince-Fiocco MA Interstitial lung disease associated with vindesine and radiation therapy for carcinoma of the lung. South Med J 1986 79:894–896.

Bradley WG, Lassman LP, Pearce GW, and Walton JN The neuromyopathy of vincristine in man: Clinical electrophysiological and pathological studies. J Neurol Sci 1970 10:107–131.

Brann M and Hacker M Neurotoxicity of intranigral injections of vincristine, vinblastine and colchine in rats. FASEB Proc 1983 42:1104.

Brady ST Basic properties of fast axonal transport and the role of fast axonal transport in axonal growth. In: Axonal Transport in Neuronal Growth and Regeneration Elam JS Ed Plenum Press, New York 1984 pp. 13–27.

Breza TS, Halprin KM, and Taylor R Photosensitivity reaction to vinblastine. Arch Dermatol 1975 111:1168–1170.

Brook J and Schreiber W Vocal cord paralysis: A toxic reaction to vinblastine (NSC-49842) therapy. Cancer Chemother Rep 1971 55:591–593.

Byrd RI, Rohrbaugh TM, Raney BB Jr, and Norris DG Transient cortical blindness secondary to vincristine therapy in childhood malignancies. Cancer 1981 47:37–42.

Canobbio L, Boccardo F, Pastoino G, Brema F, Martini C, Resasco M, and Santi L Phase II study of navelbine in advanced breast cancer. Semin Oncol 1989 16:33–36.

Carbone PP, Bono V, Frei E, III, and Brindley CO Clinical studies with vincristine. Blood 1963 21:640–645.

Casey EB, Jeliffe AM, LeQuesne PM, and Millett YI Vincristine neuropathy. Brain 1973 96:69–86.

Cassady JR, Tonnesen GL, Wolfe LC, and Sallan SE Augmentation of vincristine neurotoxicity by irradiation of peripheral nerves. Cancer Treat Rep 1980 64:963–965.

Cho ES, Lowndes HE, and Goldstein BD Neurotoxicology of vincristine in the cat. Arch Toxicol 1983 52:83–90.

Choy DSJ Effective treatment of inadvertent intramuscular administration of vincristine. JAMA 1979 241:695.

Creasy WA, Bensche KA, and Malawista SE Colchicine, vinblastine and griseofulvin: Pharmacological studies with human leukocytes. Biochem Pharmacol 1971 20:1579–1588.

Cullinan GJ, Gerzon K, Poore GA, and Todd GC Inhibition of experimental tumor systems by desacetyl vinblastine amide and congeners. In: Proceedings of the Eleventh International Cancer Congress. Casa Edirfrice Ambrosiana, Milan 1974.

Currie VE, Wong PP, Krakoff IH, and Young CW Phase I trial of vindesine in patients with advanced cancer. Cancer Treat Rep 1978 62:1333–1336.

Deconti RC and Creasey WA Clinical aspects of the dimeric Catharanthus alkaloids. In: The Catharanthus Alkaloids, Botany, Chemistry, Pharmacology and Clinical Use. Taylor WI and Farnsworth NR Eds 1975 Dekker, New York pp. 237–278.

Delaney P Vincristine induced laryngeal nerve paralysis. Neurology 1982 32:1285–1288.

Depierre A, Lemarie E, Dabouis G, Garnier G, Jacoulet P, and Dalphin JC Efficacy of navelbine in non-small cell lung cancer. Semin Oncol 1989 26–29.

DeVita VT, Canellos GP, and Moxley JH III A decade of combination chemotherapy of advanced Hodgkin's disease. Cancer 1972 30:1495–1504.

DiConstanza F, Gori S, Tonato M, Buzzi F, Crino L, Grignani F, and Davis S Vindesine and mitomycin c in chemotherapy refractory advanced breast cancer. Cancer 1986 57:904–907.

Dustin P Microtubules. Springer-Verlag, Berlin 1978.

Dustin P Microtubule poisons. In: Microtubules Justin P Ed Springer-Verlag, Berlin 1984 pp. 167–225.

Dyke RW and Nelson RL Phase I anticancer agents. Vindesine (desacetyl vinblastine amide sulfate). Cancer Treat Rev 1977 4:135–142.

Dyke RW, Nelson RL, and Brade WP Vindesine, a short review of preclinical and first clinical data. Cancer Chemother Pharmacol 1979 2:229–232.

Einhorn LH, Loehrer PJ, Williams SD, Meyers S, Gabrys T, Nattan SR, Woodburn R, Drasga R, Songer J, Fisher W, Stephens D, and Hui S Random prospective study of vindesine versus vindesine plus high-dose cisplatin versus vindesine plus cisplatin plus mitomycin c in advanced non-small cell lung cancer. J Clin Oncol 1986 4:1037–1043.

Fellous A, Ohayon R, Vacassin T, Binet S, Lataste H, Krikorian A, Couzinier JP, and Meininger V Biochemical effects of navelbine on tubulin and associated proteins. Semin Oncol 1989 16:9–14.

Frei E, Franzino A, Schnider BI, Costa G, Colsky J, Brinley CO, Hosley H, Holland JF, Gold GL, and Jonsson V Clinical studies of vinblastine. Cancer Chemother Rep 1961 12:125–129.

Ferguson PJ, Phillips JR, Selner M, and Cass CE Differential activity of vincristine and vinblastine against cultured cells. Cancer Res 1984 44:3307–3312.

Gaidys WG, Dickerman JD, Walters CL, and Young PC Intrathecal vincristine. Report of a fatal case despite CNS washout. Cancer 1983 52:799–801.

Garewal HS and Dalton WS Metoclopramide in vincristine induced ileus. Cancer Treat Rep 1985 69:1309–1311.

George MJ, Heron JF, Kerbrat P, Chauverge J, Goupli A, Lebrun D, Guastalla JP, Namer M, Bugat R, Ayme Y, Toussaint C, and Lhomme C Navelbine in advanced ovarian epithelial cancer: A study of the French oncology centers. Semin Oncol 1989 16:30–32.

Ginsberg SJ, Comis RL, and Fitzpatrick AV Vinblastine and inappropriate ADH secretion. N Engl J Med 1977 296:941.

Goldstein BD, Lowndes HE, and Cho ES Neurotoxicology of vincristine in the rat. Electrophysiological studies. Arch Toxicol 1981 48:253–264.

Gottlieb RJ and Cuttner J Vincristine induced bladder atony. Cancer 1971 28:674–679.

Gottschalk PG, Dyck PJ, and Kiely JM Vinca alkaloid neuropathy: Nerve biopsy studies in rats and in man. Neurology 1968 18:875–882.

Gout PW, Noble RL, Bruchovsky N, and Beer CT Vinblastine and vincristine-growth inhibitory effects correlate with their retention by cultured Nb2 lymphoma cells. Int J Cancer 1984 34:245–248.

Gralla RJ, Casper ES, and Kelsen DP Cisplatinum and vindesine combination chemotherapy for advanced carcinoma of the lung: A randomized trial investigating two dosage schedules. Ann Intern Med 1980 95:414–420.

Grau JJ, Grau M, Milla A, Estape J, and Mulet M Cancer chemotherapy and Raynaud's phenomenon. Ann Int Med 1983 98:258.

Green LS, Donoso JA, Heller-Bettinger IE, and Samson Axonal transport disturbances in vincristine-induced peripheral neuropathy. Ann Neurol 1977 255–262.

Griffiths JD, Stark RJ, Ding JC, and Cooper IA Vincristine neurotoxicity in Charcot-Marie-Tooth syndrome. Med J Australia 1985 143:305–306.

Guiheneuc P, Ginet J, Groleau JY, and Rojouan J Early phase of vincristine neuropathy in man. J Neurolog Sci 1980 45:355–366.

Hamel E and Lin CM Glutamate-induced polymerization of tubulin: Characteristics of the reaction and application to the large-scale purification of tubulin. Arch Biochem Biophys 1981 209:29–40.

Hancock BW and Naysmith A Vincristine induced autonomic neuropathy. Brit Med J 1975 3:207–210.

Harvey HA, Lipton A, and Lawrence BV Raynaud's phenomenon with vinblastine and bleomycin. Ann Int Med 1981 94:542–543.

Hertz R, Lipsett MB, and Moy RH Effect of vincaleukoblastine on metastatic choriocarcinoma and related trophoblastic tumors in women. Cancer Res 1960 20:1050–1053.

Himes RH, Kersey RN, Heller-Bettinger IE, and Samson FE The action of vinca alkaloids, vincristine, vinblastine and desacetyl vinblastine amide on microtubules in vitro. Cancer Res 1976 36:3798–3802.

Holland JF, Scharlane C, Gailani S, Krant MJ, Olson KB, Horton J, Shnider BI, Lynch JJ, Owens A, Carbone PP, Colsky J, Grob D, Miller SP, and Hall TC. Vincristine treatment of advanced cancer: A cooperative study of 392 cases. Cancer Res 1973 33:1258–1264.

Hurwitz RL, Mahoney DH, Armstrong DL, and Browder TM Reversible encephalopathy and seizures as a result of conventional vincristine administration. Med Pediatr Oncol 1988 16:216–219.

Hwang YF, Hamilton HE, and Sheets RF Vinblastine-induced thrombocytosis. Lancet 1969 2:1075–1076.

Ishii E, Hara T, Mizuno Y, and Veda K Vincristine-induced fever in children with leukemia and lymphoma. Cancer 1988 61:660–662.

Isreal RH and Olson JP Pulmonary edema associated with intravenous vinblastine. JAMA 1978 240:1585.

Jackson DV Jr, Rosenbaum DL, Carlisle LH, Long TR, Wells HB, and Spurr CL Glutamic acid modification of vincristine toxicity. Cancer Biochem Biophys 1984 7:245–252.

Jackson DV, Wells HB, Atkins JN, Zekan PJ, White DR, Richards F 2nd, Cruz JM and Muss HB Amelioration of vincistine neurotoxicity by glutamic acid. Am J Med 1988 84:1016–1022.

Jewkes J, Harper PG, Tobias JS, Geddes DM, Souhami RL, and Spiro SG Comparison of vincristine and vindesine in the treatment of inoperable non-small cell bronchial carcinoma. Cancer Treat Rep 1983 67:1119–1121.

Johnson FL, Bernstein ID, and Hartman JR Seizures associated with vincristine sulfate therapy. J Pediatr 1973 82:699–702.

Johnson IS Plant alkaloids. In: Cancer Medicine Holland JF and Frei E III Eds Lea and Febriger, Philadelphia 1973 pp. 840–850.

Johnson IS, Armstrong JG, Gorman M, and Burnett JP Jr The vinca alkaloids: A new class of oncolytic agents. Cancer Res 1963 23:1390–1427.

Journey GP and Goldstein MN Effect of vincristine on the fine structure of HeLa cells in mitosis. JNCI 1965 35:355–375.

Kaufman, IA, Kung FH, Koenig HM, and Giammona ST Overdoseage with vincristine. J Pediatr 1976 89:671–674.

Kaplan RS and Wiernik PH Neurotoxicity of antineoplastic drugs. Semin Oncol 1982 9:103–130.

Konitis PH, Aisner J, Sutherland JC, and Wiernik PH Possible pulmonary toxicity secondary to vinblastine. Cancer 1982 50:2771–2774.

Luce JK, Gamble JF, Wilson HE, Monto RW, Isaacs BL, Palmer RL, Coltman CA, Hewlett JS, Gehan EA, and Frei E Combined cyclophosphamide, vincristine, and prednisone therapy of malignant lymphoma. Cancer 1971 28:306–317.

Lucas VS and Huang AT Vinblastine-related pain in tumors. Cancer Treat Rep 1977 61:1735–1736.

Ludwig R, Alberts DS, Miller TP and Salmon SE Evaluation of anticancer drug schedule dependency using an in vitro human tumor clonogenic assay. Cancer Chemother Pharmacol 1984 12:135–141.

Malawista SE, Sato H, and Bensch K Vinblastine and griesofulvin reversibly disrupt the living mitotic spindle. Science 1968 160:770–772.

Mandel EM, Lewinski U, and Djaldetti M Vincristine induced myocardial infarction. Cancer 1975 36:1979–1982.

Mantel N Raynaud's phenomenon and cryoglobulinemia during chemotherapy for testicular carcinoma. Cancer Treat Rep 1982 67:317–318.

Maral P, Bourut C, and Chenue E Experimental antitumor activity of 5'-nor-anhydrovinblastine, navelbine. Cancer Lett 1984 22:49–54.

Margileth DA, Poplack DG, Pizzo PA, and Leventhal BG Blindness during remission in two patients with acute lymphoblastic leukemia: A possible complication with multi-modality therapy. Cancer 1977 39:58–62.

Margolis RL and Wilson L Microtubule treadmills—possible molecular machinery. Nature 1981 293:705–711.

Marmont AM and Damasio EE Clinical experiences with cytotoxic immunosuppressive treatment of idiopathic thrombocytopenia purpura. Acta Haemtol 1971 46:74–80.

Marmont AM, Damasio EE, and Gori E Vinblastine sulfate in idiopathic thrombocytopenia purpura. Lancet 1971 2:94

Mathe G and Reizenstein P Phase I pharmacologic study of a new vinca alkaloid: Navelbine. Cancer Lett 1985 27:285–293.

McLendon BF and Bron AJ Corneal toxicity from vinblastine. Brit J Ophthalmol 1978 62:97–99.

McLeod JG and Penny R Vincristine neuropathy: An electrophysiological and histological study. J Neurol Neurosurg Psychiatry 1969 32:297–304.

Mitchison T and Kirschner M Dynamic instability of microtubule growth. Nature 1984 312:237–242.

Mosci L Astigmatisom contro regola in un caso di causticazione corneale da vincoblastina. Annali de Ottalmologia e Clinica Oculistica 1967 93:94–100.

Neville AJ, Rand CA, and Barr RD Vinblastine-induced erythrocytotoxicity. Scand J Haematol 1982 28:32–38.

Noble RL, Beer CT, and Cutts JH Further biological activities of vincaleukoblastine—an alkaloid isolated from Vinca rosea (L). Biochem Pharmacol 1958 1:347–348.

Nordino F, Finesso M, Fiorto C, Favaro G, Fusco M, Tessari F, and Prosdocimi M General toxicity and peripheral nerve alterations induced by chronic vincristine treatment in the rabbit. Toxicol Appl Pharmacol 1988 93:433–441.

Norman M, Elinder G, and Finkel Y Vincristine neuropathy and Guillain-Barre syndrome: A case with acute lymphatic leukemia and quadriparesis. Eur J Haematol 1987 39:75–76.

Norton SW and Stockman JA Unilateral optic neuropathy following vincristine chemotherapy. J Pediat Ophthalmol Strabismus 1979 16:190–195.

Ochs S and Worth R Comparison of the block of fast axoplasmic transport in mammalian nerve by vincristine, vinblastine, and desacetyl vinblastine amide sulfate (DVA). Proc Am Assoc Cancer Res 1975 16:70.

Paulson JC and McClure WO Inhibition of axoplasmic transport by colchicine, podophyllotoxin and vinblastine: An effect on microtubules. Ann NY Acad Sci 1975 253:517–527.

Pedrazzini A, Cavalli F, Kiser J, and Goldhirsch A Early onset thrombocytopenia in the chemotherapy of testicular teratoma. Eur J Cancer Clin Oncol 1983 19:867.

Postmus PE, Mulder NH, Schipper DL, and de Vries EGE Twice weekly vindesine, a phase II study in lung cancer. J Cancer Res Clin Oncol 1987 113:99–100.

Raphelson MI, Stevens JC, and Newman RP Vincristine neuropathy with bowel and bladder atony, mimicking spinal cord compression (letter). Cancer Treat Rep 1983 67:604–605.

Ratain MJ and Vogezang NJ Phase I and pharmacological study of vinblastine by prolonged continuous infusion. Cancer Res 1986 46:4827–4830.

Ravikumar TS and Grage TB The syndrome of inappropriate ADH secretion secondary to vinblastine-bleomycin therapy. J Surg Oncol 1983 24:242–245.

Rees GJ, Slade RR, and Hopes P Reduced platelet survival following chemotherapy with vinblastine, bleomycin and cisplatinum for testicular teratoma. Eur J Cancer Clin Oncol 1982 18:1125–1129.

Reiquam CW and Prosper JC Chronic idiopathic thrombocytopenia; treatment with prednisone, 6-mercaptopurine, vincristine and fresh plasma transfusion. J Pediatr 1966 68:885–891.

Robertson GL, Bhoopalam N, and Zelkowitz IJ Vincristine neurotoxicity and abnormal secretion of ADH. Arch Int Med 1973 132:717–720.

Robertson JH and McCarthy GM Periwinkle alkaloids and the platelet-count. Lancet 1969 2:353–355.

Rosenberg RF and Caridi JG Vincristine induced megacolon. Gastrointest Radiol 1983 8:71–73.

Rosenthal RC Clinical applications of VINCA alkaloids. J Amer Vet Med Assoc 1981 179:1084–1086.

Rosenthal S and Kaufman S Vincristine neuropathy. Ann Intern Med 1974 80:733–737.

Rothberg H Raynaud's phenomenon after vinblastine-bleomycin chemotherapy. Cancer Treat Rep 1978 62:569–570.

Rhomberg WU Vindesine for recurrent and metastaic cancer of the uterine cervix: A phase II study. Cancer Treat Rep 1986 70:1455–1457.

Ripps H, Carr RE, Siegel IM, and Greenstein VC Functional abnormalities in vincristine induced night blindness. Invest Ophthalmol Vis Sci 1984 25:787–794.

Ryan JR and Emami A Vincristine neurotoxicity with residual equincavus deformity in children with acute leukemia. Cancer 1983 51:423–425.

Sahenk Z, Brady ST, and Mendell JR Studies on the pathogenesis of vincristine-induced neuropathy. Muscle & Nerve 1987 10:80–84.

Samuels ML and Howe CD Vinblastine in the management of testicular cancer. Cancer 1970 25:1009–1017.

Sanderson PA, Kuwabara T, and Cogan DG Optic neuropathy presumably caused by vincristine therapy. Am J Ophthalmol 1976 81:146–151.

Sandler SG, Tobin W, and Henderson ES Vincristine-induced neuropathy. Neurology (Minneapolis) 1969 19:367–374.

Scheulen ME and Schmidt CG Raynaud's phenomenon and cancer chemotherapy. Ann Int Med 1982 96:256.

Schochet SS, Lampert PW and Earle KM Neuronal changes induced by intrathecal vincristine sulfate. J Neuropathol Exp Neurol 1968 27:645–658.

Shulman NR, Marder VJ, and Weinrach RS Similarities between known antiplatelet antibodies and the factor responsible for thrombocytopenia in idiopathic thrombocytopenia purpura: Physiologic, serologic and isotopic studies. Ann NY Acad Sci 1965 124:499–542.

Shurin SB, Rekate HL, and Annable W Optic atrophy induced by vincristine. Pediatrics 1982 70:288–291.

Slyter H, Liwnicz B, Herrick MK, and Mason R Fatal myeloencephalopathy caused by intrathecal vincristine. Neurology 1980 30:867–871.

Smith DS, Jorlfors U, and Cameron BF Morphological evidence for the participation of microtubules in axoplasmic transport. Ann NY Acad Sci 1975 253:472–506.

Somers G, Abramow M, Witter M, and Naets JP Myocardial infarction: A complication of vincristine treatment? Lancet 1976 2:690.

Stark Db and Fletcher WS Severe tumor pain with intravenous injection of vinblastine sulfate (NSC 49842). Cancer Chemother Rep 1966 50:281–282.

Stein RS and Roth DG Myelotoxicity of vincristine-prednisone therapy in treatment of chronic myelogenous leukemia in blastic transformation. Amer J Hematol 1976 1:387–391.

Stein RS, Moran EM, Desser RK, Miller JB, Golomb HM, and Ultmann JE Combination chemotherapy of lymphomas other than Hodgkin's disease. Ann Int Med 1974 76:1258–1264.

Subar M and Muggia FM Apparent myocardial ischemia associated with vinblastine administration. Cancer Treat Rep 1986 70:690–691.

Sultan Y, Delobel J, Jeanneau C, and Caen JP Effect of periwinkle alkaloids in idiopathic thrombocytopenia purpura. Lancet 1971 1:496–497.

Sumner AJ Physiology of dying back neuropathies. In: Physiology and Pathobiology of Axons Waxman SG Ed Raven Press, New York 1978 pp. 349–359.

Sweeney MJ, Boder GB, Cullinan GJ, Culp HW, Daniels WD, Dyke RW, Gerzon K, McMahon RE, Nelson RL, Poore GA, and Todd GC Antitumor activity of deacetyl vinblastine amide sulfate (vindesine) in rodents and mitotic accumulation studies in culture. Cancer Res 1978 38:2886–2891.

Tan CTC and Aduna NS Preliminary clinical experience with leurocristine in children. Proc Amer Assoc Cancer Res 1961 3:367.

Teutsch C, Lipton A, and Harvey HA Raynaud's phenomenon as a side effect of chemotherapy with vinblastine and bleomycin for testicular carcinoma. Cancer Treat Rep 1977 61:925–926.

Thant M, Hawley RJ, and Smith MT Possible enhancement of vincristine neurotoxicity by VP-16. Cancer 1982 49:859–864.

Todd GC, Gibson WR, and Morton DM Toxicology of vindesine (desacetyl vinblastine amide) in mice rats and dogs. J Toxicol Environ Health 1976 1:843–849.

Todd GC, Griffing WJ, Gibson WR, and Morton DM Animal models for the comparative assessment of neurotoxicity following repeated administration of vinca alkaloids. Cancer Treat Rep 1979 63:35–41.

Tomiwa K, Mikawa H, Hazama F, Yazawa K, Hosoya R, Ohya T, and Nishimura K Syndrome of inappropriate secretion of antidiuretic hormone caused by vincristine therapy: A case report of neuropathology. J Neurol 1983 229:267–272.

Vogelzang NJ, Bosl, GJ, Johnson K, and Kennedy BJ Raynaud's phenomenon: A common toxicity after combination chemotherapy for testicular cancer. Ann Int Med 1981 95:288–292.

Vogl SE, Camacho FJ, Kaplan BH, and O'Donnell MR Phase II trial of vindesine in advanced squamous cell cancer of the head and neck. Cancer Treat Rep 1984 68:559–560.

Warwick OH, Alison RE, and Darte JMM Clinical experience with vinblastine sulfate. Canad Med Assoc J 1961 85:579–583.

Weiss HD, Walker MD, and Weirnik PH Neurotoxicity of commonly used antineoplastic agents. N Engl J Med 1974 291:127–133.

Wheeler JS, Siroky MB, Bell R, and Babayan RK J Urol 1983 130:342–343.

Whittaker JA and Griffith IP Recurrent laryngeal nerve paralysis in patients receiving vincristine and vinblastine. Brit Med J 1977 1:1251–1252.

Williams ME, Walker AN, Bracikowski JP, Garner L, Wilson KD, and Carpenter JT Ascending myeloencephalopathy due to intrathecal vincristine sulfate. A chemotherapeutic error. Cancer 1983 51:2041–2047.

Winter SC and Arbus GS Syndrome of inappropriate secretion of antiduiretic hormone secondary to vinblastine overdose (letter). Can Med Assoc J 1977 117:1134.

Yap HY, Blumenschein GR, Keating MJ, Hortobagyi GN, Tashima CK, and Loo TL Vinblastine given as a continuous 5-day infusion in the treatment of refractory advanced breast cancer. Cancer Treat Rep 1980 64:279–283.

Yancey RS and Talpaz M Vindesine-associated angina and ECG changes. Cancer Treat Reports 1982 66:587–589.

Young DF and Ponsner JB Nervous toxicity of the chemotherapeutic agents. In: Handbook of Clinical Neurology Vinken PJ and Bruyn GW Eds vol. 39 Elsevier, Amsterdam 1980 pp. 91–129. Biochem Pharmacol 1958 1:347–348.

CHAPTER 9

Immunologic Effects of Cancer Chemotherapy

Larry D. Grant, M.D., Paul R. Kaesberg, M.D., and William B. Ershler, M.D.

ABBREVIATIONS

ADCC	Antibody-dependent cellular cytotoxicity
ALL	acute lympocytic leukemia
ara-C	cytosine arabinoside
AZA	azathioprine
CDDP	cisplatin
Con A	concanavalin A
CTL	cytotoxic T lymphocyte
CY	cyclophosphamide
DOX	doxorubicin
DNR	daunorubicin
5-FU	5-fluorouracil
4-HC	4-hydroperoxycyclophosphamide
IgA, IgG, IgM	immunoglobulin A, G, M
IFN	interferon
IL-1, IL-2	interleukin-1, interleukin-2
LPS	lipopolysaccharide
6MP	6-mercaptopurine
MTX	methotrexate
NK	natural killer
PBL	peripheral blood lymphocyte
PG	prostaglandin
PHA	phytohemagglutinin
PWM	pokeweed mitogen
VCR	vincristine
VLB	vinblastine

INTRODUCTION

Immunotoxicity and myelotoxicity were the early findings associated with World War I mustard gas poisoning that led to the development of modern antineoplastic chemotherapy. In 1919, Krumbhaar observed that poisoning with sulfur mustard was characterized by leukopenia, bone marrow aplasia, dissolution of lymphoid tissue, and ulceration of the gastrointes-

Supported by V.A. Merit Award and PHS Award R01A6007831.

tinal (GI) tract. Bronchopneumonia in these poisoned soldiers was characterized by the absence of a leukocytic response (Krumbhaar, 1919; Calabresi and Parks, 1985). Subsequent to WWI, studies on the biological actions of the nitrogen mustards revealed that the susceptible tissues were those with rapid regenerative capacity, such as lymphoid tissue, bone marrow, and the epithelium of the GI tract (Gilman, 1963). These findings prompted the experimental treatment of lymphosarcoma in mice with nitrogen mustard and ultimately to the initial human trials in 1942 in patients with lymphoproliferative disorders (Calabresi and Parks, 1985; Gilman, 1963). Early in the studies of antineoplastic agents, their ability to reduce antibody formation by humoral immune suppression was also noted. For example, 6-mercaptopurine (6MP) inhibited specific antibody formation in rabbits immunized with human serum albumin was demonstrated by Schwartz (Schwartz and Dameshek, 1959). It is difficult to separate the antineoplastic activity of these agents from their side effects, because in most cases the mechanism by which an agent exerts its antineoplastic effect is also the mechanism of its undesired immunologic, hematologic, dermatologic, and gastrointestinal toxicities.

Myelosuppression and immunosuppression are common consequences of antineoplastic chemotherapy, and often times the antecedent of infection, (Table 9-1) (Wade and Schimpff, 1988; Wands et al., 1975; Levine et al., 1974). Immunotoxicity is a desired effect of cytotoxic therapy when used in certain lymphoproliferative disorders, organ and bone marrow transplants, and a variety of medical disorders with known immunologic components outlined in Table 9-2 (Perry and Yarbo, 1984). Nevertheless, when the antineoplastic effects are the desired end, immunosuppression is considered a therapy-related complication. Although there is some overlap, it is possible to define the differences between the myelosuppressive and immunosuppressive effects of those agents based upon the types of infections observed. The myelosuppressed patient characteristically develops bacterial infections, whereas the immunocompromised patient develops opportunistic fungal or protozoal infections, or unusually widespread or severe viral infections. These differences, however, may be less apparent in patients who are both immuno- and myelosuppressed by chemotherapy compared to patients with more clearly defined immunosuppression (e.g., acquired immunodeficiency syndrome) or myelosuppression (aplastic anemia).

Complicating our understanding of the immunosuppressive effects of the antineoplastic agents are the complex immunologic impairments that are constitutive features of the diseases in patients with solid tumors, lymphoproliferative, and myeloproliferative disorders. Therefore, the immunotoxicity of chemotherapeutic agents is expressed upon a background of variably impaired immunocompetence. These impairments have been reviewed extensively (Table 9-3) (Bast, 1982; Karavodin and Golub, 1983; Ehrke and Mihich, 1985).

Much of the research concerning the effects of chemotherapy agents upon the immune system has focused upon immunosuppression. However, work in the past decade has also emphasized the immunopotentiating aspects of the various agents.

This review will focus upon the immunomodulatory effects of commonly used chemotherapy agents and also describe the known hypersensitivity reactions seen with these agents. Human data will be emphasized with contributory animal and in vitro data mentioned where

Table 9-1. Infections Seen Commonly in Myelosuppressed or Immunosuppressed Patients

Immunosuppression
Viral – Varicella-Zoster, Cytomegalovirus, Herpes Simplex, reactivated Hepatitis B, Adenovirus, Epstein-Barr virus
Fungal – Cryptococcus, reactivated *Histoplasma capsulatum, Coccidioides immitis*
Protozoa – *Pneumocystis carinii, Toxoplasma gondii*, Cryptosporidium
Bacterial – *Listeria monocytogenes*, Salmonella, *Nocardia asteroides*, Mycobacteria, Legionella
Myelosuppression (bacterial)
Gram negative – *Escherichia coli, Klebsiella pneumoniae, Pseudomona aeruginosa*
Gram positive – *Staphylococcus aureus*

Table 9-2. Agents Used in the Treatment of Non-Malignant Disease Excluding Corticosteriods, Cyclosporin (Perry and Yarbo, 1984)

DISEASE/CONDITION	TREATMENT
Transplant	
Kidney	azathioprine, actinomycin D
Liver	azathioprine, actinomycin D
Bone marrow	cyclophosphamide
Autoimmune disease	
Rheumatoid arthritis	azathioprine, cyclophosphamide
Lupus	cyclophosphamide
Diabetes	methotrexate
AIHA	azathioprine
Glomerulonephritis	azathioprine, cyclophosphamide
ITP	vincristine
Goodpasture's Synd.	azathioprine
UC, Crohn's Disease	azathioprine
CAH	azathioprine
Pemphigus	azathioprine
Wegener's Granulomatosis	methotrexate, azathioprine, cyclophos-pham
Myeloproliferative disorders	
P. Vera	busulfan, chlorambucil, hydroxyurea
Essential thrombocythemia	busulfan
Agnogenic myeloid metaplasia	busulfan
Miscellaneous	
Hypercalcemia	mithramycin
Paget's disease	mithramycin
Psoriasis	methotrexate, hydroxyurea
Pleural effusion	nitrogen mustard, bleomycin

human data is lacking. Within a class of chemotherapeutic drugs, the immunomodulatory properties of a single prototype agent will be considered in depth. When other agents within a class have differing properties, these will be noted.

ALKYLATING AGENTS: CYCLOPHOSPHAMIDE

Introduction

Alkylating agents were the first immunosuppressive agents investigated. Hektoen and Corper (1921) demonstrated suppression of antibody formation against sheep red blood cells in nitrogen mustard-treated rabbits. We will discuss cyclophosphamide (CY), since it is the most extensively studied drug in this class, though the majority of data is from in vitro animal

Table 9-3. Immunologic Impairments Characteristic of Different Malignancies

B cell defects
1) Chronic lymphocytic leukemia
2) Multiple myeloma
3) Hodgkin's lymphoma

T cell defects
1) Hodgkin's lymphoma
2) Disseminated carcinomas
3) Kaposi's sarcoma/HIV

Granulocyte defects
1) Acute lymphoblastic leukemia
2) Acute myeloid leukemia
3) Chronic myeloid leukemia
4) Multiple myeloma

Monocyte defects
1) Carcinomas/sarcomas
2) Hodgkin's lymphoma

models. In vitro investigation of the cellular basis of immunoregulation by CY has been aided by the synthesis of 4-hydroperoxycyclophosphamide (4-HC), an analog that does not require in vivo activation. The cytotoxic activity and DNA cross-linking activity of 4-HC is equivalent to CY and in vitro 4-HC has been shown to mimic the immunomodulatory effects of CY in vivo (Shand and Howard, 1979; Diamenstein et al., 1979, 1981; Kaufman et al., 1980). It is widely accepted that CY can exert either immunosuppressive effects by damage or death of B cells, helper cells, or natural killer or immunopotentiating effects, through damaging or killing of suppressor T lymphocytes (Maguire and Ettore, 1967; Turk and Parker, 1982). High doses of CY are immunosuppressive, whereas lower doses frequently are immunopotentiating.

It is believed that CY is the most immunosuppressive of the alkylating agents in humans (Santos, 1967; Bast, 1982). However, in spite of its high immunosuppressive activity, CT has a more favorable therapeutic ratio with regard to humoral suppression than other therapy modalities, such as antimetabolites, glucocorticoids, vinca alkaloids, or radiation (Spreafico and Ancelerio, 1977).

Effects on B Cells, Humoral Immunity

In animal models CY has been shown to inhibit antibody responses when given before, during, or after antigen administration. Primary antibody responses are inhibited to a greater extent than secondary responses (Spreafico and Ancelerio, 1977). Primary antibody responses to bacterial antigens have been shown to be totally suppressed during high-dose CY treatment (3.5–7 mg/kg/d) in humans (Santos, 1970). Histopathologic studies in CY-treated animals (mice, guinea pigs) have revealed a marked reduction of B cells and depletion in lymph node follicles, medullary cords, germinal centers, and corticomedullary junctions, but a preservation of the paracortical regions (Turk and Poulter, 1972a; Turk et al., 1972b). Serum immunoglobulin levels (IgG, IgM, IgA) are reduced in patients receiving chronic low-dose CY with the greatest reduction in IgM (Fauci et al., 1971; Alepa and Zvaiffler-Sliwinski, 1979). Similarly, long-term low-dose therapy with CY (2 mg/kg/d) was found to profoundly inhibit pokeweed mitogen (PWM)-induced immunoglobulin production by human peripheral blood lymphocytes (PBL) without suppressing the proliferative response to PWM, phytohemagglutinin (PHA), or concanavalin A (Con A) (Cupps, 1982). A subsequent study revealed that in addition to suppression of activation and proliferation, the differentiation phase of B-cell maturation was suppressed by chronic low-dose CY therapy (Zhu et al., 1987). In that study, the B-cell functional parameters returned to normal within one year following CY therapy. Of interest, a single low dose of CY (300 mg/m^2) given to cancer patients was shown to potentiate the primary antibody response to keyhole limpet hemocyanin, but this effect was not seen in a study at a higher dose (1 g/m^2) (Berd et al., 1982; 1984b). Augmented antibody responses have also been seen in animal systems (Berd et al., 1983).

Cell-Mediated Immunity

Low-dose or high-dose CY therapy results in lymphopenia in humans without selective depletion of any particular lymphocyte subset (Cupps et al., 1982; Berd et al., 1984a, Berd and Mastrangelo, 1987). The in vitro generation of Con A-inducible suppressor T cells in cancer patients receiving either low-dose (300 mg/m^2) or high-dose (1 g/m^2) CY therapy has been shown to be significantly impaired (Berd, 1984a). There was no effect of CY upon PHA mitogen responses in these same patients. Precursors to human Con A induced suppressor cells have been shown to be sensitive to pretreatment in vitro with very low concentrations of 4-HC (Ozer et al., 1982). In vitro studies on human mixed lymphocyte responses also show that the differentiation of suppressor precursors into mature suppressor cells is inhibited by low doses of 4-HC (Smith et al., 1987). Mature cytotoxic or suppressor cells are very resistant to high concentrations of 4-HC (Smith et al., 1987). Note that the most susceptible human lymphocyte to 4-HC killing is the Con A-induced suppressor T cell (Ozer et al., 1982; Ozer, 1985). These 4-HC sensitive suppressor cells appear to have a T4+, T8− phenotype, which raises the possibility that the primary target of low-dose CY therapy may be a T4+ inducer cell for the typical T8+ suppressor/killer cells. This is in concordance with recent work that demonstrates that secondary mixed lymphocyte responses are nonspecifically suppressed to a lesser degree than primary mixed lymphocyte responses and that resistance to the suppression appears to be at the level of the helper inducer cell (Goekin, 1982).

Potentiation of delayed-type hypersensitivity by CY in animal systems is well established, with the critical factor being the timing of CY administration. Maximum potentiation occurs when CY is administered from three days before to one day after antigen administration. If CY is administered later (i.e., 3–5 days postantigen), the delayed type hypersensitivity response will be suppressed, since this is the time of maximal proliferation of lymphocytes (Turk and Parker, 1982; Turk, 1987). Augmentation of primary delayed-type hypersensitivity responses has been observed in humans by pretreatment with either low or high doses of CY (Berd et al., 1982, 1984b). Immunologic tolerance to specific antigens can be reversed by CY or 4-HC treatment (Polak and Turk, 1974; Polak et al., 1975; Boerrigter and Scheper, 1984). The ability of CY to break established immune tolerance and even facilitate the rejection of autologous tissue (Yoshida et al., 1979) is of great relevance to cancer immunotherapy. The hypothesis that tumor-bearing hosts initially develop immunity to their tumors but later become "tolerant" of tumor antigens has been demonstrated in a number of experimental systems (Broder and Waldmann, 1978). Thus, it is possible that CY may mediate some of its antineoplastic effect by interruption of established immunologic tolerance of existing tumor, the mechanism being selective inhibition of suppressor T-cell function.

4-HC treatment in vitro has been shown to increase natural killer (NK) function in samples from normal volunteers and increase cytotoxity against autologous leukemia cells in lymphocytes from children with acute lymphocytic leukemia (ALL) in remission (Sharma and Vaziri, 1984).

Hypersensitivity Reactions

CY rarely incite type I anaphylactic reactions (Table 9-4) (Weiss and Baker, 1987; Kim et al., 1985). Reactions have occurred with both oral and intravenous administration of the drug. With rare exception, most cases have occurred after weeks to years of CY therapy and frequently in patients with previous sensitivity to other alkylating agents (Weiss, 1984). Some investigators have demonstrated both skin reactivity and IgE antibody in patients that have

Table 9-4. Types of Hypersensitivity Reactions (Gell and Coobs, 1975)

TYPE	MAJOR SIGNS AND SYMPTOMS	MECHANISM
I	Bronochospasm, rash, angioedema, urticaria, abdominal cramping hypotension	Immunoglobolin E mediated mast cell degranulation
		Neurogenic release of vasoactive substances
		Activation of classic or alternate complement pathways, producing anaphylatoxins
		Drug binding to mast cell surface, causing degranulation
II	Hemolytic anemia	Complement-fixing antibody binds to cellular antigen
III	Deposition of immune complexes in tissues, leading to tissue injury	Antigen–antibody complexes form within the vascular system and deposit in various tissues
IV	Contact dermatitis, granuloma formation, graft rejection	Sensitized T cells react to antigen, proliferate and release lymphokines

reacted to CY (Lakin and Cahill, 1976). The latter finding is consistent with the finding that CY can stimulate IgE synthesis in animals (Weiss, 1984).

Antitumor Immunotherapy With Cyclophosphamide

Recent work in mice (Greenberg et al., 1981) and in humans (Kohler et al., 1985) has demonstrated tumor regression when CY is used as an immunopotentiating agent in conjunction with administration of stimulated lymphocytes. Work with antitumor vaccines carefully timed with CY administration have also shown some clinical responses against melanoma and renal cell carcinoma (Berd and Mastrangelo, 1987; Sahasrabudhe et al., 1986). These preliminary trials indicate that drugs in this class may eventually be selected because of their immunomodulatory action.

Summary

CY and its derivatives are unique in their inhibitory effects upon T-suppressor cell generation. Agents of other classes, including doxorubicin (DOX), vincristine (VCR), vinblastine (VLB), cytosine arabinoside (ara-C), and 5-fluorouracil (5-EU) have no effect upon the induction of the Con A suppressor cell (Ozer, 1985). Initial research focused upon the immunosuppressive effects and only in the last decade have many of the immunopotentiating effects been realized. Therefore, further research into the immunoregulatory effects of CY may ultimately lead to our characterization of this agent as a biologic response modifier as well as a direct cytotoxic agent.

CORTICOSTEROIDS

Introduction

Corticosteroids are of major importance in the therapy of allograft rejection and numerous autoimmune, allergic, and neoplastic diseases. However, despite extensive research efforts, the exact mechanisms by which corticosteroids mediate their effects are unclear (Cupps and Fauci, 1982; Behrens and Goodwin, 1988).

Animal studies have contributed greatly to our understanding of corticosteriods; however, such studies must be viewed with caution. Most importantly, there is a marked heterogeneity among species in sensitivity to corticosteroids. For example, the mouse, rat, hamster, and rabbit are considered "corticosteroid sensitive" whereas the guinea pig, ferret, monkey, and human are "corticosteroid resistant." In the corticosteroid-sensitive species, there is a marked lympholytic response to corticosteroid treatment with shrinkage of the thymus, spleen, and peripheral lymph nodes, and lymphopenia. In the corticosteroid-resistant species these effects are seen to a lesser degree or not at all (Claman, 1972). Even accounting for these species differences, one needs to use caution when interpreting early in vitro studies because often suprapharmacologic doses of corticosteroids were used (Cupps, 1982).

Mechanism of Action

Corticosteroids, like other steroid hormones, are believed to act primarily by activating specific gene transcription. Corticosteroids cross the plasma membrane and interact with a cytoplasmic receptor. The activated complex translocates to the nucleus where it signals the transcription of specific genes, the products of which are specific proteins important in cellular action (Schmidt and Hitwack, 1982; O'Malley, 1984). Corticosteroids induce the synthesis of a family of phospholipase inhibitory proteins, the lipocortins, which include inhibitory proteins for phospholipase A_2, phospholipase C, and phosphatidylinositol phospholipase C. Other mechanisms may exist, since some of the corticosteroids effects appear earlier than expected if they require protein synthesis for expression (Johnson et al., 1982). These may be attributed to nonenzymatic formation of adducts between corticosteroids and phospholipases (Hirata, 1984; Hirata et al., 1987). Inhibition of phospholipase A_2 results in a block in the breakdown of arachidonic acid, eliminating production of the substrate for the cyclooxygenase and lipooxygenase pathways.

A block in the production of these mediators of inflammation synthesized by these pathways may explain the antiinflammatory effects of corticosteroids; however, it does not explain the immunosuppressive effects. There are two mechanisms by which corticosteroids induce cellular immunosuppression. The first is by corticosteroid-mediated inhibition of production of various lymphokines (Table 9-5) (Guyre et al., 1988). Corticosteroids are less effective in inhibiting lymphokine production if administered after the initiation of a response than if given prior to antigen challenge. Corticosteroids do not inhibit the actions of cytokines (Beutler et al., 1986). Additionally, there is a frequently observed "lympholytic" effect of corticosteroids. Although most human T cells are resistant to the cytolytic effects of corticosteroids, there is a subpopulation of activated T cells which is sensitive, even at physiologic levels (Galili et al., 1980). There is a two- to threefold increase in the number of corticosteroid receptors in mitogen-stimulated lymphocytes in S and post-S phases of the cell cycle (Crabtree et al., 1980). However, despite numerous attempts, there has been no demonstrated relationship between corticosteroid receptor density or affinity and sensitivity to corticosteroids (Lippman et al., 1973; 1974; Lippman and Barr, 1977). This cytolytic response appears to be delayed in humans when compared to rodent systems (Munck and Crabtree, 1981). Corticosteroid-induced lymphocytotoxicity is mediated by two events: inhibition of proliferation and cytolysis (Wielckens et al., 1987). The reversible block in proliferation is "permissive" for cell death. Lymphoma cells are not killed shortly after the addition of corticosteroids, but rather after a latency period. Further evidence for this explanation is suggested by the observed accumulation of lymphoma cells in G1 of the cell cycle preceding cell death (Harmon et al., 1979). Note that the lytic event itself involves the inducation of an endonuclease, resulting in nuclear degradation (Wielckens et al., 1987; Compton et al., 1987).

Human lymphoma cells have been shown to be susceptible to the cytolytic effects of corticosteroids, both in vitro and in vivo (Norman and Thompson, 1977), making corticosteroids useful in treating lymphomas.

Effects on Lymphocyte "Traffic"

Corticosteroids induce rapid lymphopenia in humans and other animals by affecting lymphocyte traffic. In humans, maximal lymphopenia occurs four to six hours after 15 to 100 mg doses of prednisone, with return to baseline lymphocyte counts by 24 hr (Fauci et al., 1976). This transient lymphocytopenia seen with corticosteroid administration is caused by the redistribution of the peripheral lymphocytes into the spleen, bone marrow, and lymph nodes (Fauci and Dale, 1975a). Peripheral lymphocytes can be divided into two subpopulations, recirculating cells that leave the vascular space and enter the total body pool and nonrecirculating lymphocytes that reside within the vascular space (Perry et al., 1967). Corticosteroids cause increased migration of the recirculating lymphocytes from the vascular space, but have no effect upon the nonrecirculating cells (Fauci and Dale, 1975a). Furthermore, peripheral T cells appear to be depleted to a greater extent than peripheral B cells (Fauci, 1975b). By administering exogenous short-acting corticosteroids on alternate days, 48 hr cycles of lymphopenia four to six hr after dosing and nomalization of counts by 24 hr and throughout the "off" day is observed (Fauci et al., 1976). This characteristic cycle is seen despite months or

Table 9-5. Lymphokine Suppression by Corticosteroid Treatment

LYMPHOKINE	REFERENCE
Interleukin (IL)-1	Snyder and Unanue, 1982; Staruch and Wood, 1985
TNF/cachectin	Beutler et al., 1986
IL-2	Arya et al., 1984; Grabstein et al., 1986; Gillis et al., 1979
GM-CSF	Kelso and Munck, 1984
IL-3	Culpepper and Lee, 1985
Interferon-gamma	Arya et al., 1984; Grabstein et al., 1986; Guyre et al., 1988; Cesario et al., 1984

TNF-Tumor Necrosis Factor.
GM-CSF-Granulocyte-Macrophage Colony Stimulating Factor.

years of corticosteroid therapy. Corticosteroid administration in humans thus causes a transient lymphopenia, due to lymphocyte redistribution; and this occurs without cumulative effects, even upon chronic administration.

Humoral Immunity

Serum IgG, IgA, and to a lesser extent IgM levels are suppressed after large daily doses of corticosteroids (20–250 mg prednisone/day) (Posey, 1978). However, it has been shown that corticosteroids do not suppress specific antibody responses to a variety of antigens (Tuchinda et al., 1972). Patients taking modest doses of corticosteroids (15–20 mg prednisone/day) have normal primary antibody responses to vaccination (Kunin et al., 1959; Meuleman et al., 1985). The effect of corticosteroids on in vitro antibody production ranges from augmentation to suppression, depending on the experimental system (Cupps and Fauci, 1982). As mentioned above, peripheral B cells are relatively resistant to the effects of corticosteroids. Also, proliferative responses to PWM, (a T-dependent B cell mitogen) are less sensitive to suppression by corticosteroid treatment than the responses to "pure" T cell mitogens such as Con A or PHA (Gordon and Nouri, 1981). In fact, it is possible that the suppressive effect of corticosteroids on humoral immunity results more from its inhibitory effect on T helper cells than on any specific action on B cells.

Recent work with B cells in vitro, depleted of accessory cells, have revealed a corticosteroid inhibition of early B-cell activation events. Intermediate or late events in B-cell activation were less sensitive or even resistant to inhibition with corticosteroids. For inhibition of the early activation events to occur, corticosteroids had to be in the culture media for 24 hr prior to B-cell stimulation (Cupps et al., 1985). Thus, it appears that corticosteroids may be able to inhibit early activation of B cells in culture deprived of accessory cells, but are unable to inhibit immune responses that have been initiated or are fully developed.

Cellular Immunity

Cell-mediated immunity in humans is clearly influenced by exogenous corticosteroids. Cell-mediated immunity responses such as established delayed-type hypersensitivity are suppressed by two weeks of therapy with corticosteroids (prednisone 40 mg/d), with return to pretreatment values by two weeks posttherapy (Bovornkitti et al., 1960). Proliferative responses to the T cell mitogens Con A and PHA are markedly suppressed when lymphocytes are cultured from corticosteroid-treated humans (Fauci, 1975a, b). Both autologous and allogeneic mixed leukocyte reactions are inhibited by corticosteroid treatment (Katz and Fauci, 1979; Hahn et al., 1980). It is believed that corticosteroids induce suppression of graft rejection by inhibiting the proliferation of alloreactive T cells and their maturation into cytotoxic T cells (Keown and Stiller, 1986). T cells are activated in the presence of the lymphokines Interleukin-1 and Interleukin-2 (IL-1 and IL-2) and it is well established that corticosteroids reduce the production of these and other lymphokines (Table 9-5).

NK, K Cells

Natural killer cells cause lysis of virus-infected cells, participate in graft rejection, and conduct antitumor surveillance. Antibody-dependent cytotoxic cells (ADCC, K cells) perform functions similar to NK cells except the cytotoxicity mediated by these cells is antigen specific and requires prior sensitization.

K cells appear to be resistant to corticosteroid suppression both in vitro and in vivo in human and animal models (Parrillo and Fauci, 1979; Katz et al., 1984). In contrast, peripheral blood NK-cell activity has been shown to be suppressed both in vivo and in vitro by corticosteroid treatment (Nair and Schwartz, 1984; Holbrook et al., 1983; Onsrud and Thoroby, 1981; Parillo and Fauci, 1979). Recent work has shown that even physiologic doses of cortisol will suppress NK-cell activity in humans. This effect could be antagonized by a monoclonal antihuman corticosteroid-binding globulin antibody or by RU 486, a corticosteroid-receptor antagonist, suggesting that the effect is mediated through the corticosteroid receptor/corticosteroid-binding globulin complex (Gatti et al., 1987). The mechanisms by which corticosteroids exert their effects on NK cells are not well understood. It is possible that it is related to the corticosteroid inhibition of lymphokine production, many of which are known inducers of NK activity (Holbrook et al., 1983; Gillis et al., 1979a,b).

Summary

Corticosteroids have wide-ranging effects upon the immune system, including antibody production, T-cell proliferation and NK-cell function. Recent findings of their effects on lymphokine production and on lipocortins have resulted in a better understanding of their mechanism(s) of action. However, the interaction between immunoregulation and cytoreduction remains to be elucidated.

ANTIMETABOLITES: METHOTREXATE

Introduction

Methotrexate (MTX) is used clinically as an antineoplastic agent in the treatment of lymphocytic malignancies and several solid tumors, and as an immunosuppressive agent in the treatment of graft versus host disease associated with bone marrow transplantation, rheumatic diseases, and psoriasis (Calabresi and Parks, 1985). The dose-limiting toxicity of MTX has been shown to be primarily on the bone marrow and gastrointestinal tract (Chabner and Myers, 1985). Immunosuppressive effects reported both in vitro and in vivo have indicated that humoral immunity is suppressed to a greater extent than cell-mediated immunity (Friedman et al., 1961; Hersh et al., 1965; Mansour et al., 1978). Folinic acid, given to ameliorate the systemic toxicity of MTX treatment does not appear to prevent MTX immunosuppression (Mitchell et al., 1969). Even low-dose maintenance regimens of MTX cause serum levels of 10^{-9} to 10^{-8} M (O'Meara et al., 1985a), which affect cell-mediated and humoral immunity (Pinkerton et al., 1982; Breithaupt and Huenzlen, 1983).

Mechanism of Action

Methotrexate binds tightly to the enzyme dihydrofolate reductase and inhibits the conversion of dihydrofolate to tetrahydrofolate. This event produces an antithymidylate synthetase action, which is believed to be the primary cytotoxic mechanism (Taylor and Tattersall, 1981). However, MTX also inhibits purine biosynthesis as a consequence of thymidylate synthetase inhibition (Jackson, 1984; Allegra et al., 1986). In contrast to the cytotoxic effects, it appears that MTX-induced immunosuppression can be either totally or partially reversed by the addition of purines to in vitro cultures. In vitro MTX impairment of cytotoxic T-lymphocyte (CTL) function can be reversed 50% by the addition of hypoxanthine, whereas MTX impairment of in vitro antibody production is reversed partially by thymidine and totally by hypoxanthine addition (Boygo and Mihich, 1980; Rosenthal et al., 1988). Collectively these studies suggest that MTX inhibition of purine biosynthesis may be the major mechanism of MTX immunosuppression, in contrast to the commonly accepted antithymidylate synthetase cytotoxic mechanism. In a recent comparison of folinic acid rescue and thymidine-purine rescue, a higher therapeutic index was obtained with the latter approach (Samuels and Straw, 1984).

Effects on Lymphocytes

Methotrexate produces lymphopenia after infusion, with a nadir in the number of circulating lymphocytes at four hr after dosing. Analyses of lymphocyte subpopulations have shown a greater reduction in Ts than TH cells (O'Meara et al., 1985b). The lymphocyte proliferative responses to T-dependent B cell mitogens (Staph protein A, PWM) are suppressed more than the responses to the T cell mitogens (PHA, Con A) at MTX levels of 10^{-9} M (O'Meara et al., 1985b; Gereis et al., 1987). Methotrexate has been shown to be a potent suppressor of T-dependent antibody production in vitro and in vivo (Rosenthal et al., 1987; Heppner and Calabresi, 1976). Marked suppression of PWM-induced immunoglobulin production can be produced by 5×10^{-9} M MTX in vitro (O'Meara et al., 1985b). B-cell activation events preceding S phase are suppressed by MTX (Rosenthal et al., 1988). In vitro MTX concentrations of 10^{-9} to 10^{-8} M were found to inhibit CTL function by 50% (Boygo and Mihich, 1980). Studies of MTX on NK function have produced conflicting results. When measured in vitro, augmentation was observed (Matheson et al., 1983), whereas suppression was found in vivo (Rosenthal et al., 1987). Methotrexate induced in vitro augmentation can be blocked with exogenous thymidine (Matheson et al., 1983).

Hypersensitivity Reactions

Methotrexate can occasionally produce type I anaphylactic reactions, but these are severe only when the drug is administered at high doses (Weiss, 1984; Klimo and Ibrahim, 1981). Methotrexate-protein-IgG complexes have been demonstrated in patients who had type I reactions (da Costa et al., 1980); however, the mechanism remains incompletely understood.

Methotrexate occasionally produces a type III reaction as well. This is characterized by rapid onset of pneumonitis with local or systemic eosinophilia, hilar adenopathy, rashes, pleural effusion, and rapid recovery after drug withdrawal or corticosteroid treatment (Sostman et al., 1976). Another type III hypersensitivity reaction reported with MTX is manifested by a vasculitis with skin lesions (Weiss and Baker, 1987; Marks et al., 1984).

Methotrexate, and its related analogue trimetrexate, can occasionally cause toxic epidermal necrolysis (Doyle et al, 1983; Weiss et al., 1986). The mechanism of these skin reactions is not known, but it probably does not involve an antibody-mediated mechanism (Weiss and Baker, 1987).

Summary

Depressed humoral immunity is the most common immunosuppressive outcome of MTX therapy, however cell-mediated immunity is often severely suppressed resulting in opportunistic infections. The mechanism of this suppression appears to be different from the commonly accepted antithymidylate synthetase cytotoxic effect. With this in mind, perhaps future regimens designed to minimize the immunologic toxicity associated with MTX treatment may include both folinic acid and purine rescue.

AZATHIOPRINE

The thiopurines, azathioprine (AZA) and 6MP are among the most well-studied immunosuppressive agents. Clinically, AZA is used primarily for its immunosuppressive effect in the prevention of graft rejection and in rheumatoid arthritis (Calabresi and Parks, 1985), with 6MP being used to treat juvenile ALL.

Mechanism of Action

The thiopurines serve both as competitive inhibitor and substrate for hypoxanthine-guanine phosphoribosyl transferase and the result is the inhibition of purine synthesis. Cells that are deficient in this enzyme are not affected by thiopurines (Dalke et al., 1984). Thiopurines are cell cycle-specific agents, and thus exert most of their immunosuppressive effect during the proliferative or inductive phase of humoral and cellular immune responses. Thiopurines preferentially inhibit T-cell functions to a greater degree than B-cell functions. T and B cells differ in purine metabolism and this may be the basis of their differential susceptibility to thiopurines (Miller and Kataoka, 1985). However, despite the wide ranging immunologic effects that have been reported and the extensive clinical use of this class of drugs, the mechanism of immune suppression by thiopurines is not completely understood.

Humoral Immunity

Humoral suppression by AZA treatment in humans has been demonstrated in several studies (Levin et al., 1964; Santos et al., 1964; Swanson and Schwartz, 1967). Primary antibody responses are inhibited to a greater extent than secondary responses (Spreafico and Ancelerio, 1977). Fully differentiated antibody-forming cells are resistant to thiopurines, both in vivo and in vitro, even at high concentrations (Rollinghoff et al., 1973). T-independent antibody responses are more resistant to AZA than T-dependent responses (Rollinghoff et al., 1973; Galanaud et al., 1975). The dose–response curve for inhibition of antibody formation is hyperbolic, that is, there is progressively less inhibition of antibody formation with escalating thiopurine dosage, with a plateau in inhibition at high doses (Berenbaum, 1969). The timing of drug administration relative to antigen administration is essential to significant immunosuppression. Maximal immunosuppression is observed with drug administration within 48 hr after antigen administration (Winkelstein, 1979). Pretreatment with AZA can result in augmented antibody responses (Schwartz, 1966). Thiopurines appear to suppress IgG responses to a greater extent than IgM responses both in animal models and humans (Borel et al., 1965; Rowley et al., 1969). Azathioprine does not consistently produce lymphocytopenia nor is there preferential depletion of any lymphocyte population during AZA treatment (Bach and Strom, 1985; Pedersen and Bleyer, 1986). Human B and T lymphocyte cell lines have been shown to be sensitive to both AZA and 6MP in vitro (Ohnuma et al., 1978; Kazmers et al., 1983).

Cellular Immunity

Several lines of evidence suggest that T lymphocytes are the primary target of thiopurine treatment (Bach and Strom, 1985). These agents appear to suppress T-cell mediated responses (mixed leukocyte reactions, mitogen responses, delayed hypersensitivity, and graft rejection) more than humoral responses in humans and rodents (Spreafico and Ancelerio, 1977).

Azathioprine inhibits both PHA- and Con A-induced proliferation of human lymphocytes, but high doses of the drug are needed (Bach and Strom, 1985; Cook et al., 1983). Azathioprine inhibits PWM-induced proliferation (Brown et al., 1976), but there is no preferential effect upon B- or T-cell proliferation (Dimitriu and Fauci, 1978). Studies of lymphocytes taken from animals and humans receiving AZA have revealed conflicting results. Some authors have reported suppression of PHA responses by in vivo treatment (Page et al., 1971; Mansour and Nelson, 1979), whereas others found no change (Humphrey et al., 1972; Borella and Green, 1972).

Azathioprine inhibits the in vitro mixed leukocyte reactions (Bach and Bach, 1972; Bucy, 1988) and the development of CTL and T suppressor cells in mixed leukocyte reaction cultures. The latter effect cannot be reversed by addition of IL-2 to the cultures (Bucy, 1988). Fully differentiated CTL cells are resistant to inhibition by AZA (Rollinghoff et al., 1973; Brown et al., 1976), however the generation of CTLs is inhibited by a concentration of drug that is 300-fold less than the concentration necessary to inhibit T-dependent antibody formation (Rollinghoff et al., 1973). Natural killer cell activity has been shown to be depressed in patients undergoing AZA therapy (Lipinsky et al., 1980; Shih et al., 1982; Prince et al., 1984; Pederson and Bleyer, 1986). In Pederson and Bleyer's longitudinal study of patients with rheumatoid arthritis receiving AZA therapy, NK function was dramatically suppressed after five to eight months of treatment. Studies attempting to reverse suppression of NK activity with exogenous interferon either in vitro or in vivo have revealed conflicting results, either demonstrating augmentation (Ramsey et al., 1984; Kelley et al., 1984) or no significant effect (Moreau et al., 1983; Shih et al., 1982). The effect of AZA on antibody-dependent cell-mediated cytotoxicity is also controversial. Decreases in ADCC have been reported in patients undergoing AZA treatment (Shih et al., 1982; Prince et al., 1984; Spina, 1984), however, other investigators have reported normal ADCC function (Descamps et al., 1977; Lipinski et al., 1980). Azathioprine has been shown to induce immunological tolerance to protein antigens (Schwartz and Dameshek, 1963; Schwartz, 1966). Azathioprine and 6MP have been shown to inhibit the development of delayed hypersensitivity in numerous animal models (Borel and Schwartz, 1964; Borel et al., 1968; Dietrich and Hess, 1970). Azathioprine treatment is accompanied by a greater increase in T-cell dependent viral infections than in B-cell dependent bacterial infections (Fournier et al., 1973).

Hypersensitivity Reactions

Hypersensitivity reactions are seen rarely with AZA treatment (Saway et al., 1988). Reactions have occurred from three hr to 45 days after drug administration and have developed despite concurrent treatment with corticosteroids. Subsequent reexposure to AZA usually evokes reactions within several hours and has been life-threatening (Sloth and Thomson, 1971; Assini et al., 1986). Fever is a frequent finding and, when associated with rigors, may simulate infection (Saway et al., 1988). Musculoskeletal symptoms including myalgias or arthralgias are common (King et al., 1972; Zaltzman et al., 1984). Hypotension associated with AZA treatment can be severe and, when associated with fever, rigors, and rash, may mimic septic shock (Majors and Moore, 1985; Cunningham et al., 1982; Zaltzman et al., 1984; Rosenthal, 1986). The mechanism of AZA-related hypersensitivity reactions remains to be elucidated. No consistent laboratory abnormalities have been noted, and in some cases (e.g., pulmonary or hepatic injury) the mechanism may not be immunologic (Saway et al., 1988; Cooper et al., 1986).

Summary

The evidence for the preferential effect of thiopurines on T cells versus B cells is overwhelming (Bach and Strom 1985). However, the specific mechanism by which the thiopurines exert their immunosuppressive effects is lacking. Azathioprine serves an integral role in the prevention of graft rejection, but future work on the mechanism of its specific immunosuppressive effects may result in more widespread usage in other clinical settings.

5-FLUOROURACIL (5-FU)

Introduction

5-fluorouracil (5-FU) is useful clinically in the therapy of several types of carcinomas (Calabresi and Parks, 1985). The usual toxicities of 5-FU therapy are mucositis and myelosuppression (Calabresi and Parks, 1985); however, immunosuppression during 5-FU has been documented extensively (see below).

Mechanism

The cytotoxic activity of 5-FU is caused by the inhibition of thymidylate synthetase, resulting in a reduction in DNA synthesis by blocking the conversion of deoxyuridine-5′-phosphate (dUMP) to thymidine-5′-phosphate (TMP) (Miller and Kataoka, 1985). This is mediated by a metabolically-activated form of 5-FU: 5-fluorodeoxyuridine (FdUrd).

Humoral Immunity

In vivo 5-FU has a greater effect upon humoral responses than upon cellular immunity. Cancer patients undergoing 5-FU treatment demonstrate suppression of both primary and secondary antibody responses (Mitchell and DeConti, 1970). Somewhat in contrast to this, however, in murine models, 5-FU treatment after antigen administration suppresses primary responses to T-dependent antigens (Johnson et al., 1976; Ohta et al., 1980), but appears to have no effect on response to T-independent antigens (Merluzzi et al., 1982). In vitro, B cells appear to be relatively more sensitive to 5-FU than T cells (Ohnuma et al., 1980; Au et al., 1983; Srivastava and Alderfer, 1982; Vetvicka et al., 1986). There may be an enzymatic basis for the greater sensitivity of B cell fractions. B cells have higher levels of thymidine phosphorylase which facilitates the conversion of 5-FU to FdUrd (El-Assouli, 1985; Piper and Fox, 1982). Even among B cells there is a differential sensitivity relative to maturation and site, with the following proposed order of sensitivity: early precursors > pre-B cells > newly formed B cells in marrow/spleen > lymph node B cells (Vetvicka, 1986).

Cellular Immunity

Marked leukopenia after 5-FU treatment was recognized early as an untoward side effect of 5-FU treatment (Curreri et al., 1958). Suppression of PHA mitogenic responses in human PBLs has been reported in vivo in cancer patients undergoing 5-FU therapy and in vitro in PBLs from normal, healthy volunteers (Nordman et al., 1978; Gereis et al., 1987). Inhibition by 5-FU of the development of delayed-type hypersensitivity in man has been described by Mitchell and DeConti (1970). In murine models, 5-FU treatment appears to selectively reduce mature NK cells and spare immature NK cells (Sarneva et al., 1989; D'Adamio et al., 1988). Non-B, non-T cell lines are insensitive to 5-FU (Ohnuma et al., 1980).

Hypersensitivity Reactions

5-fluorouracil is a chemotherapeutic agent with a very low risk of hypersensitivity reactions (Weiss, 1982). Only three cases of 5-FU-associated acute type I hypersensitivity reactions have been reported (Weiss and Baker, 1987; DeBeer and Kabakou, 1979; Sridhar, 1986; Santos and Medina, 1986). In two patients the hypersensitivity reaction was severe hypotension, and another patient had angioedema. The mechanism of these reactions is not known. 5-

fluorouracil also causes a palmar-plantar dermatitis similar to cytarabine, beginning with hand-foot parasthesias and progressing to erythema, swelling, and desquamation (Weiss and Baker, 1987; Lokick and Moore, 1984; Feldman and Ajani, 1985; Atkins, 1985). This reaction was initially observed in patients receiving continuous infusion 5-FU therapy (Lokick and Moore, 1984). A recent study in dogs found no significant effect upon blood pressure, heart rate, or plasma histamine levels after 5-FU administration (Eschalier et al., 1988).

Summary

5-fluorouracil appears to suppress humoral immunity to a greater extent than cellular immunity. It would seem that this agent is appropriate for chemo-immunotherapy regimens that would maximize both the host's antitumor immunity and the chemical antineoplastic effects. At the time of writing, we are unaware of any such protocols incorporating 5-FU.

VINCA ALKALOIDS

Introduction

The vinca alkaloids VCR and VLB are used in the therapy of a wide range of malignancies. Vincristine and VLB share similar structures, only differing slightly at one position on the molecule (methyl versus formyl group) (Calabresi and Parks, 1985). However, in spite of this similarity in structure, they are quite dissimilar in biological activities including range of antitumor effect and toxic reactions (Calabresi and Parks, 1985; Chabner and Myers, 1985). The dose-limiting toxicities with each of the alkaloids differ; VCR is associated with neurotoxicity whereas VLB is limited by myelosuppression (Creasey, 1975). There is little cross-reactivity between the alkaloids in terms of these commonly observed toxicities (Calabresi and Parks, 1985). Despite their widespread usage, our understanding of the immunopharmacology of these agents is lacking (Spreafico and Vecchi, 1985). In the literature reviewed below, the two alkaloids differ significantly in their immunomodulatory effects. The reason(s) for these differences in light of their structural similarities is not clear.

Mechanism of Action

The presumed mechanism by which the vinca alkaloids exert their cytotoxic effect is through the binding to the protein tubulin and the resulting inhibition of microtubule and mitotic spindle formation (Creasey, 1975). The two alkaloids are quite similar in their rates of binding and affinity to tubulin (Owellen et al., 1972). There is some evidence that their cytotoxic functions may not be related directly to their inhibition of microtubule assembly (Noble et al., 1977).

Cellular Immunity

Both VCR and VLB inhibit the development of primary allogeneic CTL activity in vitro (Orsini et al., 1980). In vivo, it appears that CTL cells are more sensitive to VLB whereas ADCC cells (K cells) are more sensitive to VCR (Ryoyama et al., 1982). Vinblastine has been shown to inhibit suppressor T-cell development and function both in vitro and in vivo (Bianchi et al., 1985; Powderly et al., 1986; 1987; Ryoyama et al., 1982). Both VLB and VCR can, at high doses, inhibit delayed-type hypersensitivity development, homograft rejection, and established delayed type hypersensitivity (Aisenberg and Wilkes, 1964). Natural killer activity in human PBLs is minimally suppressed by VCR (Carpen, 1987). Antibody-dependent Cellular Cytotoxicity is augmented at therapeutic VLB concentrations (Ralph and

Nakoinz, 1982). Lymphocyte proliferation in response to viral antigen stimulation is reduced by VCR treatment (Gorse and Kopp, 1987). Proliferative responses to PHA are similarly suppressed by VCR (Cesario et al., 1982; 1984). Inhibition of yeast phagocytosis by PBLs is seen in vitro with VLB or VCR levels that are roughly equivalent to in vivo therapeutic levels (Athlin et al., 1985). This sensitivity of monocyte phagocytosis is in accordance with the clinical responsiveness of idiopathic thrombocytopenic purpura and autoimmune hemolytic anemia to vinca alkaloid therapy, clinical conditions in which the disease pathogenesis is related to the activity of the reticuloendothelial system.

Humoral Immunity

Vincristine appears to be more potent than VLB at suppressing in vitro antibody formation (Ryoyama et al., 1982). In vivo, both have been shown to suppress specific antibody production (Aisenberg and Wilkes, 1964; Kettman et al., 1979; Powderly, 1987, 1986). Vincristine treatment can abolish the specific antibody response to *Pseudomonas aeruginosa* immunization while preserving protective cell-mediated responses (Powderly, 1987, 1986). Thus, it appears that both in vitro and in vivo VCR preferentially affects B-cell functions and VLB preferentially affects T-cell functions (Ehrke and Mihich, 1985).

Lymphokine Effects

Interferon (IFN)-alpha and IFN-gamma, and IL-2 are key lymphokines in the activation of NK cells and mitogen- or anitgen induced lymphocyte proliferative responses. Decreased production of these mediators may contribute to the increased severity of viral infections in patients undergoing chemotherapy (Levine et al., 1974). Newcastle disease virus induced IFN-alpha production in human PBLs is suppressed by VCR (Gorse et al., 1984). Similarly, VCR suppresses PHA induced IFN-gamma and IL-2 production (Cesario et al., 1984). In contrast, other investigators have found that the production of either IFN-gamma or IL-2 in human PBLs in response to influenza A virus was not suppressed by VCR or VLB treatment (Gorse and Kopp, 1987). It is possible, therefore, that suppression of IFN or IL production by vinca alkaloid treatment depends upon the inducing agent used, but further investigation in this area is needed.

Hypersensitivity Reactions

Acute respiratory failure has been reported with VLB and mitomycin combination therapy (Kris et al., 1984; Rao et al., 1985). Whereas this reaction is uncommon, it is a recurring syndrome, which may occur as frequently as in three to four percent of all patients receiving both drugs in combination (Hoelzer et al., 1986). The clinical features are the abrupt onset of profound wheezing and an interstitial pattern on chest x-ray (Ballen and Weiss, 1988). Despite a number of reported cases in the literature, only three have been fatal (Ballen and Weiss, 1988; Rao et al., 1985). Autopsy findings in these cases suggest a type 1 hypersensitivity mechanism (Ballen and Weiss, 1988; Rao et al., 1985).

Summary

The two commonly used vinca alkaloids differ selectively in their anticancer and immunosuppressive effects. Because two structurally similar molecules can produce different immunoregulatory effects suggests that they may be useful in chemo-immunotherapy regimens that try to maximize both immunologic and antineoplastic effects. However, more research into the specific immunomodulatory activities of these agents is needed before this possibility can be realized.

ANTHRACYCLINE ANTIBIOTICS

Introduction

The anthracycline antibiotic doxorubicin (DOX) is perhaps the single most important anticancer agent. It is used in the treatment of a variety of human neoplasms including lymphomas, leukemias, and solid tumors (Bonadonna et al., 1975; Haanen and Hillen, 1975; Middleman et al., 1971; Wang et al., 1971). Although DOX differs slightly at one site from its parent compound daunorubicin (DNR), it has been shown to have a larger spectrum of activity and a higher therapeutic index both in animal models and in humans (Schwartz and Grindey, 1973; Carter, 1980). Acute toxicity includes bone marrow suppression, alopecia, and mucosal ulceration, but the long-term toxicity of DOX treatment is the cumulative dose-dependent cardiac toxicity that may result in congestive heart failure (Wang et al., 1971; Rinehart et al., 1974).

Although human research is limited, the immunosuppressive and immunopotentiating effects of the two major anthracyclines have been studied extensively in rodent models (Ehrke et al., 1982; Ehrke and Mihich, 1985).

Mechanism of Action

The cytotoxic activity of DOX is multifaceted. It may affect cell viability in a number of ways including intercalation with DNA (Carter, 1975), intracellular generation of oxygen free radicals (Bachur et al., 1978), or induction of damaging cell surface interactions (Tritton and Yee, 1982). Furthermore, DOX may induce augmentation of the host antitumor response (Ehrke et al., 1982; Ehrke and Mihich, 1985). Thus, it appears that the effect of DOX is mediated both by direct cytotoxicity and by immunomodulation of the host–tumor relationship. The relative contribution of these effects to the overall antitumor effect of DOX remains unresolved (Salazar and Cohen, 1984).

Humoral Immunity

In comparative studies of DOX and DNR in mice, DOX suppresses to a greater extent the primary antibody responses to both T-dependent and T-independent antigens. In contrast, DNR may have a greater effect upon secondary antibody responses, allograft rejection, and macrophage-mediated tumor cell killing (Bast, 1982; Ehrke and Mihich, 1985).

Cellular Immunity

In vivo or in vitro DOX treatment in murine models has been shown to enhance the development of cytotoxic activity against allogenic cells (Orsini et al., 1977; Tomazic et al., 1980). Arinaga et al. (1986) recently demonstrated a twofold higher level of cell-mediated cytotoxicity in cancer patients after one dose of DOX. Doxorubicin treatment regimens that optimize cell-mediated immunity appear to inhibit humoral responses, and conditions that augment humoral responses appear to inhibit cellular responses (Mihich and Ehrke, 1985; Ehrke et al., 1982). Treatment of mice intraperitoneally with DOX has been shown to induce both NK cell activity and macrophage cytolytic function (Santoni et al., 1980; Stoychkov et al., 1979; Salazar and Cohen, 1984). This augmentation of cellular cytotoxicity by DOX appears to be mediated by effects upon at least two cell subsets: enrichment of immature monocyte-macrophage accessory cells, and elimination of adherent regulatory T cells (Ehrke et al., 1982, 1984). In addition, other investigators have presented evidence that DOX-elicited macrophages may owe their antitumor cytostatic properties in vivo to the uptake, retention, and subsequent transfer of the drug to tumor cells (Haskill, 1981; Salazar and Cohen, 1984).

Doxorubicin has been shown to be stored in vacuoles or cytoplasmic inclusions by macrophages (Haskill, 1981; Martin et al., 1982).

The proliferative response to PHA by human PBLs is inhibited by DOX in vitro (Cesario et al., 1984; Gereis et al., 1987). In murine models DOX has been shown to inhibit the proliferative response to Con A (Rahman et al., 1986b). However, DOX has no effect in vitro or in vivo upon the activation of human PBLs into tumoricidal monocytes by liposome encapsulated immunomodulators of LPS (Hudson et al., 1988; Mace et al., 1988).

Cytokine Effects

Early studies with DOX demonstrated no effect upon IFN-alpha or beta production in human PBLs (Cesario et al., 1982). However, IFN-gamma production was subsequently shown to be reduced by DOX pretreatment (Cesario et al., 1984). DOX has no observed effect upon IL-1 secretion by human PBLs (Hudson et al., 1988). In mice, in vivo high-dose treatment (10 mg/kg) increases Con A-induced IL-2 production, whereas low-dose treatment decreases production (Hamied and Turk, 1987; Kedar et al., 1986). Similarly, DOX treatment in rats increases lymphocyte release of prostaglandin E_2 (PGE_2) (Hamied and Turk, 1987). Conditioned media from nonstimulated splenocyte cultures from DOX-treated mice appear to have increased amounts of IL-2 activity. A slight increase in PHA-induced IL-2 production has been seen in human PBLs after DOX treatment in vivo (Arinaga et al., 1986). However, both virus-induced and mitogen-induced IL-2 production in human PBLs are reduced in the presence of DOX in vitro (Gorse et al., 1987; Dupont et al., 1985).

Note that DOX promotes release of IL-1 activity (Cohen et al., 1983), which could account for the known changes in IL-2 and IFN-gamma production (Mace et al., 1988). Doxorubicin can enhance cell mediated cytotoxicity and this may occur by its effects upon PGE_2 or IL-2 production (Ehrke et al., 1986).

Hypersensitivity

Both DNR and DOX have occasionally produced severe type I reactions (Weiss and Bruno, 1981; Hatfield et al., 1981; Prados, 1981). Doxorubicin can cause erythema at the injection site that does not appear to be immune mediated, since it can occur immediately with the initial drug administration. Furthermore, erythema at the injection site does not necessarily occur with subsequent injections, and a history of such an occurrence does not preclude retreatment with DOX (Weiss, 1984).

Sudden death during DOX administration has been reported, and at least in some cases, was secondary to cardiac arrythmia (Wortman et al., 1979; Cosgriff, 1980). Dog studies have demonstrated hypotension and nonimmunologically-mediated histamine release after DOX treatment (Levandowski, 1980; Eschalier et al., 1988). This may explain some of the rare sudden deaths associated with DOX administration (Weiss, 1984).

Therapy Options

Recent work has focused on reducing the toxicity of DOX by the incorporation of the drug into liposomal delivery systems. Liposomally encapsulated DOX, in comparison with free DOX, has been associated with a decrease in toxicity and augmented or equivalent antitumor effects in animal models (Forssen et al., 1983; Gabizon et al., 1982; Rahman et al., 1985; 1986a; Herman et al., 1983). Phase I and II trials are currently in progress (Gabizon et al., 1989; Rahman et al., 1989; Treat et al., 1989).

The effect of liposamally encapsulated DOX versus free DOX treatment with regard to the immune system depends upon the immunological variable studied. Both splenic NK function and specific allogenic cytotoxicity are transiently reduced by both modalities of treatment, however specific allogenic cytotoxicity is reduced to a lesser degree (Rahman et al., 1986b; Mace et al., 1988). Both treatments produce similar elevations in peritoneal exudate NK function, with the liposomal-treated mice having a more sustained elevation in function (Mace et al., 1988). Similarly, LPS-induced tumoricidal macrophages can be recovered from both groups, with a longer period of recoverable macrophages in the liposome treated group (Mace et al., 1988).

Summary

The immunomodulatory actions of DOX have been systematically investigated, revealing stimulatory effects upon precursor monocyte-macrophage accessory cells for cytolytic function, inhibition of adherent regulatory T-cells, and increased IL-2 production which is permissive for the proliferation of activated effector T cells and activation of cytolytic macrophages (Mihich, 1985a). However, the individual contribution of each of these effects upon the overall antineoplastic activity of DOX remains to be demonstrated.

BLEOMYCIN

Introduction

Bleomycin is commonly used in the therapy of squamous cell carcinomas, genitourinary tract tumors, and lymphomas. It is a drug with little or no myelotoxicity. The most commonly seen toxicity is mucocutaneous reactions (Calabresi and Parks, 1985). Bleomycin has well-established pulmonary toxicity manifest as pneumonitis or even pseudotumors (Cooper et al., 1986; Ginsberg and Comis, 1982; McCrea et al., 1981; Scharstein et al., 1987).

Mechanism

The most likely mechanism of action involves bleomycin binding to DNA by intercalation, activating pathways that result in chain scission and fragmentation of DNA. In vitro studies indicate that bleomycin causes a build-up of cells in G_2, with many of the cells displaying chromosomal aberrations (Calabresi and Parks, 1985).

Immunologic Effects

Until recently, bleomycin was believed not to have any immunomodulatory effects of significance (Yamaki et al., 1969; Ohno et al., 1971; Lehane and Lane, 1978). Studies in rabbits and with human blood have demonstrated that treatment with bleomycin causes the release of endogenous pyrogen (Dinarello et al., 1973). Work by Parker and Turk recently demonstrated that delayed-type hypersensitivity could be potentiated by bleomycin administered at the time of or up to three days after sensitization (Parker and Turk, 1984). This is different from CY's effect of delayed-type hypersensitivity, in which there is suppression of delayed-type hypersensitivity with CY administration on day three, the time of maximal lymphocyte proliferation. In vivo or in vitro bleomycin administration has been shown to potentiate IL-2 release in vitro in mouse or rat spleen cells stimulated with suboptimal doses of Con A (Abdul Hamied et al., 1986; Abdul Hamied and Turk, 1987). No change in rat splenic lymphocyte subpopulations after bleomycin treatment was seen in the latter study (Abdul Hamied and Turk, 1987). Other workers have suggested that bleomycin may potentiate antitumor immunity in a rat model through the elimination of suppressor T-cell activity (Morikawa et al., 1985; Xu et al., 1988). With the observation that bleomycin has virtually no myelotoxicity but some immunomodulatory effects, future regimens combining bleomycin with other biologic response modifiers may be feasible.

Hypersensitivity Reactions

Bleomycin occasionally produces reactions similar to anaphylaxis (type 1 reaction), except that high fever is present frequently and urticaria and angioedema are rare (Levy and Chiarillo, 1980). Hypotension can occur and lead to shock and coma. A recent study using dogs found no change in blood pressure, heart rate, or plasma histamine levels after bleomycin administration (Eschalier et al., 1988). Reactions to bleomycin are more common in lymphoma patients, in whom the incidence varies from one to eight percent (Weiss, 1984). These reactions do not appear to be dose related, and can occur with as little as one unit of bleomycin, or after 60 cumulative units (Weiss and Bruno, 1981; Carter et al., 1983). Because of this, it is recommended that patients with lymphomas have a one unit test dose, followed by a 24 hr observation period before starting standard dosing schedules (Calabresi and Parks, 1985).

Summary

Recent investigations have revealed immunomodulatory effects of bleomycin that were not realized previously. Bleomycin may exert its immunopotentiating effects by increasing IL-2 production during lymphocyte proliferation or possibly through the reduction of suppressor T-cell function. Bleomycin has a unique mechanism of action and its toxicities do not overlap with those of other drugs (Calabresi and Parks, 1985). In view of these facts and the drug's potential immunomodulatory role, bleomycin may serve as an integral role in future combination chemo-immunotherapy protocols.

CISPLATIN

Introduction

Cisplatin (CDDP) is frequently used singly or in combination therapy for various neoplasms, including carcinomas of the testis, ovary, bladder, oropharynx, and certain lymphomas and childhood neoplasms (Calabresi and Parks, 1985). The literature on the immunopharmacology of CDDP is rather sparse, but there is some indirect evidence that the drug has immunomodulatory functions which may contribute to its cytoreductive effects.

Mechanism

The primary mechanism by which CDDP exerts its antitumor effect is by binding to DNA and inhibiting nucleotide synthesis (Pascoe and Roberts, 1974). However, concomitant activation or restoration of host antitumor immune defenses by CDDP has been proposed by some authors (Rosenberg, 1975).

Humoral Immunity

Inhibition of the primary antibody response in rodents to T-dependent antigen has been observed (Kahn and Hill, 1971; Berenbaum, 1971). No study has been undertaken to analyze the effect of CDDP on T-independent antigens.

Cellular Effects

The administration of CDDP in animals results in lymphopenia and cellular depletion of the thymus and spleen with relative sparing of lymph nodes (Thompson and Gale, 1971). In cancer patients undergoing CDDP therapy, a reduction in the number of T helper cells is seen with an increase in the number of T suppressor/cytotoxic cells. Normalization of the numbers of the two lymphocyte subpopulations occurs by four to six months after therapy (Onsrud et al., 1986). Cisplatin treatment of rodents resulted in decreased mitogen-induced proliferative responses in vitro (Wierda and Pazdernik, 1979; Howle et al., 1971). Suppression of the PHA response has also been observed in humans receiving CDDP (Kahn and Hill, 1973). The suppression in humans appears to be transient, beginning within minutes after drug infusion and with recovery by one to two days after stopping treatment. In vitro investigations on human PBLs with CDDP concentrations similar to therapeutic levels have demonstrated that exposure to the drug for 24 hr results in mitogenic suppression, whereas one hr exposure results in little or no suppression (Howle et al., 1971; Kleinerman and Zwelling, 1982). However, simultaneous addition of PHA and CDDP in vitro results in suppression of the PHA response by human PBLs (Vancurova et al., 1986). The response to the T cell mitogen Con A is more sensitive to suppression than the response to the B cell mitogen LPS. This differential sensitivity has been interpreted as indirect evidence that T cells may be more sensitive to platininum compounds (Wierda and Pazdernik, 1979). Cisplatin also has been shown to be more inhibitory of the proliferation of human leukemic T cells than B cells (Ohnuma, 1978).

Immunopotentiation with CDDP has also been reported. Marked enhancement (up to 300%) of spontaneous monocyte-mediated cytotoxicity has been reported after in vitro treatment of human mononuclear cells (Kleinerman et al., 1980b). Cisplatin added at the beginning of mixed lymphocyte reactivity cultures, under suboptimal stimulatory conditions (such as might be present in tumor bearing hosts) results in augmentation of the response. No effect or slight inhibition was seen when optimal in vitro sensitization conditions were used (Spreafico and Vecchi, 1985; Schlaefli et al., 1983). Cisplatin has no effect upon mature T cell effector function (Schlaefli et al., 1983). In vitro exposure of human leukocytes has been reported to increase NK activity (Spreafico and Vecchi, 1985). Similar increases in NK activity have been found in tumor bearing patients after CDDP treatment (Kleinerman et al., 1980a). In addition, rodents treated with CDDP were found to have enhanced NK cell function (Lichtenstein and Pende, 1986; Sodhi and Singh, 1988; Woolley et al., 1988).

Hypersensitivity Reactions

Hypersensitivity reactions to CDDP are well-established, with reported incidence rates ranging from one to 25% of cases (Weiss and Bruno, 1981; Weiss, 1984). The type 1 hypersensitivity reactions are manifest by anxiety, pruritus, cough, dyspnea, diaphoresis, angioedema, vomiting, bronchospasm, rash, urticaria, and hypotension (Weiss and Baker, 1987). There are a few cases of associated hemolytic anemia, but this reaction occurs to a far lesser degree than the type 1 reaction described above (Weiss, 1984). There have been no reported deaths with CDDP hypersensitivity reactions.

Conclusions

Although there is little published work on the immunoregulatory effects of CDDP, it appears that immunosuppression with this agent is transient and observed mostly at very high doses, whereas immunopotentiation may involve restoration or actual stimulation of certain activities in vivo and vitro. Also, there has been recent evidence that its antineoplastic effect may involve immunomodulation of the host's immune system in addition to its action on tumor cell proliferation (Spreafico and Vecchi, 1985).

Summary

Many antineoplastic drugs have been investigated for their immunomodulatory activities. Under conditions of normal use (i.e., maximum tolerated doses), most agents are immunosuppressive and can result in increased incidence of infections. Under other conditions, however, many of those agents are immunopotentiatory, either directly or by inhibition of suppressor cells. This may open new avenues for the treatment of malignancies with lower doses of these drugs.

REFERENCES

Adbul Hamied TA and Turk JL Enhancement of interleukin-2 release in rats with treatment with bleomycin and Adriamycin in vivo. Cancer Immunol Immunother 1987 25:245–249.

Abdul Hamied TA, Parker D, and Turk JL Potentiation of the release of interleukin-2 by bleomycin. Immunopharmacol 1986 12:127–134.

Aisenberg AC and Wilkes BM Studies on the suppression of immune responses by the periwinkle alkaloids vincristine and vinblastine. J Clin Invest 1964 43:2394–2403.

Alepa FP and Zvaiffler-Sliwinski AJ Immunologic effects of cyclophosphamide treatment in rheumatoid arthritis. Arthritis Rheum 1979 13:754–760.

Allegra CJ, Fine RL, Drake JC, and Chabner BA The effect of methotrexate on intracellular folate pools in human MCF-7 breast cancer cells: Evidence for direct inhibition of purine metabolism. J Biol Chem 1986 261:6478–6485.

Arinaga S, Akiyoshi T, and Tsuji H Augmentation of the generation of cell-mediated cytotoxicity after a single dose of Adriamycin in cancer patients. Cancer Res 1986 46:4213–4216.

Arya SK, Wong-Staal F, and Gallo RC Dexamethasone-mediated inhibition of human T cell growth factor and gamma interferon messenger RNA. J Immunol 1984 133:273–276.

Assini J, Hamilton R, and Strosberg J Adverse reactions to azathioprine mimicking gastroenteritis. J Rheumatol 1986 13:1117–1118.

Athlin L, Domellof L, and Norberg B The phagocytosis of yeast cells by blood monocytes. Effects of therapeutic concentrations of Vinca alkaloids. Eur J Clin Pharmacol 1985 29(4):471–476.

Atkins JN Fluorouracil and the palmar-plantar erythrodysesthesia syndrome. Ann Intern Med 1985 102(3):419.

Au R, Rustum YM, Minowada J, Levenson CH, and Siravastava BIS Differential selectivity of 5-fluorouracil and its analogs, beta-D-4′ hydroxyforafur and 5′-deoxy-5-fluorouridine, in cultured human lymphocytes and mouse L1210 leukemia. Biochem Pharmacol 1983 32541–32546.

Bach JF and Strom TB The mode of action of immunosuppressive agents. 2nd Ed Research Monographs in Immunology Vol 9 Elsevier, Amsterdam 1985.

Bach MA and Bach JF Activities of immunosuppressive agents in vitro. II. Different timing of azathioprine and methotrexate in inhibition and stimulation of mixed lymphocyte reaction. Clin Exp Immunol 1972 11:89–98.

Bachur NR, Gordon SL and Gee MV A general mechanism for microsomal activation of quinone anticancer agents to free radicals. Cancer Res 1978 1745–1750.

Ballen KK and Weiss ST Fatal acute respiratory failure following vinblastine and mitomycin administration for breast cancer. Am J Med Sci 1988 295:558–560.

Behrens TW and Goodwin JS Glucocorticosteroids. In: Handbook of Exp Pharm 85: The Pharmacology of Lymphocytes Bray MA, Morley J Eds Springer-Verlag, Berlin, New York 1988 pp. 425–439.

Berd D, Mastrangelo MJ, Engstrom PF, Paul A, and Maguire HC Augmentation of the human immune response by cyclophosphamide. Cancer Res 1982 42:4862–4866.

Berd D, Maguire HC, and Mastrangelo MJ Augmentation of delayed type hypersensitivity to tumor-associated antigens by treatment with autologous tumor cell vaccine preceded by cyclophosphamide. Proc Amer Soc Clin Oncol 1983 2:56.

Berd D, Maguire HC, and Mastrangelo MJ Impairment of concanavalin A-inducible suppressor activity following administration of cyclophosphamide to patients with advanced cancer. Cancer Res 1984a 44:1275–1280.

Berd D, Maguire HC, and Mastrangelo MJ Potentiation of human cell-mediated and humoral immunity by low dose cyclophosphamide. Cancer Res 1984b 44:5439–5443.

Berd D and Mastrangelo MJ Elimination of immune suppressor mechanisms in humans by oxaphosphorines. Meth Find Exptl Clin Pharmacol 1987 9:569–577.

Berenbaum MD Dose-response curves for agents that impair cell reproductive integrity. Br J Cancer 1969 23:426–445.

Berenbaum MD Immunosuppression by platinum diamines. Br J Cancer 1971 25:208–211.

Beutler B, Krochin N, Milsark IW, Leudke C, and Cerami C Control of cachectin (tumor necrosis factor) synthesis: Mechanisms of endotoxin resistance. Science 1986 232:977–980.

Bianchi ATJ, Hussarts-Odijk LM, Bril H, de Ruiter H, and Benner R The long lasting state of specific nonresponsiveness induced by I.V. immunization with alloantigens is due to generation of recirculating suppressor T cells. Adv Exp Med Biol 1985 186:521–530.

Boerrigter GH and Scheper RJ Local administration of the cytostatic drug 4-hydroperoxy-cyclophosphamide (4-HPCY) facilitates cell-mediated immune reactions. Clin Exp Immunol 1984 58:161–166.

Bonadonna G, Delenar MD, Monfardini S, and Milani F Combination chemotherapy with adriamycin in malignant lymphoma. In: Adriamycin Review Ghent M Staquet eds European Press Medikon, 1975 pp. 200–215.

Borel Y and Schwartz R Inhibition of immediate and delayed hypersensitivity in rabbit by 6-mercaptopurine. J Immunol 1964 92:754–761.

Borel Y, Fauconnet M, and Miescher PA Effect of 6-mercaptopurine (6-MP) on different classes of antibody. J Exp Med 1965 122:263–275.

Borel Y, Fauconnet M, and Miescher PA The effect of 6-mercaptopurine (6-MP) and methotrexate (MTX) on passive delayed hypersensitivity reactions. Int Arch Allergy 1968 33:583–592.

Borella L and Green AA Sequestration of PHA-responsive cells (T-lymphocytes) in the bone marrow of leukemic children undergoing long-term immunosuppressive therapy. J Immunol 1972 109:927–932.

Boygo D and Mihich E Reversal of the in vitro methotrexate suppression of cell-mediated immune response by folinic acid and thymidine plus hypoxanthine. Cancer Res 1980 40:650–654.

Bovornkitti S, Kangsadal P, and Sathirapat P Reversion and reconversion rate of tuberculin skin reactions in correlation with the use of prednisone. Dis Chest 1960 38:51–55.

Breithaupt H and Huenzlen E High dose methotrexate for osteosarcoma: Toxicity and clinical results. Oncology 1983 40:85–89.

Broder S and Waldmann TA The suppressor-cell network in cancer. N Engl J Med 1978 299:1335–1341.

Brown TE, Ahmed A, Filo RS, Knudsen RC, and Sell KW The immunosuppressive mechanism of azathioprine. I. In vitro effect on lymphocyte function in the baboon. Transplantation 1976 21:27–35.

Bucy RP The effects of immunosuppressive pharmacological agents on the induction of cytotoxic and suppressor T lymphocytes in vitro. Immunopharmacol 1988 15:65–72.

Calabresi P and Parks RE Antiproliferative agents and drugs used for Immunosuppression. In: Goodman and Gilman's The Pharmacological Basis of Therapeutics Gilman AG, Goodman LS, Rall TW, and Murad F Eds 7th ed. MacMillan, 1985 pp. 1247–1307.

Carpen O The role of microtubules in human natural killer cell-mediated cytotoxicity. Cell Immunol 1987 106(2):376–386.

Carter SK Adriamycin-A review. JNCI 1975; 55:1265–1267.

Carter SK. The clinical evaluation of analogs. III. Anthracyclines. Cancer Chemother Pharmacol 1980 4:5.

Carter JJ, McLaughlin ML and Bern MM Bleomycin-induced fatal hyperpyrexia. Am J Med 1903 74:523–525.

Cesario TC, Slater LM, Kaplan HS, and Tilles JG Therapeutic concentrations of antineoplastic agents diminish interferon yields. Proc Soc Exp Biol Med 1982 171:92–97.

Cesario TC, Slater LM, Kaplan HS, Gupta S, and Gorse GJ Effect of antineoplastic agents on gamma-interferon production in human peripheral blood mononuclear cells. Cancer Res 1984 44:4962–4966.

Chabner BA and Myers CE Clinical pharmacology of cancer chemotherapy. In: Principles and Practice of Oncology DeVita VT, Hellman S, Rosenberg SA, Eds J.B. Lippincott, 1985 pp. 288–296.

Claman HN Corticosteroids and lymphoid cells. N Engl J Med 1972 287:388–397.

Cohen S, Salazar D, and Wicher J Adriamycin-induced activation of NK activity may initially involve LAF production. Cancer Immunol Immunother 1983 15:188.

Compton MM, Caron LAM, and Cidlowski JA Glucocorticoid action on the immune system. J Steroid Biochem 1987 27:201–208.

Cook JD, Lai W, and McGrane B The effect of sub-optimal concentrations of mitogens on the immunosuppressive action of azathioprine and prednisolone on human lymphocytes in vitro. J Immunopharmacol 1983 5:257–275.

Cooper C, Cotton D, Minihane N, and Cawley M Azathioprine hypersensitivity manifesting as acute focal hepatocellular necrosis. J R Soc Med 1986 70:171–173.

Cooper JAD, White DA, and Matthay RA Drug-induced pulmonary disease: Part 1, cytotoxic drugs. Am Rev Respir Dis 1986 133:321–340.

Cosgriff TM Doxorubicin and ventricular arrythmia Ann Intern Med 1980 92:434–435.

Crabtree GR, Munck A, and Smith KA Glucocorticoids and lymphocytes. II. Cell cycle-dependent changes in glucocorticoid receptor content. J Immunol 1980 125:13–17.

Creasey WA Vinca alkaloids and colclicine. In: Antineoplastic and Immuno-suppressive agents. II Sartorelli AC, Johns DG Eds Springer-Verlag, New York 1975 pp. 670–694.

Culpepper JA and Lee F Regulation of IL-3 expression by glucocorticoids in cloned murine T lymphocytes. J Immunol 1985 135:3191–3197.

Cunningham T, Barraclough D, and Muirden K Azathioprine induced shock. Br Med J 1982 283:623–624.

Cupps TR and Fauci AS Corticosteroid regulation in man. Immunol Rev 1982 65:134–155.

Cupps TR, Edgar LC, and Fauci AS Suppression of human B lymphocyte function by cyclophosphamide. J Immunol 1982 128:2453–2457.

Cupps TR, Gerrard TL, Falkoff RJM, Whalen G, and Fauci AS Effects of in vitro corticosteroids on B cell activation, proliferation, and differentiation. J Clin Invest 1985 75:754–761.

Curreri AR, Ansfield FJ, McIver FA, Waisman HA, and Heidelberger C Clinical studies with 5-fluorouracil. Cancer Res 1958 18:478–484.

daCosta M, Isacoff W, Rothenberg SP and Perwaiziqbal M Protein-methotrexate-IgG complexes in the serum of patients receiving high-dose antifolate therapy. Cancer 1980 46(1):471–474.

D'Adamio L, Cannarile L, Migliorati G, and Riccardi C In vitro generation of natural killer cells from SJL/J bone marrow precursors. J Biol Regul Homeostat Agents 1988 2:71–76.

Dalke AP, Kazmers IS, and Kelley WN Hypoxanthine-guanine phosphoribosyltransferase-independent toxicity of azathioprine in human lymphoblasts. Biochem Pharmacol 1984 33:2692–2695.

DeBeer R and Kabakow B Anaphylactoid reaction associated with intravenous administration of 5-fluorouracil. NY State J Med 1979 79:1750–1751.

Descamps B, Gagnon R, Van Der Gaag R, Meyer O, and Crosnier J Influence of azathioprine and prednisone in vivo treatment of lymphocyte-dependent antibody-mediated cytotoxicity (LDAC) in 57 human renal allograft recipients. Transplant Proc 1977 9:981–984.

Diamenstein T, Willinger E, and Reiman J T-suppressor cells sensitive to cyclophosphamide and to its in vitro active derivative 4-hydroperoxycyclophosphamide. Control of the mitogenic response of murine splenic B cells to dextran sulfate. J Exp Med 1979 150:1571–1576.

Diamenstein T, Klos M, Hahn H, and Kaufmann SHE Direct in vitro evidence for different susceptibilities to 4-hydroperoxy-cyclophosphamide of antigen-primed T cells regulating humoral and cell mediated immune responses to sheep erythrocytes: A possible explanation for the inverse action of cyclophosphamide on humoral and cell mediated immune responses. J Immunol 1981 126:1717–1719.

Dietrich FN and Hess R Hypersensitivity in mice. I. Induction of contact sensitivity to oxalone and inhibition by various chemical compounds. Int Arch Allergy 1970 38:246–255.

Dimitriu A and Fauci AS Activation of human B lymphocytes. XI. Differential effects of azathioprine on B lymphocytes and lymphocyte subpopulations regulating B cell function. J Immunol 1978 121:2335–2339.

Dinarello CA, Ward SB, and Wolff SM Pyrogenic properties of bleomycin (NSC-125066). Cancer Chemother Rep 1973 57:393–398.

Doyle LA, Berg C, Bottino G, and Chabner B. Erythema and desquamation after high-dose methotrexate. Ann Intern Med 1983 98:611–612.

Dupont E, Huygen K, Schandene L, Vandercruys M, Palfliet K, and Wybran J Influence of in vivo immunosuppressive drugs on production of lymphokines. Transplantation 1985 39:143–147.

Ehrke MJ and Mihich E Immunoregulation by cancer chemotherapeutic agents. In: The Reticuloendothelial System: A Comprehensive treatise JW Hadden, A Szentivanyi Eds Plenum Press, New York Vol. 8, 1985 pp. 309–347.

Ehrke MJ, Cohen SA, and Mihich E Selective effects of Adriamycin on murine host defense systems. Immunological Rev 1982 65:55–78.

Ehrke MJ, Ryoyama K, and Cohen SA Cellular basis for Adriamycin-induced augmentation of cell-mediated cytotoxicity in culture. Cancer Res 1984 44:2497–2504.

Ehrke MJ, Maccubbin D, Ryoyama K, Cohen SA, and Mihich E Correlation between Adriamycin-induced augmentation and of cell-mediated cytotoxicity in mice. Cancer Res 1986 46:54–60.

El-Assouli SM The molecular basis for the differential sensitivity of B and T lymphocytes to growth inhibition by thymidine and 5-fluorouracil. Leukemia Res 1985 9:391–398.

Eschalier A, Lavarenne J, Burtin C, Renoux M, Chapuy E, and Rodriguez M Study of histamine release induced by acute administration of antitumor agents in dogs. Cancer Chemother Pharmacol 1988 21:246–250.

Fauci AS Corticosteroids and circulating lymphocytes. Transplant Proc 1975b 7:37–40.

Fauci AS, and Dale DC The effect of hydrocortisone on the kinetics of normal human lymphocytes. Blood 1975a 46:235–243.

Fauci AS, Wolff SM, and Johnson JS Effect of cyclophosphamide on immune response in Wegener's granulomatosis. N Engl J Med 1971 285:1493–1496.

Fauci AS, Dale DC, and Balow JE Glucocorticosteroid therapy: Mechanisms of action and clinical considerations. Ann Intern Med 1976 84:304–315.

Feldman LD and Ajani JA Fluorouracil-associated dermatitis of the hands and feet. JAMA 1985 254:3479.

Forssen EA and Tokes ZA Improved therapeutic benefits of doxorubicin by entrapment in anionic liposomes. Cancer Res 1983 43:546–550.

Fournier C, Bach MA, Dardenne M, and Bach JF Selective action of azathioprine on T cells. Transplant Proc 1973 5:523–526.

Friedman RM, Buckler CG, and Baron S The effect of aminopteroylglutamic acid in the development of skin hypersensitivity and on antibody formation in guinea pigs. J Exp Med 1961 114:173–183.

Gabizon A, Dagan A, Goren D, Barenholtz Y, and Guks Z Liposomes as in vivo carriers of Adriamycin: Reduced cardiac uptake and preserved antitumor activity in mice. Cancer Res 1982 42:4734–4739.

Gabizon A, Sulkes A, Peretz T, Druckman S, Goren D, Amselem S, and Barenbholtz Y Liposome-associated Doxorubicin: Preclinical pharmacology and exploratory clinical phase. In: Liposomes in the Therapy of Infectious Disease and Cancer Lopez-Berestein G, Fidler IS Eds AR Liss, New York 1989 pp. 391–402.

Galanaud P, Crevon MC, and Dormaont J Effect of azathioprine on in vitro antibody response. Differential effect on B cell involved in thymus-dependent and independent responses. Clin Exp Immunol 1975 22:139–152.

Galili N, Galili U, and Klein E. Human T lymphocytes become glucocorticoid-sensitive upon immune activation. Cell Immunol 1980 50:440–444.

Gatti G, Cavallo R, Sartori ML, del Ponte D, Masera R, Salvadori A, Carignola R, and Angeli A Inhibition by cortisol of human natural killer (NK) cell activity. J Steroid Biochem 1987 26(1):49–58.

Gell PGH and Coombs RRA Clinical aspects of immunology. Gell GH, Coombs RRA Eds Blackwell Scientific Publications, Oxford 1975.

Gereis M, Burford-Mason AP, and Watkins SM Suppression of in vitro peripheral blood lymphocyte mitogenesis by cytotoxic drugs commonly used in the treatment of breast cancer: A comparative study. Agents and Actions 1987 22:324–329.

Gilman A The initial clinical trial of nitrogen mustard. Am J Surg 1963 105:574–578.

Gillis S, Crabtree GR, and Smith KA Glucocorticoid-induced inhibition of T-cell growth factor production. I. The effect of mitogen induced lymphocyte proliferation. J Immunol 1979a 123:1624–1631.

Gillis S, Crabtree GR, and Smith KA Glucocorticoid-induced inhibition of T-cell growth factor production. II. The effect of the in vitro generation of cytolytic T cells. J Immunol 1979b 123:1632–1638.

Ginsberg SJ and Comis RL The pulmonary toxicity of antineoplastic agents. Semin Oncol 1982 9:34–51.

Goekin N Activity of Con A-induced suppressor cells in human MLR: Differential effects on primary MLR, secondary MLR and memory cell precursors. J Immunol 1982 128:2081–2086.

Gordon D and Nouri AME Comparison of the inhibition by glucocorticosteroids and cyclosporin A of mitogen stimulated human lymphocyte proliferation. Clin Exp Immunol 1981 44:287–294.

Gorse GJ and Kopp WC Modulation by immunosuppressive agents of peripheral blood mononuclear cell responses to influenza A virus. J Lab Clin Med 1987 110:592–601.

Gorse GJ, Slater LM, Kaplan HS, Tilles JG, and Cesario TC Inhibition of interferon yield by vincristine. Proc Soc Exp Biol Med 1984 175(3):309–313.

Grabstein K, Dower S, Gillis S, Urdal D, and Larsen A Expression of interleukin 2, interferon-gamma and the IL-2 receptor by human peripheral blood lymphocytes. J Immunol 1986 136:4503–4508.

Greenberg PD, Cheever MA, and Fefer A Eradication of disseminated murine leukemia by chemoimmunotherapy with cyclophosphamide and adoptively transferred immune syngeneic LY-1-2-lymphocytes J Exp Med 1981 154:952–963.

Guyre PM, Girard PM, and Manganiello PD Glucocorticoid effects on the production and actions of immune cytokines. J Steroid Biochem 1988 30:89–93.

Haanen C and Hillen G Combination chemotherapy with doxorubicin in "bad risk" leukemia patients. In: Adriamycin Review. Ghent, European Press Medixon 1975 pp. 193–199.

Hahn BH, MacDermott RP, Jacobs SB, Pletscher LS, and Beale MG Immunosuppressive effects of low doses of glucocorticoids: Effects on autologous and allogeneic mixed leukocyte reactions. J Immunol 1980 124:2812–2817.

Hamied TAA and Turk JL Enhancement of interleukin-2 release in rats by treatment with bleomycin and adriamycin in vivo. Cancer Immunol Immunother 1987 25:245–249.

Harmon JM, Norman MR, Fowles BJ, and Thompson EB Dexamethasone induces irreversible G1 arrest and death of a human lymphoid cell line. J Cell Physiol 1979 98:267–278.

Haskill JS Adramycin-activated macrophages as tumor growth inhibitors Cancer Res 1981 41(5):3852–3856.

Hatfield AK, Harder L, and Abderhalden RT Chronic urticarial reactions caused by doxorubicin-containing regimens. Cancer Treat Rep 1981 65:353–354.

Hektoen L and Corper HJ The effect of mustard gas (Dichloroethyl-sulfide) on antibody formation. J Infect Dis 1921 28:279–283.

Heppner GH and Calabresi P Selective suppression of humoral immunity by antineoplastic drugs Ann Rev Pharmacol Toxicol 1976 16:367–379.

Herman E, Rahman A, Ferrans V, Vick J, and Schein P Prevention of chronic doxorubicin toxicity in beagles by liposomal encapsulation. Cancer Res 1983 43:5427–5432.

Hersh EM, Carbone P, Wong VG, and Freireich EJ Inhibition of the primary immune response in man by antimetabolites. Cancer Res 1965 25:997–1001.

Hirata F, Stracke ML, and Schiffmann E Regulation of prostaglandin formation by glucocorticoids and their second messenger, lipocortins. J Steroid Biochem 1987 27:1053–1056.

Hirata F Roles of lipomodulin, a phospholipase inhibitory protein in immunoregulation. Adv Inflammation Res 1984 7:71–78.

Hoelzer KL, Harrison BR, Luedke SW, and Luedke DW Vinblastine-associated pulmonary toxicity in patients receiving combination therapy with mitomycin and cisplatin. Drug Intell Clin Pharm 1986 20:287–289.

Holbrook NJ, Cox WI, and Horner HC Direct suppression of natural killer activity in human peripheral blood leukocyte cultures by glucocorticoids and its modulation by interferon. Cancer Res 1983 43:4019–4025.

Howle JA, Thompson HS, Stone AE, and Gale GR Cis-dichlorodiammineplatinum(II): Inhibition of nucleic acid synthesis in lymphocytes stimulated with phytohemagglutinin. Proc Soc Exp Biol Med 1971 137:820–825.

Hudson MM, Snyder JS, Jaffe N, and Kleinerman E In vitro and in vivo effect of adriamycin therapy on monocyte activation by liposome-encapsulated immunomodulators. Cancer Res 1988 48:5256–5263.

Humphrey GB, Nesbit ME, Chary KKN, and Krivit W Impaired lymphocyte transformation in leukemic patients after intensive therapy. Cancer 1972 29:402–406.

Jackson RC Biological effects of folic acid antagonists with antineoplastic activity. Pharmacol Ther 1984 25:61–82.

Johnson LK, Longnecker JP, and Baxter JD Glucocorticoid action: A mechanism involving nuclear and non-nuclear pathways. Br J Dermatol 1982 (suppl) 23:6–23.

Johnson RK, Garibjanian BT, Houchens DP, Kline I, Gaston MR, Syrkin AB, and Goldin A Comparison of 5-flurouracil and ftorafur. I. Quantitative and Qualitative differences in toxicity to mice. Cancer Treat Rep 1976 60:1335–1345.

Kahn A and Hill JM Immunosuppression with cis-platinum (II) diamminodichloride: Effect on antibody plaque-forming spleen cells. Infect Immun 1971 4:320–321.

Kahn A and Hill JM Suppression of lymphocyte blastogenesis in man following cis-platinum diamminodichloride administration. Proc Soc Exp Biol Med 1973 142:324–326.

Karavodin LM and Golub SH Immunocompetence in cancer patients. In: Basic and Clinical Tumor Immunology Herberman RB Ed Martinus Nijhoff, Boston 1983 pp. 215–256.

Katz P and Fauci AS Autologous and allogeneic intercellular interactions: Modulation by adherent cells, irradiation, and in vitro or in vivo corticosteroids. J Immunol 1979 123:2270–2277.

Katz P, Zaytoun AM, and Lee JH The effects of in vivo hydrocortisone on lymphocyte mediated cytotoxicity. Arthritis Rheum 1984 27:72–78.

Kaufmann SHE, Hahn H, and Diamenstein T Relative susceptibilities of T cell subsets involved in delayed type hypersensitivity of sheep red blood cells to the in vitro action of 4-hydroperoxycyclophosphamide. J Immunol 1980 125:1104–1108.

Kazmers IS, Daddona PE, Dalke AP, and Kelley WN Effect of immunosuppressive agents on human T and B lymphoblasts. Biochem Pharmacol 1983 32:805–810.

Kedar E, Bercowitz, Katz-Gross A, and Chriqui-Zeira E Stimulatory and suppressive effects of anticancer drugs and x-irradiation on the production of interleukin-2 by murine lymphoid cells. Immunopharmacol 1986 11:61–65.

Kelly AP, Schooley RT, Rubin RH, and Hirsh MS Effect of interferon alpha on natural killer cell cytotoxicity in kidney transplant recipients. Clin Immunol Immunopathol 1984 32:20–28.

Kelso A and Munck A Glucocorticoid inhibition of lymphokine secretion by alloreactive T lymphocyte clones. J Immunol 1984 133:784–791.

Keown PA and Stiller CR Control of rejection of transplanted organs. Adv Intern Med 1986 31:17–46.

Kettman J, Skarval H, and Mathews M Delayed-type hypersensitivity in the mouse: Effect of vinblastine on sensitization by sheep red blood cells. Immunopharmacology 1979 2:73–82.

Kim HC, Kesarwala HH, Colvin M, and Saidi P Hypersensitivity reaction to a metabolite of cyclophosphamide. J Allergy Clin Immunol 1985 76:591–594.

King J, Laver M, Fairley K, and Ames G Sensitivity to azathioprine. Med J Aust 1972 2:939–941.

Kleinerman ES, Zwelling LA, and Muchmore AV Enhancement of naturally occurring human spontaneous monocyte-mediated cytotoxicity by cis-diammino-dichloroplatinum(II). Cancer Res 1980b 40:3099–3102.

Kleinerman ES, Zwelling LA, and Muchmore AV Enhancement of naturally occurring human spontaneous monocyte-mediated cytotoxicity by cis-diammino-dischloroplatinum(II). Cancer Res 1980b 40:3099–3102.

Kleinerman ES and Zwelling LA The effect of cis-diammino-dichloroplatinum(II) on immune function in vitro and in vivo. Cancer Immunol Immunother 1982 12:191–196.

Klimo P and Ibrahim E Anaphylactic reaction to methotrexate in high doses as adjuvant treatment of osteogenic sarcoma. Cancer Treat Rep 1981 65:725.

Kohler PC, Hank JA, Exten R, Minkhoff DZ, Wilson DG, and Sondel PM Clinical response of a patient with diffuse histiocytic lymphoma to adoptive chemoimmunotherapy using cyclophosphamide and alloactivated haploidentical lymphocytes. A case report and phase I trial. Cancer 1985 55:552–560.

Kris MG, Pablo D, Gralla RJ, Burke MT, Prestifilippo J, and Lewin D Dyspnea following vinblastine or vindesine administration in patients receiving mitomycin plus vinca alkaloid combination therapy. Cancer Treat Rep 1984 68:1029–1031.

Krumbhaar EB Role of the blood and bone marrow in certain forms of gas poisoning. I. JAMA 1919 72:39–41.

Kunin CM, Schwartz R, Yaffe S, Knapp J, Fellers FX, Janeway CA, and Finland M Antibody response to influenza virus vaccine in children with nephrosis: Effects of cortisone. Pediatrics 1959 23:54–62.

Lakin JD and Cahill RA Generalized urticaria to cyclophosphamide: Type I hypersensitivity to an immunosuppressive agent. J Allergy Clin Immunol 1976 58:160–171.

Lehane DE and Lane M The immunopharmacology of bleomycin in man. In: Bleomycin. Current Status and New Developments. Cater SK and Crooke ST Eds Academic Press, New York 1978 pp. 143–150.

Levandowski RA Doxorubicin and the heart. Ann Intern Med 1980 92:866–867.

Levin RJ, Landy M, and Frei E The effect of 6-mercaptopurine on the immune response in man. N Engl J Med 1964 271:16–22.

Levine AS, Schimpff SC, Graw RG, and Young RC Hematologic malignancies and other marrow failure states: Progress in the management of complicating infections. Semin Hematol 1974 11:141–202.

Levy RL and Chiarillo S Hyperpyrexia, allergic-type response and death occurring with low-dose bleomycin administration. Oncology 1980 37:316–317.

Lichtenstein AK and Pende D Enhancement of natural killer cell cytotoxicity by cis-diamminedichloroplatinum (II) in vivo and in vitro. Cancer Res 1986 46:639–644.

Lipinski M, Tursz, T, Kreis H, Finaley Y, and Amiel JL Dissociation of natural killer cells activity and antibody-dependent cell-mediated cytotoxicity in kidney allograft recipients receiving high dose immunosuppressive therapy. Transplantation 1980 29:214–218.

Lippman ME, Halterman RH, Leventhal BG, Perry S, and Thompson EB Glucocorticoid-binding protein in human adult lymphoblastic leukemia. J Clin Invest 1973 52:1715.

Lippman ME, Perry S, and Thompson EB Cytoplasmic glucocorticoid-binding protein in glucocorticoid-unresponsive human and mouse leukemic cell lines. Cancer Res 1974 34:1572–1576.

Lippman ME and Barr R Glucocorticoid receptors in purified subpopulations of human peripheral blood lymphocytes. J Immunol 1977 118:1977–1981.

Lokick JJ and Moore C Chemotherapy-associated palmar-plantar erythrodyesthesia syndrome. Ann Intern Med 1984 101:798–800.

Mace K, Mayhew E, Mihich E, and Ehrke MJ Alterations in murine host defense functions by adriamycin or liposome-encapsulated adriamycin. Cancer Res 1988 48:130–136.

Maguire HC and Ettore VL Enhancement of dinitrochlorobenzene (DNCB) contact sensitization by cyclophosphamide in the guinea pig. J Invest Dermatol 1967 48:39–43.

Majors G and Moore P Profound circulatory collapse due to azathioprine. J R Soc Med 1985 78:1052–1053.

Mansour A and Nelson DS Effect of treatment with azathioprine on the responses of rat lymphocytes to phytohemagglutinin. Aust J Exp Biol Med Sci 1979 57:115–125.

Mansour A, Herderson JA and Nelson DS Effect of methotrexate on the response of rat lymphocytes to phytohaemagglutin. Clin Exp Immunol 1978 34:393–401.

Marks CR, Willkens RF, Wilske KR, and Brown PB Small vessel vasculitis and methotrexate. Ann Intern Med 1984 100:916.

Martin F, Caignard A, Olsson O, Jeannin JF, and Leclerc A Tumoricidal effect of macrophages exposed to Adriamycin in vivo or in vitro. Cancer Res 1982 42:3851–3857.

Matheson DS, Green B, and Hoar DI The influence of methotrexate and thymidine on the human natural killer function in vitro. J Immunol 1983 131:1619–1621.

McCrea ES, Diaconis JN, and Wade JC Bleomycin toxicity simulating metastatic nodules to the lungs. Cancer 1981 48:1096–1100.

Merluzzi VJ, Last-Barney K, Susskind BM, and Faanes RB Recovery of humoral and cellular immunity by soluble mediators after 5-fluorouracil-induced immunosuppression. Clin Exp Immunol 1982 50:318–326.

Meuleman J and Katz P The immunologic effects, kinetics, and use of glucocorticoids. Med Clin N America 1985 69:805–816.

Middleman E, Luce J, and Frei E Clinical trials with adriamycin. Cancer 1971 28:844–850.

Mihich E Immunomodulation by adriamycin. Sci Rep Res Inst Tohoku Univ 1985a 32:10–13.

Mihich E and Ehrke MJ Immunomodulation by anticancer compounds. In: Advances in Immunopharmacology 3 Chedid L, Hadden JW, Spreafico F, Dukor P, and Willoughby Eds Pergamon Press, Oxford 1985 pp. 257–265.

Miller FR and Kataoka T Interactions of antimetabolites with tumors and the immune system. In: Biological Responses in Cancer, Vol. 3, Immunomodulation by Anticancer Drugs Mihich E and Sakurai Y Eds Plenum Press, New York 1985 pp. 33–70.

Mitchell MS, Wade ME, DeConti RC, Bertino JR, and Calabresi P Immunosuppressive effects of cytosine arabinoside and methotrexate in man. Ann Intern Med 1969 70:535.

Mitchell MS and DeConti RC Immunosuppression by 5-fluorouracil. Cancer 1970 26:884–889.

Moreau JF, Soulillou JP, Ythier A, Hegaret A, and Fauconnie R Decrease in natural killer cell activity in kidney allograft recipients. Ann Immunol (Inst Pasteur) 1983 134C:191–205.

Morikawa K, Hosokawa M, Hamada J, Sugawara M, and Kobayashi H Host-mediated therapeutic effects produced by appropriately timed administration of bleomycin on a rat fibrosarcoma. Cancer Res 1985 45:1502–1506.

Munck A and Crabtree GR Glucocorticoid-induced lymphocyte death. In: Cell Death in Biology and Pathology Bowen ID, Lockshin RA eds Chapman and Hall, London, 1981 pp. 329–359.

Nair MPN and Schwartz SA Immunomodulatory effects of corticosteroids on natural killer and antibody-dependent cellular cytotoxic activities of human lymphocytes. J Immunol 1984 132:2876–2882.

Noble RL, Gout PW, Wijicik LL, Hebden F, and Beer CT The distribution of [^{3}H] vinblastine in tumor and host tissues of Nb rats bearing a transplantable lymphoma which is highly sensitive to the alkaloid. Cancer Res 1977 37:1455–1460.

Nordman E, Saarimaa H, and Toivand A The influence of 5-flurouracil on cellular and humoral immunity in cancer patients. Cancer 1978 41:64–69.

Norman MR and Thompson EB Characterization of a glucocorticoid-sensitive human lymphoid cell line. Cancer Res 1977 37:3785–3791.

Ohno R, Nishiwaki H, Kawashima K, Uetani T, Hirano M, Miura M, and Yamada K Lack of immunosuppressive effect of bleomycin on the primary response of mice to sheep red blood cells. Gann Monogr Cancer Res 1971 62:267–274.

Ohta Y, Sueki K, Kitta K, Takemoto K, Hideo I, and Yagi Y Comparative studies on the immunosuppressive effect among 5′-deoxy-5-fluorourdine, ftorafur, and 5-fluorouracil. Gann 1980 71:190–196.

Ohnuma T, Arkin H, and Holland JF Differences in chemotherapeutic susceptibility of human T-, B-, and non-T, non-B lymphoctyes in culture. Recent results. Cancer Res 1980 75:61–67.

Ohnuma T, Arkin H, Minowada J, and Holland JF Differential chemotherapeutic susceptibility of human T-lymphocytes and B-lymphocytes in culture. JNCI 1978 60:749–752.

O'Malley BW Steroid action in eucaryotic cells. J Clin Invest 1984 74:307–312.

O'meara, A, Headon B, and Reen DJ Effect of methotrexate on the immune response of children with acute lymphatic leukemia. Immunopharmacol 1985a 9:33–38.

O'meara A, Brazil J, and Reen DJ The effect of methotrexate on in vitro immunoglobulin production. J Immunopharm 1985b 7:235–245.

Onsrud M and Thorsby E Influence of in vivo hydrocortisone on some human blood lymphocyte populations. Scand J Immun 1981 13:573–579.

Onsrud M, Bosnes V, and Grahm I cis-platin as adjunctive to surgery in early stage ovarian carcinoma: Effects on lymphoid cell subpopulations. Gynecol Oncol 1986 23:323–328.

Orsini F, Pavelic Z, and Mihich E Increased primary cell mediated immunity in culture subsequent to adriamycin or daunorubicin treatment of spleen donor mice. Cancer Res 1977 37:1719–1726.

Orsini F, Eppolito C, Ehrke MJ, and Mihich E Inhibition by selected anticancer agents of the development of primary cell-mediated immunity against allogeneic tumor cells in culture. Cancer Treat Rep 1980 64:211–218.

Owellen RJ, Owens AH, and Donigian DW The binding of vincristine, vinblastine and colchicine to tubulin. Biochem Biophys Res Comm 1972 47:685–691.

Ozer H Effects of aklylating agents on immunoregulatory mechanisms. In: Biological Responses in Cancer, Vol 3 Mihich E and Sakuri Y eds Plenum Press, New York 1985, pp. 95–130.

Ozer H, Cowens JW, Colvin M, Nussbaum-Blumenson A, and Sheedy D In vitro effects of 4-hydroperoxycyclophosphamide on human immunoregulatory T subset function. I. Selective effects on lymphocyte function in T-B cell collaboration. J Exp Med 1982 155:276–290.

Page D, Posen G, Stewart T, and Harris J Immunological detection of renal allograft rejection in man. Increased deoxynucleic acid synthesis by peripheral lymphoid cells. Transplantation 1971 12:341–347.

Pascoe JM and Roberts JJ Interactions between mamamalian cell DNA and inorganic platinum compounds. I. DNA interstrand cross-linking and cytotoxic properties of platinum(II) compounds. Biochem Pharmacol 1974 23:1345–1357.

Parker D and Turk JL Potentiation of T-lymphocyte function by bleomycin. Immunopharmacol 1984 7:109–113.

Parrillo JE and Fauci AS Mechanisms of glucocorticoid action on immune processes. Ann Rev Pharmacol Toxicol 1979 19:179–201.

Pedersen BK and Beyer JM A longitudinal study of the influence of azathioprine on natural killer cell activity. Allergy 1986 41:286–289.

Perry MC and Yarbo JW Beneficial effects of chemotherapy. In: Toxicity of Chemotherapy Perry MC and Yarbo JW eds Grune & Stratton, Orlando 1984.

Perry S, Irvin GL, and Whang J Studies of lymphocyte kinetics in man. Blood 1967 29:22–28.

Pinkerton CR, Welshman SG, and Bridges JM Serum profiles of methotrexate after its administration in children with ALL. Br J Cancer 1982 45:300–303.

Piper AA and Fox RM Biochemical basis for the differential sensitivity of human T- and B-lymphocyte lines to 5-fluorouracil. Cancer Res 1982 42:3753–3760.

Polak L and Turk JL Reversal of immunological tolerance by cyclophosphamide through inhibition of suppressor cell activity. Nature 1974 249:654–656.

Polak L, Geleick H, and Turk JL Reversal of contact sensitization with cyclophosphamide. Immunology 1975 29:939–942.

Posey WC, Nelson HS, and Pearlman DS The effects of acute corticosteroid therapy for asthma on serum immunoglobulin levels. J Allergy Clin Immunol 1978 62:340–348.

Powderly WG, Pier GB, and Markham RB In vitro T cell-mediated killing of Pseudomonas aeruginosa. IV: Nonresponsiveness in polysaccharide immunized BALB/c mice is attributable to vinblastine-sensitive suppressor T cells. J Immunol 1986 137:2025–2030.

Powderly WG, Pier GB, and Markham RB In vitro T cell-mediated killing of pseudomonas aeruginosa. V. Generation of bactericidal T cells in nonresponder mice. J Immunol 1987 138:2272–2277.

Prados M Hypersensitivity reactions to adriamycin: Two case reports. J LA State Med Soc 1981 133:154–155.

Prince HE, Ettenger RB, Dorey FJ, Fine RN, and Fahey JL Azathioprine suppression of natural killer activity and antibody-dependent cellular cytotoxicity in renal transplant recipients. J Clin Immunol 1984 4:312–318.

Rahman A, White G, More N, and Schein PS Pharmacological, toxicological, and therapeutic evaluation in mice of doxorubicin entrapped in cardiolipin liposomes. Cancer Res 1985 45:796–803.

Rahman A, Fumagalli A, Barbieri B, Schein PS, and Cabazza AM Antitumor and toxicity evaluation of free doxorubicin and doxorubicin entrapped in cardiolipin liposomes. Cancer Chemother Pharmacol 1986a 16:22–27.

Rahman A, Ganjei A, and Neefe JR Comparative immunotoxicity of free doxorubicin and doxorubicin encapsulated in cardiolipin liposomes. Cancer Chemother Pharmacol 1986b 16:28–34.

Rahman A, Roh JK, and Treat J Preclinical and clinical pharmacology of doxorubicin entrapped in cardiolipin liposomes. In: Liposomes in the Therapy of Infectious Disease and Cancer. Lopez-Berestein G and Fidler IS Eds AR Liss, New York 1989 pp. 367–389.

Ralph P and Nakoinz I Augmentation of macrophage antibody-dependent killing of tumor targets by microtubule inhibitors. Cell Immunol 1982 70:321–329.

Ramsey KM, Djeu JY, and Rook AH Decreased circulating large granular lymphocytes associated with depressed natural killer cell activity in renal transplant recipients. Transplantation 1984 38:351–356.

Rao SX, Ramaswamy G, Levin M, and McCravey JW Fatal acute respiratory failure after vinblastine-mitomycin therapy in lung carcinoma. Arch Intern Med 1985 145:1905–1907.

Rinehart JJ, Louis RP, and Baleerzak SP Adriamycin cardiotoxicity in man. Ann Intern Med 1974 81:475–478.

Rollinghoff M, Schrader J, and Wagner H Effect of azathioprine and cytosine arabinoside on humoral and cellular immunity in vitro. Clin Exp Immunol 1973 15:261–269.

Rosenberg B Possible mechanisms for antitumor activity of platinum coordination complexes. Cancer Chemother Rep 1975 59:589–598.

Rosenthal E Azathioprine shock. Postgrad Med J 1986 62:677–678.

Rosenthal GJ, Germolec DR, Lamm KR, Ackermann MF, and Luster MI Comparative effects on the immune system by methotrexate and trimetrexate. Int J Immunopharmacol 1987 9:793–801.

Rosenthal GJ, Weigand GW, Germolec DR, Blank JA, and Luster MI Suppression of B-cell function by methotrexate and trimetrexate. Evidence for inhibition of purine biosynthesis as a major mechanism of action. J Immunol 1988 141:410–416.

Rowley MJ, Mackay IR, and Mckenzie IFC Antibody production in immunosuppressed recipients of renal allografts. Lancet 1969 2:708–710.

Ryoyama K, Mace K, Ehrke MJ, and Mihich E The differential sensitivity of T cell immune functions to vincristine and vinblastine. Int J Immunopharmacol 1982 4:187–193.

Sahasrabudhe DM, et al. Specific immunotherapy with suppressor function inhibition for metastatic renal cell carcinoma. J Biol Resp Mod 1986 5:581–594.

Salazar D and Cohen SA Multiple tumoricidal effector mechanisms induced by adriamycin. Cancer Res 1984 44:2561–2566.

Samuels LL and Straw JA Improved therapeutic index with high dose methotrexate: Comparison of thymidine-purine rescue with citrovorum factor rescue in mice. Cancer Res 1984 44:2278–2284.

Santoni A, Riccardi C, Sorci V, and Herberman RB Effects of adriamycin on the activity of mouse natural killer cells. J Immunol 1980 124:2329–2335.

Santos AM and Medina FS Anaphylactic reaction following IV administration of 5-fluorouracil. Cancer Treat Rep 1986 70:1346–1354.

Santos GW Immunosuppressive drugs. Fed Proc 1967 26:907–913.

Santos GW, Owens AH, and Sensenbrenner LL Effects of selected cytotoxic agents on antibody production in man, a preliminary report. Ann NY Acad Sci 1964 114:404–423.

Santos GW, Burke PJ, Sensenbrenner LL, and Owens AM Rationale for the use of cyclophosphamide as an immunosuppressant for marrow transplantation in man. In: Pharmacological Treatments in Organ and Tissue Transplantation Bertelli A and Monaco AP Eds Excerpta Medica, Amsterdam 1970 p. 24.

Sarneva M, Vujanovic NL, Van den Brink MR, Herberman RB, and Hiserodt JC Lymphokine-activated killer cells from bone marrow progenitor cells. Cell Immunol 1989 118:448–457.

Saway PA, Heck LW, Bonner JR, and Kirklin JK Azathioprine hypersensitivity: Case report and review of the literature. Am J Med 1988 84:960–964.

Scharstein R, Johnson JF, Cook BA and Stephenson SR Bleomycin nodules mimicking metastatic osteogenic sarcoma. Am J Pediatr Hematol Oncol 1987 9(3):219–221.

Schlaefli E, Ehrke MJ, and Mihich E The effects of dichloro-trans-dihydroxy-bis-isopropyl-amine platinum IV on the primary cell-mediated cytotoxic response. Immunopharmacology 1983 6:107–122.

Schmidt TJ and Hitwack G Activation of the glucocorticoid-receptor complex. Phys Rev 1982 62:1131–1192.

Schwartz HS and Grindey GB Adriamycin and daunorubicin: A comparison of anti-tumor activities and tissue uptake in mice following immunosuppression. Cancer Res 1973 33:1837–1844.

Schwartz R and Dameshek W Drug-induced immunological tolerance. Nature 1959 185:1682–1683.

Schwartz RS and Dameshek W The role of antigen dosage in drug-induced immunologic tolerance. J Immunol 1963 90:703–710.

Schwartz RS Specificity of immunosuppression by antimetabolites. Proc Fed Am Soc Exp Biol 1966 25:165–168.

Shand FL and Howard JG Induction of in vitro reversible immunosuppression and inhibition of B cell receptor generation by defined metabolites of cyclophosphamide. Eur J Immunol 1979 9:17–21.

Sharma B and Vaziri ND Augmentation of human natural killer cell activity by cyclophosphamide in vitro. Cancer Res 1984 44:3258–3261.

Shih WWH, Ellison GW, Myers LW, Durkos-Smith D, and Fahey LL Locus of selective depression of human natural killer cells by azathioprine. Clin Immunol Immunopathol 1982 23:672–681.

Sloth K and Thomsen A Acute renal insufficiency during treatment with azathioprine. Acta Med Scand 1971 189:145–148.

Spina CA Azathioprine as an immunomodulating drug: Clinical applications. Clin Immunol Allergy 1984 4:415–446.

Spreafico F and Ancelerio A Immunosuppressive agents. In: Immunopharmacology Hadden JW, Coffey RG and Spreafico F Eds Plenum Press, New York 1977 pp. 245–278.

Spreafico F and Vecchi A The immunomodulatory activity of certain cancer chemotherapeutic agents. In: Biological Responses in Cancer, Vol 3, Immunomodulation by Anticancer Drugs Mihich E and Sakurai Y Eds Plenum Press, New York 1985 pp. 131–154.

Smith JJ, Mihich E, and Ozer H In vitro effects of 4-hydroperoxycyclophosphamide on human immunoregulatory T subset function. Meth Find Exptl Clin Pharmacol 1987 9:555–568.

Snyder DS and Unanue ER Corticosteroids inhibit murine macrophage la expression and interleukin 1 production. J Immunol 1982 129:1803–1805.

Sodhi A and Singh SM Increased capacity of lymphocytes to lyse tumor cells in vitro and production of lymphotoxins after cisplatin treatment. Int J Immunopharmacol 1988 10:753–761.

Sostman HD, Matthay RA, Putman CE, and Smith GJW Methotrexate-induced pneumonitis. Medicine 1976 55:371–388.

Sridhar KS Allergic reaction to 5-fluorouracil infusion. Cancer 1986 58:862–864.

Srivastava BIS and Alderfer JL Differential cytotoxicity of some fluorinated derivatives against human leukemic cell lines. Proc Amer Assoc Cancer Res 1982 23:216.

Staruch MJ and Wood DD Reduction of serum interleukin-1-like activity after treatment with dexamethasone. J Leukocyte Biol 1985 37:193–207.

Stoychkov JN, Schultz RM, Chirigos MA, Paulidis NA and Goldin A Effects of adriamycin and cyclophosphamide treatment on induction of macrophage cytotoxic function in mice. Cancer Res 1979 39:3014–3017.

Swanson HA and Schwartz RS Immunosuppressive therapy. The relation between clinical response and immunologic competence. N Engl J Med 1967 277:163–170.

Taylor IW and Tattersall MH Methotrexate cytotoxicity in cultured human leukemic cells by flow cytometry. Cancer Res 1981 41:1549–1558.

Thompson HS and Gale GR Cis-Dichlorodiamminoplatinum(II): Hematopoietic effects in rats. Toxicol Appl Pharmacol 1971 19:602–609.

Tomazic V, Ehrke MJ, and Mihich E Modulation of the cytotoxic response against allogeneic tumor cells in culture by adriamycin. Cancer Res 1980 40:2748–2755.

Treat J, Greenspan AR, and Rahman A Liposome encapsulated doxorubicin: Preliminary results of Phase I and Phase II trials. In: Liposomes in the Therapy of Infectious Disease and Cancer Lopez-Berestein G Fidler IS eds AR Liss, New York 1989 pp. 353–365.

Tritton TR and Yee G The anticancer agent adriamycin can be cytotoxic without entering cells. Science 1982 217:248–250.

Tuchinda M, Newcomb RW and De Vald BL Effect of prednisone treatment on the human immune response to keyhold limpet hemocyanin. Int Arch Allergy 1972 42:533–544.

Turk JL Enhancement of the delayed-type hypersensitivity reaction by oxaphosphorines. Meth Find Exptl Clin Pharmacol 1987 9:605–610.

Turk JL and Parker D Effect of cyclophosphamide on immunological control mechanisms. Immunol Rev 1982 65:99–113.

Turk JL and Poulter LW Selective depletion of lymphoid tissue by cyclophosphamide. Clin Exp Immunol 1972a 10:285–296.

Turk JL, Parker D, and Poulter LW Functional aspects of the selective depletion of lymphoid tissue by cyclophosphamide. Immunology 1972b 23:493–501.

Vancurova M, Prochazkova J, and Krejsek J Monitoring of effects of cis-diamminodichloroplatinum(II). Part III. Effect of platinum complexes on PHA-stimulated proliferation of human peripheral mononuclear cells in vitro. Neoplasma 1986 33:345–353.

Vetvicka V, Kincade PW, and Witte PL Effects of 5-fluorouracil on B lymphocyte lineage cells. J Immunol 1986 137:2405–2410.

Wade JC and Schimpff SC Epidemiology and prevention of infection in the compromised host. In: Clinical Approach to Infection in the Compromised Host Rubin RH and Young LS Eds Plenum Press, 1988.

Wands JR, Chura CM, Roll FJ, and Maddrey WC Serial studies of hepatitis associated antigen and antibody in patients receiving anti-tumor chemotherapy for myeloproliferative and lymphoproliferative disorders. Gastroenterology 1975 68(1):105–112.

Wang JJ, Cortes E, Sinks LF, and Holland JF Therapeutic effect and toxicity of adriamycin in patients with neoplastic disease. Cancer 1971 28:837–843.

Wierda D and Pazdernik TL Suppression of spleen lymphocyte mitogenesis in mice injected with platinum compounds. Eur J Cancer 1979 15:1013–1023.

Weiss RB Hypersensitivity reactions to cancer chemotherapy. Semin Oncol 1982 9:5–13.

Weiss RB Hypersensitivity reactions to cancer chemotherapy. In: Toxicity of Chemotherapy Perry MC and Yarbro JW Eds, Grune and Stratton, Inc., Orlando 1984 pp. 101–123.

Weiss RB and Bruno S Hypersensitivity reactions to cancer chemotherapeutic agents. Ann Intern Med 1981 94:66–72.

Weiss RB, James WD, Major WB, Porter MB, Allegra CJ, and Curt GA Skin reactions induced by trimetrexate, an analog of methotrexate. Invest New Drugs 1986 4:159–163.

Weiss RB and Baker JR Hypersensitivity reactions from antineoplastic agents. Cancer Metastasis Rev 1987 6:413–432.

Wielckens K, Delfs T, Muth A, Freese V, and Kleeberg HJ Glucocorticoid-induced lymphoma cell death: The good and the evil. J Steroid Biochem 1987 27:413–419.

Winkelstein A The effects of azathioprine and 6MP on immunity. J Immunopharmacol 1979 1:429–454.

Woolley JL, Lau BH, Ruckle HC, and Torrey RR Phagocytic and natural killer cytotoxic responses of murine transitional cell carcinoma to postsurgical immunochemotherapy. J Urol 1988 140:660–663.

Wortman JE, Lucas VS, Schuster E, Thiele D, and Logue GL Sudden death during doxorubicin administration. Cancer 1979 44(2):1588–1591.

Xu ZY, Hosokawa M, Morikawa K, Hatakeyama M, and Kobayashi H Overcoming suppression of antitumor immune reactivity in tumor bearing rats by treatment with bleomycin. Cancer Res 1988 48:6658–6663.

Yamaki H, Tanaka N, and Umezawa H Effects of several tumor-inhibitory antibiotics on immunological responses. J Antibiot 1969 22:315–321.

Yoshida S, Nomoto K, Himeno K, and Takeya K Immune response to syngeneic or autologous testicular cells in mice. I. Augmented delayed footpad reaction in cyclophosphamide-treated mice. Clin Exp Immunol 1979 38:211–217.

Zaltzman M, Kallenback J, Shapiro T, Lewis M, Fritz V, Reef H, and Zwi S Life threatening hypotension associated with azathioprine therapy: A case report. S Afr Med J 1984 65:306.

Zhu LP, Cupps TR, Whalen G, and Fauci AS Selective effects of cyclophosphamide therapy on activation, proliferation, and differentiation of human B cells. J Clin Invest 1987 79:1082–1090.

CHAPTER 10

Toxicity of Biological Response Modifiers

Garth Powis, D.Phil., and Miles P. Hacker, Ph.D.

INTRODUCTION

Agents that modify the host's biological response to tumor with resultant therapeutic effects (biological response modifiers, BRMs) (Vanky and Argou 1980) were among the earliest agents used to treat cancer. In 1891 Coley reported the use of bacterial cell filtrates to treat human cancer and reported some striking transient responses (Coley, 1891). The treatment was, however, highly toxic. Although the reason for the response was not known at the time we now conclude that it was probably due to stimulation of the body's own immunological defenses against the tumor as well as hyperthermia, which can slow tumor growth, caused by a pyretic effect of the bacterial extracts. A number of nonspecific immune stimulants such as Bacillus Calmette-Guérin (BCG) continued to find a limited use in cancer therapy but the modern era of BRM therapy began in the early 1970s with the clinical testing of crude human interferon (INF) obtained from the buffy coat layers of blood (Panem, 1985). Problems of production, purity, and cost continued and seriously hampered the studies of INF until in the early 1980s when recombinant DNA technology allowed the production of high-quality material and extensive trials became possible. A number of BRMs have now undergone clinical trial as antitumor agents including INF α, β, and γ, interleukin-2 (IL-2) and tumor necrosis factor (TNF)-α. These are the agents that are more correctly designated cytokines, endogenous substances that affect cellular response to tumor. Interleukin-2 is a lymphokine, because it specifically affects immune function. There are other BRMs that are not naturally occurring and they will not be covered here. They include: tamoxifen, aminoglutethamide, flavone acetic acid, and low-dose cyclophosphamide. Overall, the antitumor responses seen with the cytokines have been disappointing and they have not fulfilled their early expectations. However, they are clearly capable of mediating significant tumor regression in a small number of patients but not without considerable toxicity. The challenge now is how to use cytokines to benefit the majority of cancer patients and how to decrease their toxicity.

INTERFERONS

Introduction

Interferons are a family of proteins first discovered in 1957 by Isaacs and Lindenmann as activity in cell supernatant fluids and animals that had the capability to block the replication of a broad range of viruses through the activation of mRNA and protein synthesis in responding cells. Although original studies showed "species specificity" for the INFs with, for example, chick INF having no activity on calf cells and vice versa (Tyrell, 1959), more recent studies have shown there is some cross-species activity (Rubinstein et al., 1981). In addition to antiviral activity the INFs have been shown to have hormone-like activity (Blalock and

Stanton, 1980), immunoregulatory properties (Sonnefeld et al., 1977), and growth regulatory activity (Paucker et al., 1962). The latter two points suggested INF use as antitumor agents.

There are three families of INFs, designated INF-α, INF-β, INF-γ (Stewart et al., 1980). Interferon-α, a protein of 166 amino acids, is produced by lymphocytes and macrophages that have been induced with viruses, foreign nucleic acids, synthetic polymers, bacteria, bacterial components, tumor cells, and heterologous cells. Human DNA encodes for at least 17 different INF-α subtypes and at least eight are naturally expressed (Allen and Fantes, 1980; Goeddel et al., 1980). The genes for INF-α are located in one region of human chromosome 9 (Owerbach et al., 1981). Interferon-β is produced by fibroblast and epithelial cells that have been induced by foreign nucleic acids. Human DNA encodes for at least two INF-β subtypes, both of which are expressed naturally (Sehgal, 1982; Tavernier et al., 1981). The gene for at least one INF-β is located in close proximity to the INF-α genes on chromosome 9 (Owerbach et al., 1981). Interferon-β is composed of 166 amino acids and is distinguished from INF-α by being a glycoprotein (Tavernier et al., 1981). INF-γ differs considerably from the other INFs. It is a glycoprotein composed of 145 amino acids (Devos et al., 1982) and is produced by T lymphocytes that have been stimulated with mitogens or with foreign antigens to which they have previously been sensitized. Only one genetic sequence for INF-α has been identified in human DNA (Devos et al., 1982; Gray et al., 1982) and is located on chromosome 12 (Degrave et al., 1982). Interferon-αs and INF-βs show considerable homology and have probably been generated by divergent evolution from a common ancestral INF gene (Miyata and Hayashida, 1982). They interact with the same cell surface receptor encoded on chromosome 21 (Aguet and Mogensen, 1983) and appear to exert many similar biological effects. Interferon-γ does not share significant homology to the other INFs (Devos et al., 1982; Gray et al., 1982), except perhaps in its secondary structure (Degrado et al., 1982), and interacts with a unique receptor encoded on chromosome 6 (Aguet and Mogensen, 1983). There is some evidence that INF-α exerts its antiviral activity by a different mechanism to INF-α and INF-γ (Dianzani et al., 1978).

Interferons have growth inhibitory effects on normal and tumor cells in vitro and in vivo. Interferon-β and INF- α can cause tumor cell lysis at relatively high INF concentrations and low cell concentrations (Ito and Buffet, 1981; Tyring et al., 1982), whereas combinations of INF-α and INF-γ or INF-β have potent lytic effects even at low INF concentrations (Tyring et al., 1984). However, the major effect of INFs on cell growth appears to be the prolongation of time of passage through the cell cycle (Balkwill and Taylor-Papdimitrious, 1978; Lundbald and Lundgren, 1981; Mataresse and Rossi, 1977). Interferons have been shown to have antitumor activity in animals against a variety of spontaneous neoplasms (Came and Moore, 1971; Gresser et al., 1969), virally induced neoplasms (Atanasiu and Chany, 1960; Lampson et al., 1963), and transplantable tumors (Gresser and Tovey, 1978). The mechanisms of antitumor activity in vivo include a direct antiproliferative effect on the tumor as well as immunomodulatory effects mediated by cytotoxic effector cells, such as natural killer (NK) cells, cytotoxic T cells, and activated macrophages (Einhorn et al., 1978; Lindahl et al., 1972; Schultz et al., 1978). Studies in animals suggest that INFs may be more effective antitumor agents when combined with each other (Fleischmann et al., 1979; 1980), with conventional chemotherapeutic agents (Chirigos and Pearson, 1973; Gresser et al., 1969), with gamma-irradiation (Namba et al., 1984), or with colony stimulating factor-1 which blocks INF-mediated myelosuppression (Korean et al., 1986).

Mechanisms of Activity

At the cellular level INF acts by gene activation leading to the decreased synthesis of some proteins and the synthesis of some new proteins. There are four enzyme systems that are induced that interfere with viral protein synthesis and that may be involved in the antiproliferative activity of the INFs. These are: 2′,5′-oligoadenylate synthetase, which synthesizes oligonucleotides that can activate endoribonuclease to cleave both viral and cellular RNA (Chebath et al., 1987); a protein kinase that phosphorylates proteins PI and elongation initiation factor EIF2α that in turn inhibits t-RNA binding to the ribosome (Samuel, 1986; Senn, 1984); a 2′,5′-phosphodiesterase that catalyzes t-RNA degradation (Samuel, 1986; Senn, 1984); and indoleamine 2,3-dioxygenase that degrades intracellular tryptophan (Byrne et al., 1986). At the cellular level there is activation of NK cells, the killer cell, and lymphokine activated killer (LAK) cells, all of which show direct cytotoxic activity towards a variety of cultured and primary tumor cells. Other aspects of immune function that are stimulated by INFs are human-leucocyte-associated antigen class 1 expression, activation of B cells, and augmentation of other lymphokines such as IL-2 and TNF.

Clinical Uses

Early studies of INFs antitumor activity in the 1970s was restricted by the limited availability, the purity (generally less than 1%), and specific activity (around 10^6 U/mg protein) of INF material. The advent of genetic engineering in the early 1980s permitted INFs to be produced by recombinant DNA technology in large amounts for human testing with high purity (more than 99%) and high specific activity (2×10^5 U/mg protein) (Goeddel et al., 1980).

Most complete clinical studies to date of INF have used leukocyte and recombinant INF-α. Clinical trials of INF-β and INF-γ are currently in progress (Goldstein and Laszlo, 1988). The best responses to INF have occurred in hematological malignancies, in particular hairy cell leukemia, a rare form of leukemia characterized by pancytopenia and splenomegaly (Quesada et al., 1986). Response rates over 80% have been reported in a number of trials using low doses of INF of 2×10^6 U/m^2 (subcutaneously) trice weekly (Goldstein and Laszlo, 1988). Lymphoma responds better to high doses of INF, and response rates over 50% have been reported (Bunn et al., 1984; Goldstein and Laszlo, 1986). Chronic myeloid leukemia is also highly responsive to high-dose INF therapy (Billiau, 1986). Juvenile laryngeal papillomatosis (Göbel et al., 1981; Haglund et al., 1981) shows response rates that approach 90%. However, long-term studies of patients with juvenile laryngeal papillomatosis have shown that the tumor can reoccur following withdrawal of INF therapy or even with continued INF therapy (Goepfert et al., 1982). Multiple myeloma, Kaposis sarcoma, carcinoid tumors, renal cancer, and melanoma are moderately responsive to INF therapy whereas lung, colon, breast cancer, and other bulky tumors have proven unresponsive (Goldstein and Laszlo, 1988; Spiegel, 1987). The general characteristics of INF therapy are that continuous dosing is more efficacious than intermittent dosing, a delayed response of eight to 12 weeks is the rule rather than the exception, and like many chemotherapeutic agents INF is more active in patients with minimal tumor bulk (Spiegel, 1987). An important question for any of the BRMs is what dose is necessary to give the maximum antitumor effect. The "optimum biological response modifying" dose may not correspond to the maximum tolerated dose (Foon et al., 1985). In patients with hairy cell leukemia, lower INF-α doses of 3×10^6 U compared to 5×10^6 U or less frequent treatment twice or three times a week produce the same clinical benefit of less toxicity (Berneman et al., 1986). In multiple myeloma, doses varying from two to 100×10^6 U produce similar clinical benefit but with much more toxicity at the higher doses (Constanzi, 1987). Increasing doses of INF-α above 0.5 mg/m^2/d has been shown to block the tumoricidal properties of monocytes from cancer patients (Kleinerman et al., 1986). It is, unfortunately, difficult to decide which immunological function is relevant to measure to determine the "optimum biological response modifying" dose. The main use of INF in cancer in the future will probably be in an adjuvant setting or as part of combination therapy. Interferon-α has also been given to patients with a variety of viral infections (Dekonig et al., 1982; Sundmacher et al., 1978), and to treat hepatitis B (Greenberg et al., 1976), hepatitis C

(Di Besceglie et al., 1989), and multiple sclerosis (Jacob et al., 1985). Interferon inducers have been used in patients with Reye's syndrome (Guggenheim and Baron, 1977), multiple sclerosis (Bever et al., 1986), and Guillain-Barré syndrome (Bever et al., 1986).

Pharmacokinetics

Intramuscular (IM) and subcutaneous INF-α (Bornemann et al., 1985; Wills et al., 1984) and nonglycosylated INF-γ (Gutterman et al., 1984) are well-absorbed with peak plasma or serum concentrations occurring one to eight hr postinjection. Peak plasma concentrations following these routes of administration are an order of magnitude or more less than when the same dose is given intravenously (IV). The absorption of INF-β from muscle or skin gives barely detectable serum concentrations (Quesada et al., 1982). Serum concentrations of INF following IV administration decline rapidly in a biexponential manner for INF-α, with a terminal half-life of four to 16 hr (Shah et al., 1984; Smith et al., 1985) and mono-exponentially for INF-α with a half-life of about 30 min (Gutterman et al., 1984; Kurzrock et al., 1985). The apparent volume of distribution for both INF-α and INF-γ is from 12 to 40 liters (Gutterman et al., 1984; Kurzrock et al., 1985; Shah et al., 1984; Wills et al., 1984). Interferon-α does not readily cross the blood–brain barrier after IV, IM, or subcutaneous administration and concentrations in the cerebrospinal fluid (CSF) are only 0.1% those in the plasma (Smith et al., 1982). Only a trace or no INF has been found in the CSF after continuous daily infusions of up to 100×10^6/U m^2 of lymphoblastoid INF, a dose that may eventually lead to cerebral coma (Rohatiner et al., 1982; Smith et al., 1985). It is possible, therefore, that local high concentrations of INF are reached in certain parts of the brain or that an INF breakdown product or metabolite is responsible for the neurotoxicity. Animal studies have shown that INF-α is filtered through the renal glomeruli by luminal endocytosis followed by proximal tubular resorption and during this time there is proteolytic degradation by lysosomal enzymes (Bino et al., 1982; Bocci et al., 1984). Very little INF-α is excreted unchanged in the urine. The liver plays only a minor role in the catabolism of INF-α (Bocci et al., 1983). Interferon-β and INF-γ undergo much less renal catabolism than INF-α and liver catabolism may be the predominant pathway for the elimination of INF-β and INF-γ A both of which are glycosylated proteins (Bocci et al., 1985; 1982).

Toxicity

Because INF is a natural substance there was a hope that it would prove to be less toxic than conventional chemotherapy. This has not proved to be the case. Nearly all patients receiving INF-α experience toxicity. Interferon-γs toxicity appears to be dose related and fever and chills develop in nearly all patients at doses greater than 1×10^6 U/m^2. This can usually be controlled with aspirin, acetaminophen, and, if necessary, meperidine hydrochloride. Initially there was reluctance to use powerful inhibitors of prostaglandin synthesis such as aspirin and indomethacin because of the fear this might abrogate the antitumor and antiviral activity of INF (Laszlo et al., 1983; Pottahil et al., 1980). Acetaminophen, which is an analgesic and antipyretic but a weak inhibitor of prostaglandin synthetase (Van Arman et al., 1985), was preferred. This view is now changing (Aoki et al., 1984; Sarkar and Gupta, 1982). The dose-limiting toxicity of INF-α is an influenza-like syndrome with myalgia, anorexia, rigors, lassitude, and depression (Smedley and Wheeler, 1983). The severity of these symptoms increase with dose and show a decreased incidence over time (Spiegel, 1987). The symptoms are rapidly reversible within a few days of discontinuing treatment. Other toxicities may occur but are rarely dose limiting including leucopenia, thrombocytopenia and anemia, nausea and vomiting, and increased hepatic enzyme levels (Silver et al., 1985; Spiegel, 1987). These toxicities are all rapidly reversible when INF therapy is discontinued. Administering INF-α in the evening may produce fewer side effects (Abrams et al., 1985). The toxicities of

INF-α encountered in 1403 patients receiving $2 \times 10 \times 10^6$ U/m^2 subcutaneous from a survey by Spiegel are shown in Table 10-1.

Interferon-β produces severe chills and other toxicities similar to INF-α but apparently with less neurotoxicity (Bogdahn et al., 1985; Liberati et al., 1988) although prolonged infusions do produce some neurotoxicity (Brown et al., 1987). Interferon-γ causes fever, headache, fatigue, myelosuppression, and hepatitis (Gonzales et al., 1989; Lane et al., 1989).

The mechanisms of INF toxicity are not known. Many of the effects are nonspecific and probably in part mediated by inflammatory prostaglandin synthesis. Interferons have been shown to induce the formation of inflammatory prostaglandins in vitro (Fuse et al., 1982; Yaron et al., 1977). Prostaglandin synthetase inhibitors including acetaminophen, aspirin, and steroids may give symptomatic relief. It has been suggested that the symptoms of INF toxicity reflect the normal pathophysiological effects of high levels of endogenous INF produced acutely during virus infections or chronically during active autoimmune processes (Scott, 1988). Because of the species specificity of INF there are few animal models in which to study human INF toxicity. The chimpanzee is the only animal species in which the side effects of human INF have been reproduced (Schellekens et al., 1984).

Central Nervous System Toxicity

At lower doses of INF-α up to 10×10^6 U/m^2 mild central nervous system (CNS) toxicity consisting of somnolence and confusion occurs in about one-third of patients (Spiegel, 1987). More severe CNS effects have been described with high doses of INF-α including lethargy, somnolence, confusion, loss of taste and smell, and overall mental and motor slowing (Mattson et al., 1983; Rohatiner et al., 1983; Smedley et al., 1983). In patients receiving INF-α at $> 20 \times 10^6$ U/m^2 per day, psychotic reactions, auditory and visual hallucinations, and occasional seizures have been reported (Creagan et al., 1984; Diercks et al., 1985; Eggermont et al., 1985; Kirkwood et al., 1985). The incidence and severity of CNS toxicity decreases with time and tolerance appears to develop. The CNS toxicity resolves in one to two weeks after INF-α treatment is discontinued (Spiegel, 1987). Older patients experience more CNS toxicity than younger patients. Patients with preexisting neurologic dysfunction are at increased risk for severe INF-α toxicity (Adams et al., 1988). Bocci (1988) has summarized the neurotoxicity caused by different schedules of administration of INF as: IV bolus (daily administration) < IM < subcutaneous < continuous (weekly) IV infusion. This relationship appears to hold true for INF-α and INF-β. Interferon-γ may produce no serious neurologic toxicity except for complaints of headache at doses of up to 2 mg IV twice or three times weekly (Panitch et al., 1986).

The neuropsychiatric effects of high- and low-dose INF-α have been compared by Mattson

Table 10-1. Toxicities of Interferon-α_{2b}*

TOXICITY	PERCENT
Flu-like symptoms	96
Nausea/vomiting	42
Other gastrointestinal symptoms	24
Central nervous system	33
Cardiovascular	12
Skin	6
Respiratory	6
Alopecia	6
Weight loss	6
Hepatic	<1

*Taken from a survey of 1403 patients, the majority receiving INF-α_{2b} to 10 × 106 U/m2 subcutaneously, three times a week (Speigel, 1987). Any severity of toxicity is recorded.

et al. (1983; 1984) with patients receiving either 800 $\times$ 10^6 U over five days by continuous IV infusion followed by 6 $\times$ 10^6 U by IM injection thrice weekly or 6 $\times$ 10^6 U daily. Both regimens resulted in progressive mental and motor slowing with memory loss and changes in psychomotor behavior. The degree of dysfunction was influenced by INF-α dose and the greatest changes were seen between eight and 10 days in patients receiving the high dose IFN-α and between the third and fourth weeks in patients receiving the low doses. The clinical and psychometric abnormalities disappeared within two weeks of discontinuing INF-α treatment. EEG changes have been described in patients receiving both high- and moderate-dose INF-α (Mattson et al., 1983; Rohatiner et al., 1983; Smedley et al., 1983). The changes, which include slowing of the alpha rhythm and the appearance of diffuse slow theta, then delta waves, are suggestive of encephalopathy and can be observed even in patients with no clinical evidence of CNS toxicity (Rohatiner et al., 1983). It is not possible to state whether INF-α has intrinsically lower neurotoxicity than INF-β or INF-γ (Bocci, 1988). The lower apparent neurotoxicity of INF-β compared to INF-γ could be due to a much lower bioavailability of INF-γ following IM or subcutaneous administration (Grunberg et al., 1987; Chang et al., 1985; Hawkins et al., 1984) and INF-βs higher turnover rate or decreased transfer through the circumventricular organs of the brain (Bocci, 1988).

Mechanisms of CNS Toxicity

The mechanism for the CNS toxicity of INF-α is not known. It has been suggested, however, that INF-α may have widespread neurochemical activity (Färkkilä et al., 1988; Rohatiner and Färkkilä, 1988). Interferon-γ decreases CSF 5-hydroxyindoleacetic acid concentrations, suggesting an effect on central serotonergic neurotransmission (Färkkilä et al., 1988). Interferon will compete for membrane receptors with neurotropic hormones such as thyrotropin (Maheshware et al., 1979). Intracerebral injection of leukocyte INF-α into mice produces endorphin-like effects, including decreased motor activity and naloxone-reversible catalepsy (Blalock and Smith, 1981). Adams et al. (1984) have shown that metaclopramide, a dopamine antagonist, and methylphenidate, a dopamine agonist, both reverse some of the neuropsychiatric effects of leukocyte INF-α in cancer patients. Although these findings are apparently contradictory the authors suggested that the hypersomnia caused by INF is due to an effect of INF on the reticular activating system (RAS) or interference with the RAS connections of the frontal lobes.

Immunogenic Potential of INF

It was originally hoped that recombinant human INF would not be clinically immunogenic. However, serum-neutralizing antibodies have been detected in 25% of patients receiving INF-α_{2a} (Roche, Nutley, NJ) with particularly high rates in patients with renal carcinoma (44%) and Kaposi's sarcoma (34%) (Hri et al., 1987). Interferon-α_{2b} (Schering, Kenilworth, NJ) is much less immunogenic and indicates only a 2.5% incidence of serum-neutralizing antibodies (Spiegel, 1987). These two recombinant INF-αs differ by one amino acid in the primary structure and are purified by different methodologies. It is not known why the differences in immunogenicity exist and what the consequences for therapeutic response or toxicity are.

TUMOR NECROSIS FACTOR

Introduction

Tumor necrosis factor was discovered in 1975 by Carswell et al. (1975) as a soluble factor in the serum of animals infected with BCG and injected with bacterial endotoxin or lipopolysaccharide. Initially TNF appeared to be preferentially cytotoxic for tumor cells and was named for its ability to cause hemorrhagic necrosis of transplantable solid tumors. Tumor necrosis factor was later shown to be identical to a factor called cachectin produced by macrophages in response to bacterial lipopolysaccharide, and was termed TNF-α (Beutler and Cerami, 1986). TNF-β is produced by lymphocytes and is identical to lymphotoxin, a cytotoxic product of lymphocytes (Aggarwal et al., 1987). TNF-α and TNF-β have 52% structural homology (Aggarwal et al., 1987). TNF-α is a protein with 157 amino acid residues whereas TNF-β is a glycoprotein with 148 or 171 amino acid residues (Aggarwal et al., 1987). Unlike the INFs, TNF is nonspecies-specific (Fransen et al., 1986a). Recombinant human TNF-α and TNF-β have been available since 1984 (Gray et al., 1984; Pennica et al., 1984). Clinical studies have employed exclusively TNF-α.

TNF-α is the major endotoxin inducible secretory protein in macrophages (Beutler et al., 1985a). It has been claimed to be a primary mediator of endotoxin-mediated shock in vivo (Beutler et al., 1985) and to have cachectic activity (Cerami et al., 1985). Tumor necrosis factor has been shown to induce tumor cell lysis both in vivo and in vitro (Oettgen, 1987; Spriggs et al., 1987) and displays multifunctional immunoregulatory activity on T and B cell lymphocytes and on NK and LAK cells (Fiers et al., 1988). TNF-α probably plays a major role in the host's defense against infections and possibly in the immune response against cancer. The clinical antitumor activity of TNF-α has proved to be disappointing and its use has been accompanied by considerable toxicity.

Toxicity

TNF-α is usually administered by short daily IV infusion for five days repeated at two or three week intervals or as one to five day continuous infusions at daily doses of around 100 to 250 $\mu g/m^2$. The pattern of toxicity is the same for both schedules of administration (Aboulafia et al., 1989; Childs et al., 1989; Creaven et al., 1989; Feinberg et al., 1988; Moritz et al., 1989; Niederle et al., 1988; Ozaki et al., 1989; Savona et al., 1988; 1989; Sherman et al., 1988; Spriggs et al., 1988; Steinmetz et al., 1988). All patients experience fever and chills but this can usually be adequately treated with acetaminophen, indomethacin, or meperidine hydrochloride (Aboulafia et al., 1989; Childs et al., 1989; Kahn et al., 1989; Moritz et al., 1989). Other constitutive toxicities due to TNF-α are headache, nausea and vomiting, fatigue and athralgia. These toxicities are dose dependent and at high TNF-α doses profound prostatration can be a limiting toxicity (Feinberg et al., 1988; Steinmetz et al., 1988). Nearly all studies have reported pronounced hypotension caused by TNF-α which can be dose limiting (Creaven et al., 1989; Feinberg et al., 1988; Spriggs et al., 1988; Steinmetz et al., 1988; Zamkoff et al., 1988). Hematological toxicities of TNF-α are leukopenia and thrombocytopenia, which are rapidly reversible when TNF-α administration is discontinued (Feinberg et al., 1988; Sherman et al., 1988). Mild hepatic (Childs et al., 1989; Zukiwski et al., 1989) and pulmonary toxicity (Kuei et al., 1989) have also been reported (Childs et al., 1989; Zukiwski et al., 1989) and seizures have been seen in patients with a prior history of cerebral infarction (Savona et al., 1988). When given subcutaneously, TNF-α can cause severe skin ulceration (Zamkoff et al., 1988). Metabolic effects of TNF-α administration in cancer patients have been noted with an increase in serum triglycerides, very low-density lipoprotein (VLDL), and a decrease in serum high-density lipoprotein (HDL) (Feinberg et al., 1988; Sherman et al., 1988; Zamkoff et al., 1988). TNF-α causes the efflux of amino acids from muscle and produces anabolic and catabolic changes in liver and skeletal muscle protein metabolism characteristic of the cachexia seen in cancer patients (Warren et al., 1987).

Mechanisms of Toxicity

Very little is known of the mechanisms of TNF-α antitumor activity or its toxicity. TNF-α appears to induce a classical acute inflammatory response in the tumor which leads to disruption of the tumor's blood supply (Palladino et al., 1987). The inflammation of the vascular endothelium induced by TNF-α is not limited to the tumor vascular bed but can also be seen in other organs (Patton et al., 1987). Studies in animals suggest that multiple organ damge by TNF-α may be mediated by neutrophils (Mallick et al., 1989). TNF-α is thought to cause release of polyunsaturated fatty acids, which would explain the synthesis of prostaglandins and leukotrienes by many cell types after TNF-α treatment (Kettelhut et al., 1987). Events preceding TNF-α-induced death in rats including hypotension, acidosis, and hypoglycemia can be prevented by indomethacin or ibuprofen, both arachidonic acid cyclooxygenase inhibitors, without affecting the cytotoxic action of TNF-α on malignant cells (Kettelhut et al., 1987). This suggests that it may be possible clinically to separate antitumor activity and toxicity. Tumor-bearing mice can be made resistant to the toxic effects of TNF by repeated nonlethal dosing (Fraker and Norton, 1988). Unfortunately there is also a decrease in therapeutic efficacy so that there is no net gain in the therapeutic index of TNF. This work suggests that it may be difficult to separate the toxic and therapeutic effects TNF-α in cancer patients.

INTERLEUKIN-2

Introduction

Interleukin-2 was originally described as T cell growth factor based on the ability of this protein to promote mitosis in mitogen or antigen-stimulated T lymphocytes in vitro (Morgan et al., 1976). This glycoprotein, having a molecular weight of 15 kD, is produced by phytohemagglutinin-activated T cells (Grimm and Rosenberg, 1982) and appears to be able to mediate a number of immunologic functions. For example, administration of IL-2 to nude mice will enhance autoantibody production and induce specific helper T cell subsets (Stotter et al., 1980; Reimann and Diamanstein, 1981). Immune function can also be enhanced to some extent in mice or rats following exposure to either irradiation or cyclophosphamide (Clason et al., 1982; Merluzzi et al., 1981).

The impetus for clinical studies with IL-2 came from a number of experimental studies which clearly demonstrated that systemically administered IL-2 could mediate tumor regression. The antitumor activity of long-term cultured T lymphocytes could be augmented by systemic IL-2 administration following inoculation of mice with the cultured T cells (Cheever et al., 1982; Donohue et al., 1984). Further, it has been shown that the systemic administration of high-dose IL-2 can result in the regression of established pulmonary or hepatic metastases when given as a single agent (Rosenberg et al., 1987) or in combination with activated lymphocytes (Lafreniere and Rosenberg, 1985).

Given the efficacy of IL-2 as a single agent or as part of an adoptive immunotherapy protocol in the experimental system, initial Phase I studies were begun at the National Cancer Institute (Lotze et al., 1984; 1985). The limiting factor for these studies was the supply of IL-2 which at that time was obtained from the Jurkat cell line. A total of 12 patients were entered into the study and were administered IL-2 a single IV bolus or 24 hr infusion weekly for four weeks. Once the gene for human IL-2 had been successfully transfected into and expressed by *Escherichia coli* (Taniguchi et al., 1983; Rosenberg et al., 1984), vast quantities of IL-2 were purified, and large-scale human studies could begin.

Mechanism of Action

The in vivo activity of IL-2 has been ascribed to several possible mechanisms. IL-2 is critical to the development on cytotoxic lymphocytes and death of tumor target cells probably through its effect of helper T cells. Differentiation of normal blood lymphocytes into LAK cells having broad-spectrum cytotoxicity selective for neoplastic cells is facilitated by IL-2. Activation and proliferation of NK cells which appear to be quite important in the immune surveillance system occurs in the presence of IL-2. Natural killer cells can also be stimulated by IL-2 into becoming LAK cells. Finally, IL-2 has been shown to induce the production of secondary lymphokines, activate T cell proliferation and autoregulate further IL-2 production. Any or all of these experimental observations could account for the antitumor activity of IL-2.

Clinical studies have demonstrated a striking fall in circulating lymphocytes immediately after cessation of a 24 hr infusion of IL-2. Within 24 hr after stopping the infusion there is a rebound in the lymphocytes well above baseline levels (Lotze et al., 1985; Ettinghausen et al., 1987). Cells obtained during the rebound effect show a marked increase in in vitro proliferation and cytotoxic responses when activated by IL-2. These cells are able to mediate direct destruction of NK-sensitive and resistant target cells and their activity is enhanced by the presence of IL-2 in the culture (Rosenstein et al., 1986). Patients who completed the entire four week IL-2 protocol had even more striking immunobiological changes. The absolute lymphocyte count increased with each course of therapy and the in vitro cytotoxicity of lymphocytes taken from these patients increased >100-fold in the number of lytic units of killer cell activity (Sondel et al., 1988). The mechanism of the immediate fall in leukocytes is not understood but the functional studies performed on the peripheral lymphocytes suggest strongly that systemically administered IL-2 has marked immunomodulatory activity.

Kinetics

Initial clinical studies were done using IL-2 obtained from the Jurkat cell line and compared the half-lives of IL-2 given as a single IV bolus injection (administered over a 5 min period) to a 24 hr continuous IV infusion (Lotze et al., 1985). In this study, IV bolus resulted in a biphasic clearance pattern with the initial half-life of five to seven min and a secondary half-life of 30 to 120 min. Continuous infusion produced significantly lower peak plasma levels but resulted in a more prolonged period of measurable plasma levels of IL-2. Plasma levels dropped rapidly following cessation of the IL-2 infusion. Similar results were reported for recombinant IL-2 (Lotze et al., 1985). Atkins et al. (1986) found only a single half-life of 20 to 25 min when IL-2 was administered as a single IV bolus injection. The authors correlated the difference in plasma kinetics compared to those of Lotze et al. (1985; 1986) with the lack of improved lymphocyte function in their study.

More recently, Thompson et al. (1987) studied the effect of subcutaneous injection and a two or 24 hr IV infusion on the pharmacokinetic and immunomodulatory activity of IL-2. Although the data were not analyzed for true half-life values, they clearly show that the two hr infusion resulted in the higher peak plasma levels but the clearance of IL-2 was rapid. The 24 hr infusion resulted in a lower but more prolonged levels of IL-2. Finally, the subcutaneous route increased the clearance time but had dramatically lowered plasma levels compared to either infusion protocol.

The other route of IL-2 administration investigated thus far is an intraperitoneal (IP) injection (Urba et al., 1989; Stewart et al., 1990). The primary goal of both studies was to determine the feasibility of treating intra-abdominal masses with IP IL-2. When administered IP every eight hr for five days, following a priming regimen of IV IL-2 every eight hr for three days, IL-2 levels were 10 to 100-fold higher in the peritoneum than the plasma and were maintained at levels well above those required to generate and maintain LAK cells in vitro.

Toxicity

In the initial Phase I studies IL-2 was administered as a single IV bolus injection to patients who had failed previous therapeutic regimens. Up to one million U/kg were given with the resulting toxicities being related to the dose of IL-2 administred. The most frequent side effects included fevers as high as 40.2°C, malaise, headache, nausea, vomiting, diarrhea, and an occasional pruritic rash (Lotze et al., 1985). For the most part the symptoms were manageable with a variety of medications such as indomethacin or acetaminophen and, occasionally, an antihistamine or antiemetic. Other, less frequent toxicities included mild alterations of liver function tests, microscopic hematuria and eosinophilia. No persistent toxicities were encountered in this study and all abnormal hematological and clinical chemistry values returned to baseline ranges within one week following cessation of IL-2. Similar toxicities were encountered when IL-2 was administered as a 24 hr infusion at doses of 10,000 U/kg/hr. Although these toxicities were manageable and readily reversible upon cessation of therapy, single doses of IL-2 had little immunomodulatory activity.

As stated above the activation of immune cells appears to occur only after multiple injections of IL-2, thus as large quantities of recombinant IL-2 became available, multiple treatment protocols were begun. Atkins et al. (1986) administered IL-2 as weekly IV bolus injections and found effects similar to those reported by Lotze et al. (1985). However, they also reported that four of 17 patients developed a transient hypotension with systolic blood pressure of approximately 90 mmHg and one patient required IV saline and pressor support for severe hypotension and myocardial ischemia. Similar toxicities have been reported by others using intensive IL-2 administration (doses of $1–3 \times 10^6$ U/m²/d) when the protein is given for four to seven consecutive days as an IV bolus or as a continuous infusion (Kohler et al., 1987).

As the dose of IL-2 is increased up to 10^7 u/m²/d renal insufficiency, severe hypotension, and fluid retention become dose limiting (Lotze et al., 1986; Rosenberg et al., 1987). Pulmonary edema is common and some patients may require ventilatory support during the acute crisis. Fortunately such episodes are usually reversible but may require seven days for complete recovery to occur. Treatment of these toxicities may include the use of pressors to maintain blood pressure and diuretics to increase urinary output and decrease fluid retention.

The mechanism of IL-2 edema, hypotension, and pulmonary distress are not understood but may be related to increased capillary leakage, which has been demonstrated in murine models (Rosenstein et al., 1986). Whereas not established clinically, the laboratory and hemodynamic alterations observed with IL-2 are similar to those reported for endotoxic or gram negative septic shock (Belldegrun et al., 1987; Ognibene et al., 1986). Although dexamethasone can prevent much of IL-2 induced toxicity there is a concern about the effect of dexamethasone on the immunomodulatory activity of IL-2.

Kozeny et al. (1988) examined the effects of IV bolus IL-2, given every eight hr for five days at a dose of 10^5 μm/kg, on renal function, acid-base status, and calcium/phosphrous balance in eight patients. All patients developed a reversible capillary leak syndrome, prerenal azotemia, hypophosphatemia, hypocalcemia, hypomagnesemia, and respiratory alkalosis. No defects in renal calcium, magnesium, phosphorous, net acid excretion, or glycosuria were noted. From this study it was concluded that IL-2 induces vascular permeability and respiratory alkalosis but does not cause renal tubular dysfunction. Thus little, if any long-term effect on renal function is expected and should not be a limiting factor in IL-2 therapy.

A prospective study on the development of IL-2-related pruritus was conducted by Gaspari et al. (1987) in which punch skin biopsies were obtained before and upon completion of five days of IL-2 therapy (IV injections every eight hrs at dosages of 30,000–100,000 U/kg). All patients developed an eruption that was characterized by macular erythema, with burning and pruritus of the skin beginning two to three days after initiation of therapy. The eruption resolved with desquamation of the affected areas, localized primarily to the head and neck, within 48 to 72 hr after cessation of IL-2 administration. No specific histologic changes, other than an accumulation of DR+/Leu-4+ lymphoid cells surrounding the blood vessels of the papillary dermis, were detected in the biopsies. The authors ascribe this skin response to a cutaneous manifestation of the capillary leak syndrome discussed above.

A less frequently mentioned side effect of IL-2 administration is the development of neuropsychiatric changes that are dose and time dependent (Denicoff et al., 1987). Behavioral problems appeared in 22 out of 44 patients beginning at the end of IL-2 treatment (patients received 30,000–100,000 U/kg every 8 hr for 5 days) and consisted of mild-to-severe behavioral and cognitive changes, hallucinations, and delusions. The rate of recovery from these toxicities was usually quite rapid with only two of 22 affected patients expressing behavioral changes for more than four days after cessation of IL-2 administration. The mechanism of this toxicity is unknown. Lymphokines have been shown to increase neuroendocrine secretion (Denicoff et al., 1987), neuropsychiatric changes (Adams et al., 1984; Rohatiner et al., 1983), and alter vascular permeability of perhaps the blood–brain barrier (Rosenstein et al., 1986).

Given that ovarian cancer is primarily a local disease of the peritoneal cavity, locoregional therapy has been the focus of multiple clinical trials (Brenner 1986). An obvious extension of the clinical investigations with IL-2 was to study the effect of this lymphokine on ovarian carcinoma. To date, only a limited number of Phase I studies have been completed but the data accumulated thus far indicate that IP IL-2 is far better tolerated than IV IL-2. Beller et al. (1989) treated five women with relatively low doses of IL-2 and found only mild toxicities. Two patients developed transient asymptomatic episodes of hypotension, three patients had an aggravation of preexisting peripheral neuropathy induced by prior exposure to cisplatin, one patient had impaired renal function and was taken off study, and fever and anemia occurred in eight and five patients, respectively. All patients remained ambulatory and required no intensive care. At higher doses of IP IL-2 more severe toxicities were encountered (Chapman et al., 1989). The major dose-limiting toxicity was diarrhea resulting in hypovolemia in five of seven patients. In addition, fever, nausea, vomiting, neuropsychiatric changes, and azotemia were reported. Using a dose range similar to that reported by Chapman et al. (1989), Stewart et al. (1990) found the dose-limiting toxicity to be nausea and abdominal pain secondary to ascites accumulation with significant weight gain. Other toxic effects included decreased performance status, fever, diarrhea, and anemia.

Conclusion

The cytokine BRMs are a unique class of agents to treat cancer. They are normal constituents of the body that are used to fight against invading organisms and tumor cells. Modern technology has allowed us to prepare large amounts of these agents in a highly purified form and to use them for the treatment of cancer. The clinical use of these agents has been bedeviled by questions of the appropriate dose and schedule to obtain the maximum biological response without excessive toxicity. The toxicities of the agents appear to be those that they mediate pathophysiologically. Because we can give, biologically speaking, enormous doses of these agents we should not be surprised to see an intensification of these toxicities. Interestingly, the formation of antibodies to the agents does not appear to be a factor in toxicity, although it may limit therapeutic effectiveness. We do not know why the symptoms, such as fever, chills, and lassitude, should be associated with the agents and what role they play in fighting disease normally. The challenge for the future use of cytokines is to determine which mechanisms mediate tumor cell regression and which mechanisms mediate toxicity and to learn how the cytokines should be given to maximize tumor effectiveness in the face of their biological toxicity.

REFERENCES

Aboulafia D, Miles SA, Saks SR, and Mitsuyasu RT Intravenous recombinant tumor necrosis factor in the treatment of AIDS-related Kaposi's sarcoma. J Acquir Immune Defic Syndr 1989 2:54–58.

Abrams PG, McClamrock, and Foon KA Evening administration of alpha interferon. N Engl J Med 1985 312:443–444.

Adams F, Quesada JR, Jordan U, and Gutterman JU Neuropsychiatric manifestations of human leukocyte interferon therapy in patients with cancer. JAMA 1984 252:938–941.

Adams F, Femandez F, and Marligit G Interferon-induced organic mental disorders associated with unsuspected preexisting neurologic abnormalities. J Neurooncol 1988 6:355–359.

Aggarwal BB, Aiyer RA, Pennica D, Gray PW, and Goeddel DV Human tumor necrosis factors: Structure and receptor interactions. In: Tumor Necrosis Factor and Related Cytotoxins Ciba Foundation Symposium, John Wiley, Chichester, UK 1987 131:39–51.

Aguet M and Mogensen KE Interferon receptors. In: Interferons Gresser I Ed Volume 5, Academic Press, New York 1983 pp. 1–22.

Allen G and Fantes KH A family of structural genes for human lymphoblastoid (leukocyte-type) interferon. Nature 1980 287:408–411.

Aoki N, Maruyama Y, Ohno Y, and Azuma Y Indomethacin augments inhibitory effects of interferons on lympho-proliferative response. Immunol Lett 1984 7:321–324.

Atanasiu P and Chany C Action d'un interferon provenant de cellules malignes sur l'infection experimentale du hamster nouveau-ne par le virus du polyme. CR Acad Sci Paris 1960 251:1687–1689.

Atkins MB, Gould JA, Allegretta M, Li JJ, Dempsey RA, Rudders RA, Parkinson DR, Reichlin S, and Mier JW Phase I evaluation of recombinant interleukin 2 in patients with advanced malignant disease. J Clin Oncol 1986 4:1380–1391.

Balkwill F and Taylor-Papdimitrious J Interferons affect both G_1, and S + G_2 in cells stimulated from quiescence to growth. Nature 1978 274:798–800.

Belldegrun A, Webb DE, and Austin HA Effects of interleukin 2 on renal function in patients receiving immunotherapy for advanced cancer. Ann Intern Med 1987 106:817–822.

Beller UB, Chachoua A, Speyer JL, Sorich J, Dugan M, Liebes L, Hayes R, and Beckman EM Phase IB study of low-dose intraperitoneal recombinant interleukin 2 in patients with refractory advanced ovarian cancer: Rationale and preliminary report. Gynecol Oncol 1989 34:407–412.

Berneman ZN, Gastl G, Gangji D, Van Camp B, Jochmans K, Aulitzky J, Flament J, Peetermans ME, and Huber C Treatment of hairy-cell leukemia with recombinant alpha$_2$-interferon. Eur J Cancer Clin Oncol 1986 22:987–990.

Beutler B and Cerami A Cachectin and tumour necrosis factor as two sides of the same biological coin. Nature (Lond) 1986 320:584–588.

Beutler B, Mahoney J, Le Trang N, Pekala P, and Cerami A Purification of cachectin, a lipoprotein lipase suppressing hormone secreted by endotoxin induced RAW 264.7 cells. J Exp Med 1985 161:984–995.

Beutler B, Milsark IW, and Cerami AC Passive immunization against cachectin/tumor necrosis factor protects mice from lethal effect of endotoxin. Science (Wash DC) 1985 229:869–871.

Bever CT Jr, Salazar AM, Neely E, Ferraraccio BE, Rose JW, McFarland HF, Levy HB, and McFarland DE Preliminary trial of poly ICLC in chronic progressive multiple sclerosis. Neurology (NY) 1986 36:494–498.

Billiau A Bsf-2 is not just a differentiation factor. Nature 1986 324:415.

Bino T, Edery H, Gertler A, and Rosenberg H Involvement of the kidney in catabolism of human leukocyte interferon. J Gen Virol 1982 59:39–45.

Blalock JE and Stanton GJ Common pathways of interferon and hormonal action. Nature 1980 283:406–408.

Blalock JE and Smith EM Human leukocyte interferon: Potent endorphin-like opioid activity. Biochem Biophys Res Commun 1981 101:472–478.

Bocci V Central nervous system toxicity of interferons and other cytokines. J Biol Reg Homeostat Agents 1988 2:107–118.

Bocci V, Pacini A, Bandinelli L, Pessini GP, Muscettola M, and Paulesu L The role of liver in the catabolism of human α- and β-interferon. J Gen Virol 1982 60:397–400.

Bocci V, Maunsboch AB, and Mogensen EK Autoradiographic demonstration of human ^{125}I-interferon alpha in lysosomes of rabbit proximal tubule cells. J Submiscrosc Cytol 1984 16:753–757.

Bocci V, Mogensen KE, Muscettola M, Pacini A, Paulesu L, Pessina GP, and Skiftas S Degradation of human ^{125}I-interferon alpha by isolated perfused rabbit kidney and liver. J Lab Clin Med 1983 101:857–863.

Bocci V, Pacini A, Pessina GP, Paulesu L, Muscettola M, and Lunghetti G Catabolic sites of human interferon-gamma. J Gen Virol 1985 66:887–891.

Bogdahn U, Fleischer B, Hilfenhaus J, Rothig HJ, Krauseneck P, Mertens HG, and Przuntek H Interferon-beta in patients with low-grade astrocytomas. A Phase I study. J Neurooncol 1985 3:125–130.

Bornemann LD, Spiegel HE, Dziewanowska ZE, Krown SE, and Colburn WA Intravenous and intramuscular pharmacokinetics of recombinant leukocyte A interferon. Eur J Clin Pharmacol 1985 28:467–471.

Brenner DE Intraperitoneal chemotherapy: A review. J Clin Oncol 1986 4:1135–1147.

Brown TD, Koeller J, Beougher K, Goland J, Bonnem EM, Spiegel RJ, and Von Hoff DD A Phase I clinical trial recombinant DNA gamma interferon. J Clin Oncol 1987 5:790–798.

Bunn PA, Foon KA, Ihde DC, Longo DL, Eddy J, Winkler CF, Veach SR, Zeffren J, Sherwin S, and

Oldham R Recombinant leukocyte A interferon: An active agent in advanced cutaneous T-cell lymphomas. Ann Intern Med 1984 101:484–487.

Byrne G, Lehmann LK, Kirschbaum JG, Borden EC, Lee CM, and Brown RR Induction of tryptophan degradation in vitro and in vivo: A gamma interferon stimulated activity. J Interferon Res 1986 6:389–396.

Came PE and Moore DH Inhibition of spontaneous mammary carcinoma of mice by treatment with interferon and poly I:C. Proc Soc Exp Biol Med 1971 137:304–305.

Carswell EA, Old LJ, Kassel RL, Green S, Fiore N, and Williamson B An endotoxin-induced serum factor that causes necrosis of tumors. Proc Natl Acad Sci USA 1975 72:3666–3670.

Cerami A, Ikeda Y, Trang N, Hotez PJ, and Beutler B Weight loss associated with an endotoxin-induced mediator from peritoneal macrophages: The role of cachectin (tumor necrosis factor). Immunol Lett 1985 11:173–177.

Chang AYC, Pandya KJ, Asbury RF, Carignan J, Woll J, Storer B, Merritt JA, and Bennett JM Phase I study of recombinant beta interferon ser (rINF-β ser) in cancer patients by subcutaneous (SC) injection. Proc Amer Soc Clin Oncol 1985 4:226.

Chapman PB, Kolitz JE, Gragilove JL, Merluzzi VJ, Engert A, Bradley KM, and Mertelsmann R A phase I trial of intraperitoneal recombinant interleukin 2 in patients with ovarian carcinoma. Invest New Drugs 1989 6:179–188.

Chebath J, Benech P, Hovanessian A, Galabru J, and Revel M Four different forms of interferon induced 2′5′ oligo(A)synthetase identified by immunoblotting in human cells. J Biol Chem 1987 262:3852–3857.

Cheever MA, Greenberg PD, and Fefer A Augmentation of the antitumor therapeutic efficacy of long term cultured T lymphocytes by in vivo administration on purified interleukin 2. J Exp Med 1982 155:968–980.

Childs B, Kemeny N, Kelsen D, and Rosado K A Phase II trial of recombinant tumor necrosis factor (RTNF) in patients advanced colorectal carcinoma. Proc Annu Meet Am Soc Clin Oncol 1989 8:A743.

Chirigos MA and Pearson JW Cure of murine leukemia with drug and interferon treatment. JNCI 1973 51:1367–1368.

Clason AE, Duarte AJS, Kupiec-Weglinski JW, Williams JN, Wang BS, Strom TB, and Tilney NL Restoration of allograft responsiveness in B rats by interleukin 2 and/or adherent cells. J Immunol 1982 129:252–259.

Coley WB Contributions to the knowledge of sarcoma. Ann Surg 1891 14:199–220.

Constanzi J The use of alpha-2 interferon in the treatment of multiple myeloma. 4th Intern Symposium on Therapy of Acute Leukemias, Roma Feb 7–12 1987 Abstract No 314 p. 297.

Creagan ET, Ahmann DL, Green SJ, Long HJ, Rubin J, Schutt AJ, and Dziewanowski ZE Phase II study of recombinant leukocyte A interferon (rINF A) in disseminated malignant melanoma. Cancer 1984 54:2844–2849.

Creaven PJ, Brenner DE, Cowens JW, Huben RP, Wolf RM, Takita H, Arbuck SG, Razack MS, and Proefrock AD A Phase I clinical trial of recombinant human tumor necrosis factor given daily for five days. Cancer Chemother Pharmacol 1989 23:186–191.

Degrado WF, Wasserman ZR, and Chowdhry V Sequence and structural homologies among type I and type II interferons. Nature 1982 300:379–381.

Degrave S, Derynck R, Tavernier J, Haegeman G, and Fiers W Nucleotide sequence of the chromosomal gene for human fibroblast ($beta_1$) interferon and the flanking regions. Gene 1982 14:137–143.

Dekonig EWG, van Bijsterveld OP, and Cantell K Combination therapy for dendritic keratitis with human leukocyte interferon and trifluorothymidine. Br J Opthalmol 1982 66:509–512.

Denicoff KD, Rubinow DR, Papa MZ, Simpson C, Seipp CA, Lotze MT, Chang AE, Rosenstein D, and Rosenberg SA The neuropsychiatric effects of treatment with interleukin 2 and lymphokine activated killer cells. Ann Int Med 1987 107:293–300.

Devos R Cheroutre H, Taya Y, Degrave W, Van Heuverswyn H, and Fiers W Molecular cloning of human immune interferon cDNA and its expression in eukaryotic cells. Nucleic Acids Res 1982 10:2487–2501.

Di Besceglie AM, Martin P, Kassianides C, Lisker-Melman M, Murray L, Waggoner J, Goodman Z, Banks SM, and Hoofnagle JH Recombinant interferon-alpha therapy for chronic hepatitis C. N Engl J Med 1989 321:1506–1510.

Dianzani F, Salter L, Fleischmann WR Jr, and Zucca M Immune interferon activates cells more slowly than does virus-induced interferon. Proc Soc Exp Biol Med 1978 159:94–97.

Diercks RA, Michotte A, Schmedding E, Ebinger G, Ebinger G, Degeeter T, and Van Camp B Unilateral seizures in a patient with hairy cell leukemia treated with interferon. Clin Neurol Neurosurg 1985 87–93.

Donohue JH, Rosenstein M, Chang AE, Lotze MT, Robb MT, and Rosenberg SA The systemic administration of purified interleukin 2 enhances the ability of sensitized murine lymphocyte cell lines to cure a disseminated syngeneic lymphoma. J Immunol 1984 132:2123–2128.

Eggermont AM, Weimar W, Marquet RL, Lameris JD, and Jeekel J Phase II trial of high-dose recombinant leukocyte alpha-2 interferon for metastatic colorectal cancer without previous systemic treatment. Cancer Treat Rep 1985 69:185–187.

Einhorn S, Blomgren H, and Strander H Interferon and spontaneous cytotoxicity in man. II. Studies in patients receiving exogenous leukocyte interferon. Acta Med Scand 1978 204:477–483.

Ettinghausen SE, Moore JG, White DE, Platanias L, Young NS, and Rosenberg SA Hematologic effects of immunotherapy with lymphokine activated killer cells and recombinant interleukin 2 in cancer patients. Blood 1987 69:1654–1660.

Färkkilä M, Iivanainen M, Harkonen M, Laakso J, Mattson K, Niranen A, Larsen TA, and Cantell K Effect of interferon-γ on biogenic amine metabolism, electrocephalographic recordings, and transient potentials. Clin Neuropharmacol 1988 11:63–67.

Feinberg B, Kurzrock R, Talpaz M, Blick M, Saks S, and Gutterman JU A Phase I trial of intravenously-administered recombinant tumor necrosis factor-alpha in cancer patients. J Clin Oncol 1988 6:1328–1334.

Fiers W, Beyaert R, Brouckaert P, Everaerdt B, Haegeman C, Suffys P, Tavernier J, and Vanhaesebroeck B TNF: Its potential as an antitumor agent. Dev Biol Stand 1988 69:143–151.

Fleischmann WR Jr, Georgiades JA, Osborne LC, and Johnson HM Potentiation of interferon activity by mixed preparations of fibroblast and immune interferon. Infect Immun 1979 26:248–253.

Fleischmann WR Jr, Kleyn KM, and Baron S Potentiation of antitumor effect of virus-induced interferon by mouse immune interferon preparations. JNCI 1980 65:963–966.

Foon KA, Sherwin SA, Abrams PG, Stevenson HC, Holmes P, Maluish AE, Oldham RK, and Heberman RB A Phase I trial of recombinant gamma in patients with cancer. Cancer Immunol Immunother 1985 20:193–197.

Fraker DL and Norton JA Tumor necrosis factor toxicity parallels therapeutic efficacy in mice tolerant to tumor necrosis factor. Proc Am Assoc Cancer Res 1988 29:A1711.

Fransen L, Ruysschaert M-R, Van der Heyden J, and Fiers W Recombinant transformed cell lines. Cell Immunol 1986 100:260–267.

Fuse A, Mahmud I, and Kuwata T Mechanism of stimulation by human interferon of prostaglandin synthesis in human cell lines. Cancer Res 1982 42:3209–3214.

Gaspari AA, Lotze MT, Rosenberg SA, Stern JB, and Katz SI Dermatologic changes associated with interleukin 2 administration. JAMA 1987 258:1624–1629.

Göbel U, Arnold W, Wahn V, Treuner J, Jürgens H, and Cantell K Comparisons of human fibroblast and leukocyte interferon in the treatment of severe laryngeal papillomatosis in children. Eur J Pediatr 1981 137:175–176.

Goeddel DV, Yelverton E, Ullrick A, Heynecker HL, Miozzari G, Holmes R, Seeburg PH, Tabor JM, Gross M, Familleti PC, and Pestka S Human leukocyte interferon produced by E. coli is biologically active. Nature 1980 287:411–416.

Goepfert H, Sessions RB, Gutterman JU, Cangiv A, Dichtel WJ, and Sulek M Leukocyte interferon in patients with juvenile laryngeal papilomatosis. Ann Otol Rhinol Laryngol 1982 9:431–436.

Goldstein D and Laszlo J Interferon therapy in cancer: From imaginon to interferon. Cancer Res 1986 45:4315–4329.

Goldstein D and Laszlo J The role of interferon in cancer therapy: A current perspective. Cancer 1988 38:258–277.

Gonzales R, Robinson W, Adlakha A, Lamb R, Rovira D, Ferguson J, Saks S, and Bunn P Efficacy and toxicity of gamma interferon in chronic myelogenous leukemia. Proc Amer Soc Clin Oncol 1989 8:A815.

Gray PW, Leung DW, Pennica D, Yelverton E, Najarian R, Simonsen CC, Derynck R, Sherwood PJ, Wallace DM, Berger SL, Levinson AD, and Goeddel DV Expression of human immune interferon cDNA in E. coli and monkey cells. Nature 1982 295:503–508.

Gray PW, Aggarwal BB, Benton CV, Bringmen TS, Henzel WJ, Jarrett JA, Leung DW, Moffat B, Ng P, Svedersky LP, Palladino MA, and Nedwin GE Cloning and expression of cDNA for human lymphotoxin, a lymphokine with tumor necrosis activity. Nature (Lond) 1984 312:721–724.

Greenberg HV, Pollard RB, Lutwick LI, Gregory PB, Robinson WS, and Merigan TC Effect of human leukocyte interferon on hepatitis B virus infection in patients with chronic active hepatitis. N Engl J Med 1976 295:517–522.

Gresser I, Coppey J, and Bourali C Interferon and murine leukemia. VI. Effect of interferon on preparations on the lymphoid leukemia of AKR mice. JNCI 1969 43:1083–1089.

Gresser I, Maury C, and Tovey MG Efficacy of combined interferon cyclophosphamide therapy after diagnosis of lymphoma in AKR mice. Eur J Cancer 1978 14:97–99.

Grimm EA and Rosenberg SA Production and properties of human IL-2. In: Isolation Characterization and Utilization of T Lymphocyte Clones Fathman CG and Fitch FW Eds Academic Press Inc, Orlando FL 1982 pp. 57–82.

Grunberg SM, Kempf RA, Venturi CL, and Mitchell MS Phase I study of recombinant β-interferon given by four-hour infusion. Cancer Res 1987 47:1174–1178.

Guggenheim MA and Baron S Clinical studies of an interferon inducer, polyriboinosinic-polyribocytidylic acid (Poly (1) Poly (C)) in children. J Infect Dis 1977 136:50.

Gutterman JU, Rosenblum MG, Rios A, Fritsche HA, and Quesada JR Pharmacokinetic study of partially pure gamma-interferon in cancer patients. Cancer Res 1984 44:4164–4171.

Haglund S, Lundquist PG, Cantell K, and Strander H Interferon therapy in juvenile laryngeal papillomatosis. Arch Otolaryngo 1981 107:327–332.

Hawkins MJ, Krown SE, Borden Mathilde Krim EC, Real FX, Edwards BS, Anderson SA, Cunningham-Rundles S, and Oeltgen HF American cancer society Phase I trial of naturally produced β-interferon. Cancer Res 1984 44:5934–5938.

Hri LM, Campion M, and Dennin RA Incidence and clinical significance of neutralizing antibodies in patients receiving recombinant interferon-alpha-2b by intramuscular injection. Cancer 1987 59:668–674.

Isaacs A and Lindenmann J Virus interference. I. The interferon Proc R Soc Lond (Biol) 1957 147:258–267.

Ito M and Buffet RF Cytocidal effect of purified human fibroblast interferon on tumor cells in vitro. JNCI 1981 66:819–825.

Jacob L, O'Malley JA, Freeman A, Ekes R, and Reese RA Intrathecal interferon in the treatment of multiple sclerosis: Patient follow-up. Arch Neurol 1985 42:841–847.

Kahn JO, Kaplan LD, Volberding PA, Ziegler JL, Crowe S, Saks SR, and Abrams DI Intralesional recombinant tumor necrosis factor-alpha for AIDS-associated Kaposi's sarcoma: A randomized double-blind trial. J Acquir Immune Defic Syndr 1989 2:217–223.

Kettelhut I, Fiers W, and Goldbert AL The toxic effects of Tumor Necrosis Factor in vivo and their prevention by cyclooxygenase inhibitors. Proc Natl Acad Sci USA 1987 84:4273–4277.

Kirkwood JM, Ernstoff MS, and Davis CA Comparison of intramuscular and intravenous recombinant alpha-2 interferon in melanoma and other cancers. Ann Intern Med 1985 103:32–36.

Kleinerman ES, Kurzrock R, Wyatt D, Quesada JR, Gutterman JU, and Fidler IJ Activation or suppression of the tumericidal properties of monocytes from cancer patients following treatment with human recombinant gamma-interferon. Cancer Res 1986 46:5401–5405.

Kohler PC, Hank JA, Moore KH, Storer B, Bechhofer R, and Sondel PM Phase I clinical evaluation of recombinant interleukin 2. In: Cellular Immunology of Cancer Truitt RL, Gale RP, and Bortin MM, Eds Alan Liss Publishing, New York 1987 pp. 161–172.

Koren S, Klimpel GR, and Fleischmann WR Jr Treatment of mice with macrophage colony stimulating factor (CSF-1) prevents the in vivo myelosuppression induced by murine alpha, beta, and gamma interferons. J Biol Respir Modif 1986 5:481–489.

Kozeny GA, Nicolas JD, Creekmore S, Sticklin L, Hano JE, and Fisher RI Effects of interleukin 2 immunotherapy on renal function. J Clin Oncol 1988 6:1170–1176.

Kuei JH, Tashkin DP, and Figlin RA Pulmonary toxicity of recombinant human tumor necrosis factor. Chest 1989 96:334–338.

Kurzrock R, Rosenblum MG, Sherwin SA, Rios A, Talpay M, Quesada JR, and Gutterman JU Pharmacokinetics single-dose tolerance and biological activity of recombinant gamma-interferon in cancer patients. Cancer Res 1985 45:2866–2872.

Lafreniere R and Rosenberg SA Successful immunotherapy of experimental hepatic metastases with lymphokine activated killer cells and recombinant IL-2. Cancer Res 1985 45:3735–3741.

Lampson GP, Tytell AA, Nemes MM, and Hilleman MR Purification and characterization of chick embryo interferon. Proc Soc Exp Biol Med 1963 112:468–478.

Lane HC, Davey RT, Sherwin SA, Masur H, Rook AH, Manischewitz JF, Quinnan GV, Smith PD, Easter ME, and Fauci AS A Phase I trial of recombinant human interferon-gamma in patients with Kaposis sarcoma and the acquired immunodeficiency syndrome (AIDS). J Clin Immunol 1989 9:351–361.

Laszlo J, Huang AT, Brenckman WD, Jeffs C, Koren H, Cianciolo G, Metzgar R, Cashdollar W, Cox E, Buckley CE III, Tso CY, and Lucas YS Jr Phase I study of pharmacological and immunological effects of human lymphoblastoid interferon given to patients with cancer. Cancer Res 1983 43:4458–4466.

Liberati AM, Biscottini B, Fizzotti M, Schippa M, DeAngelis V, Senatore M, Vittori O, Teggia L, Natali R, and Palmisang L A Phase I study of human natural interferon-beta in cancer patients. J Interferon Res 1988 9:339–345.

Lindahl P, Leary P, and Gresser I Enhancement by interferon of the specific cytotoxicity of sensitized lymphocytes. Proc Natl Acad Sci USA 1972 69:721–725.

Lotze MT, Matory YL, Ettinghausen SE, Rayner AA, Sharrow SO, Seipp CAY, Custer MC, and Rosenberg SA In vivo administration of purified interleukin 2.2. Half-life, immunologic effects and expansion of peripheral lymphoid cells in vivo with recombinant IL-2. J Immunol 1984 135:2865–2875.

Lotze MT, Frana LW, Sharrow SO, Robb RJ, and Rosenberg SA In vivo administration of purified human interleukin 2.1. Half-life, and immunologic effects of the Jurkat cell line-derived interleukin 2. J Immunol 1985 134:157–166.

Lotze MT, Chang AE, Seipp CA, Simpson C, Vetto JT, and Rosenberg SA High-dose recombinant IL-2 in the treatment of patients with disseminated cancer. Responses, treatment-related morbidity and histologic findings. JAMA 1986 256:3117–3124.

Lundbald D and Lundgren E Block of a glioma cell line in S by interferon. Int J Cancer 1981 27:749–754.

Maheshware RK, Lazo PS, and Friedman RM Enhancement of interferon activity by a membrane glycoprotein related to the thyrotropin receptor. In: Interferon: Properties and Clinical Uses 1979 pp. 387–396.

Mallick AA, Ishizaka A, Stephens KE, Hatherill JR, Tazelaar HD, and Raffin TA Multiple organ damage caused by tumor necrosis factor and prevent by prior neutrophil depletion. Chest 1989 95:1114–1120.

Mataresse GP and Rossi GB Effect of interferon on growth and division cycle of friend erythroleukemic murine cells in vitro. J Cell Biol 1977 75:344–354.

Mattson V, Niiranen A, Iivanainen M, Färkkilä M, Bergström L, and Holsti LR Neurotoxicity of interferon. Cancer Treat Rep 1983 67:958–961.

Mattson K, Niiranen A, Laaksonen R, and Cantell K Psychometric monitoring of interferon neurotoxicity. Lancet 1984 275–276.

Merluzzi VJ, Kenney RE, Schmid FA, Choi YS, and Faanes RB Recovery of in vitro cytotoxic T-cell response in cyclophosphamide treated mice by injection of mixed-lymphocyte culture supernatants. Cancer Res 1981 41:3663–3665.

Miyata T and Hayashida H Recent divergence from a common ancestor of human INF-alpha genes. Nature 1982 295:165–168.

Morgan DA, Ruscetti RW, and Gallo R Selective in vitro growth of lymphocytes from normal human bone marrows. Science 1976 193:1007–1008.

Moritz T, Niederle N, Baumann J, May D, Kurschel E, Osieka R, Kempeni J, Schlick E, and Schmidt CG Phase I study of recombinant human tumor necrosis factor alpha in advanced malignant disease. Cancer Immunol Immunother 1989 29:144–150.

Namba M, Yamamoto S, Tanaka H, Kanamori T, Nobuhara M, and Kimoto T In vitro and in vivo studies on potentiation of cytotoxic effects of anticancer drugs or cobalt 60 gamma ray by interferon on human neoplastic cells. Cancer 1984 54:2262–2267.

Niederle N, Moritz T, Kurschel E, Osieka R, Opalka B, Schlick E, and Schmidt CG Recombinant human tumor necrosis factor alfa (TNF) in the treatment of advanced malignancies: A Phase I study. Proc Am Assoc Cancer Res 1988 29:A1717.

Oettgen HF Tumor necrosis factor: Discovery, development, and initial study in cancer patients. Int Congr Ser 1987 776:60–69.

Ognibene FP, Rosenberg SA, Skibber J, Shelhamer JH, Lotze MT, and Parillo JE Interleukin 2 hemodynamics mimic septic shock. Crit Care Med 1986 14:352.

Owerbach D, Rutter WJ, Shows B, Gray P, Goeddel DV, and Lawn RM Leukocyte and fibroblast interferon genes are located on human chromosome 9. Proc Natl Acad Sci USA 1981 78:3123–3127.

Ozaki Y, Oyama T, and Kume S Exacerbation of toxic effects by endotoxin contamination of recombinant human tumor necrosis factor. Cancer Chemother Pharmacol 1989 23:231–237.

Palladino MA Jr, Shalaby MR, Kramer SM, Ferraiolo BL, Baughman RA, Deleo AB, Crase D, Marafino B, Aggarwal BB, Figari IS, Liggett D, and Patton JS Characterization of the antitumor activities of human tumor necrosis factor-alpha and the comparison with other cytokines: Induction of tumor specific immunity. J Immunol 1987 138:4023–4032.

Panem S The interferon crusade. Brookings Institute, Washington, DC 1985.

Panitch HS, Haley AS, Hirsch RL, and Johnson KPA A trial of gamma interferon in multiple sclerosis. Neurology (NY) 1986 36:285.

Patton JS, Crase D, McCabe J, Crase D, Hanson S, Chen AB, and Liggett D Development of tolerance to the gastrointestinal effects of high doses of recombinant tumor necrosis factor-α in rodents. J Clin Invest 1987 80:1587–1596.

Paucker K, Cantell K, and Henle W Quantitative studies on viral interference in suspended L-cells. III. Effect of interfering viruses and interferon on the growth rate of cells. Virology 1962 17:324–334.

Pennica D, Nedwin GE, Haywick JS, Seeburg PH, Derynck R, Palladino MA, Kohr WJ, Aggarwal BB, and Goeddel DV Human tumor necrosis factor: Precursor structure cDNA cloning expression and homology to lymphotoxin. Nature (Lond) 1984 312:724–729.

Pottathil R, Chandrabose KA, Cuatrecasas P, and Lang DJ Establishment of the interferon-mediated antiviral state: Role of fatty acid cyclooxygenase. Proc Natl Acad Sci 1980 77:5437–5440.

Quesada JR, Gutterman JU, and Hersh EM Clinical and immunological study of beta interferon by intramuscular route in patients with metastatic breast cancer. J Interferon Res 1982 2:593–599.

Quesada JR, Gutterman JU, and Hersh EM Treatment of hairy cell leukemia with alpha interferons. Cancer 1986 57:1678–1680.

Reimann J and Diamanstein T Interleukin 2 allows the in vivo induction of anti-erythrocyte autoantibody production in nude mice associated with the injection of rat erythrocytes. Clin Exp Immunol 1981 43:641–644.

Rohatiner AZS and Färkkilä M Neurotoxicity of interferon therapy. In: Interferon Treatment of Neurologic Disorders Smith RA Ed Dekker, New York 1988 pp. 135–145.

Rohatiner AZS, Balkwill FR, Griffin DB, Malpas JS, and Lister TA A Phase I study of human lymphoblastoid interferon administered by continuous intravenous infusion. Cancer Chemother Pharmacol 1982 9:97–102.

Rohatiner AZS, Prior PF, Burton AC, Smith AT, Balkwill FR, and Lister TA Central nervous system toxicity of interferon. Br J Cancer 1983 47:419–422.

Rosenberg SA, Grimm EA, McGrogan M, Doule M, Kawasaki E, Koths K, and Mark D Biological activity of recombinant human interleukin 2 produced in E. coli. Science 1984 223:1412–1415.

Rosenberg SA, Lotze MT, Muul LM, Chang AE, Avis FP, Leitman WM, Linehan WM, Robertson CN, Lee RE, Rubin JT, Seipp CA, Simpson CG, and White DE A progress report on the treatment of 157 patients with advanced cancer using lymphokine activated killer cells and interleukin 2 or high dose interleukin 2 alone. N Engl J Med 1987 316:889–897.

Rosenstein M, Ettinghausen SE, and Rosenberg SA Extravasation of intravascular fluid mediated by systemic administration of recombinant IL-2. J Immunol 1986 137:1735–1742.

Rubenstein S, Familleti PC, and Pestka S Conventional assays for interferons. J Virol 1981 37:755.

Samuel C Molecular mechanisms of interferon action. In: Clinical Applications of Interferons and Their Inducers Stringfellow D Ed Edition 2 Marcel Dekker, New York 1986 pp. 1–18.

Sarkar FH and Gupta SL On the inhibition of interferon action by inhibitors of fatty acid cyclooxygenase. Virology 1982 123:448–451.

Savona S, Mittelman A, Gaffney E, Skelos S, Coombe N, Wood D, Arlin Z, Ahmed T, Puccio C, Ashikari R, and Nadler P Toxicity of a 5-day continuous infusion of recombinant human tumor necrosis factor (RHTNF). Proc Am Soc Clin Oncol 1989 8:A733.

Savona S, Mittelman A, Singh B, Nadler P, Gaffney E, Skelos S, Coombe N, Ahmed T, and Arlin Z Neurotoxicity induced by continuous infusion of recombinant tumor necrosis factor in patients with advanced cancer. Proc Am Soc Clin Oncol 1988 7:A658.

Schellekens H, de Reus A, and Meide PH The chimpanzee as a model to test the side effects of human interferons. J Med Primatol 1984 13:235–245.

Schultz RM, Chirigos MA, and Heine UI Functional and morphologic characteristics of interferon-treated macrophages. Cell Immunol 1978 35:84–91.

Scott GM Toxic effects of interferons. In: Clinical Aspects of Interferons Revel PM Ed Kluwer, Boston, Dev Med Virol 1988 4:245–258.

Sehgal PB The interferon genes. Biochem Biophys Acta 1982 695:17–33.

Senn CC Biochemical pathways in interferon action. Pharmacol Ther 1984 24:235–257.

Shah I, Bond J, Samson M, Young J, Robinson R, Bailey R, Lerner AM, and Prasad AS Pharmacokinetics and tolerance of intravenous and intramuscular recombinant alpha-2 interferon in patients with malignancies. Am J Hematol 1984 17:363–371.

Sherman ML, Spriggs DR, Arthur KA, Imamura K, Frei E, and Kufe DW Recombinant human tumor necrosis factor administered as a five-day continuous infusion in cancer patients: Phase I toxicity and effects on lipid metabolism. J Clin Oncol 1988 6:344–350.

Silver HKB, Connors JM, and Salinas FA Prospectively randomized toxicity study of high-dose versus low-dose treatment strategies for lymphoblastoic interferon. Cancer Treat Rep 1985 69:743–750.

Smedley HM and Wheeler T Toxicity of INF. In: Interferon and Cancer Sikora K Ed Plenum Press, New York 1983 pp. 203–210.

Smedley HM, Katrak M, Sikora K, and Wheeler T Neurological effects of recombinant human interferon. Br Med J 1983 286:262–264.

Smith RA, Kingsbury D, Alksne J, James H, and Cantell K Distribution of interferon in cerebrospinal fluid after systemic intrathecal and intraventricular administration. Ann Neurol 1982 12:81.

Smith RA, Norris F, Palmer D, Bernhardt, and Wills RJ Distribution of alpha interferon in serum and cerebrospinal fluid after systemic administration. Clin Pharmacol 1985 Ther 37:85–88.

Sondel PM, Kohler PC, Hank JA, Moore KA, Rosenthal NS, Sosman JA, Bechhofer R, and Storer B Clinical and immunological effects of recombinant interleukin 2 given by repetitive weekly cycles to patients with cancer. Cancer Res 1988 48:2561–2567.

Sonnenfeld G, Mandel AD, and Merigan TC The immunosuppressive effect of type II mouse interferon preparations on antibody production. Cell Immunol 1977 34:193–206.

Spiegel RJ The alpha interferons: Clinical overview. Semin Oncol 1987 14:1–12.

Spriggs DR, Sherman ML, Frei E, and Kufe DW Clinical studies with tumour necrosis factor. Ciba Found Symp 1987 131:206–227.

Spriggs DR, Sherman ML, Michie H, Arthur KA, Imamura K, Wilmore D, Frei E, and Kufe DW Recombinant human tumor necrosis factor administered as a 24-hour intravenous infusion. A Phase I and pharmacologic study. JNCI 1988 80:1039–1044.

Steinmetz T, Schaadt M, Gahl R, Schenk V, Diehl V, and Pfreundschuh M Phase I study of 24-hour continuous intravenous infusion of recombinant human tumor necrosis factor. J Biol Response Mod 1988 7:417–423.

Stewart JA, Belinson JL, Moore AL, Dorighi JA, Grant BW, Branda RF, Haugh LD, and Albertini RJ Phase I trial of intraperitoneal rIL-2 in patients with ovarian cancer: I. Clinical toxicity and IL-2 kinetics. Cancer Res 1990 in press.

Stewart WE II, Blalock JE, Burke DC, Chany C, Dunnick JK, Falcoff E, Friedman RM, Galasso GJ, Joklik WK, Vilcek JT, Youngner JS, and Zoon KC Interferon nomenclature. Nature 1980 286:110.

Stotter H, Rude E, and Wagner H T-cell factor (interleukin 2) allows in vivo induction of helper Tcells against heterologous erythrocytes in athymic (nu/nu) mice. Eur J Immunol 1980 10:719–722.

Sundmacher R, Cantell Y, Skoda R, Hallermann C, and Neumann-Haefelin D Human leukocyte and fibroblast interferon in a combination therapy of dentritic keratitis. Albrecht Von Graefes Arch Klin Exp Opthalmol 1978 208:229–233.

Taniguchi T, Matsui H, Fujita T, Takaoka C, Kashima N, Yashimoto N, and Hamura J Structure and expression of a cloned cDNA for human interleukin 2. Nature 1983 302:305–307.

Tavernier J, Derynck R, and Fiers W Evidence for a unique human fibroblast interferon (INF-beta$_1$) chromosomal gene, devoid of intervening sequences. Nucleic Acids Res 1981 9:461–471.

Thompson JA, Lee DJ, Cox WW, Lindgren CG, Collins C, Neraas KA, Dennin RA, and Fefer A Recombinant interleukin 2 toxicity, pharmacokinetics and immunomodulatory effects in a phase II trial. Cancer Res 1987 47:4202–4207.

Tyrell DAJ Interferon produced by cultures of calf kidney cells. Nature 1959 184:452–453.

Tyring S, Klimpel GR, Fleischmann WR Jr, and Baron S Direct cytolysis by partially-purified preparations of immune interferon. Int J Cancer 1982 30:59–64.

Tyring S, Klimpel GR, Brysk M, Gupta V, Stanton GJ, Fleischmann WR Jr, and Baron S Eradication of cultured human melanoma cells by immune interferon and leukocytes. JNCI 1984 73:1067–1073.

Urba WJ, Clark JW, Steis RG, Bookman MA, Smith JW II, Beckner S, Maluish A, Rossio JL, Rager H, Ortaldo JR, and Longo DL Intraperitoneal lymphokine activated killer cell/interleukin 2 therapy in patients with intra-abdominal cancer: Immunologic considerations. JNCI 1989 81:602–612.

Van Arman CG, Armstrong DAJ, and Kim DH Antipyretics. Pharmacol Ther 1985 29:1–48.

Vanky F and Argov S Human tumor-lymphocyte interaction in vitro. VII. Blastogenesis and generation of cytotoxicity against autologous tumor biopsy cells are inhibited by interferon. Int J Cancer 1980 26:405–411.

Warren RS, Starnes F, Gabrilove J, Oettgen H, and Brennan MF The effects of tumor necrosis factor on protein and amino acid metabolism in man: A possible contribution to cachexia. 1987 Joint Annual Meeting of the Association of Head and Neck Oncologists of Great Britain British Association of Surgical Oncology Society of Head and Neck Surgeons and Society of Surgical Oncology, London April 25–30 1987 p. 158.

Willis RJ, Dennis S, Spiegel HE, Gibson DM, and Nadler PI Interferon kinetics and adverse reactions after intravenous intramuscular and subcutaneous injection. Clin Pharmacol Ther 1984 35:722–727.

Yaron M, Yaron I, Gurari-Rotman D, Revel M, Lindner H, and Zor V Stimulation of prostaglandin E production in cultured human fibroblasts by poly(I)-poly(C) and human interferon. Nature 1977 267:457–459.

Zamkoff K, Newman N, Rudolph A, and Poiesz B A Phase I study of subcutaneously administered recombinant tumor necrosis (RTNF) in patients with advanced malignancy. Proc Am Soc Clin Oncol 1988 7:A259.

Zukiwski A, Wallace S, Gutterman J, Saks S, and Mavligit G Hepatic arterial infusion of recombinant tumor necrosis factor (RTNF) in patients with metastatic carcinoma to the liver. Proc Am Soc Clin Oncol 1989 8:A476.

Index